www.harcourt-international.com

Bringing you products from all Harcourt Health Sciences companies including Baillière Tindall, Churchill Livingstone, Mosby and W.B. Saunders

▶ **Browse** for latest information on new books, journals and electronic products

▶ **Search** for information on over 20 000 published titles with full product information including tables of contents and sample chapters

▶ **Keep up to date** with our extensive publishing programme in your field by registering with eAlert or requesting postal updates

▶ **Secure online ordering** with prompt delivery, as well as full contact details to order by phone, fax or post

▶ **News** of special features and promotions

If you are based in the following countries, please visit the country-specific site to receive full details of product availability and local ordering information

USA: www.harcourthealth.com

Canada: www.harcourtcanada.com

Australia: www.harcourt.com.au

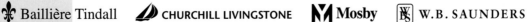

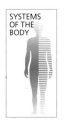

SYSTEMS
OF THE
BODY

THE DIGESTIVE SYSTEM

SYSTEMS
OF THE
BODY

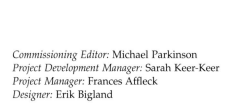

Commissioning Editor: Michael Parkinson
Project Development Manager: Sarah Keer-Keer
Project Manager: Frances Affleck
Designer: Erik Bigland

THE DIGESTIVE SYSTEM

Margaret E. Smith PhD DSc

Professor of Experimental Neurology, Division of Medical Sciences, Medical School,
University of Birmingham, Birmingham, UK

Dion G. Morton MD DSc

Reader in Surgery, Academic Department of Surgery,
University Hospital Birmingham, Birmingham, UK

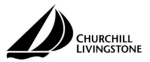

CHURCHILL
LIVINGSTONE

EDINBURGH LONDON NEW YORK PHILADELPHIA ST LOUIS SYDNEY TORONTO 2001

CHURCHILL LIVINGSTONE
An imprint of Harcourt Publishers Limited

© Harcourt Publishers Limited 2001

 is a registered trademark of Harcourt Publishers Limited

The right of M. E. Smith and D. Morton to be identified as authors
of this work has been asserted by them in accordance with the
Copyright, Designs and Patents Act 1988

First published 2001

ISBN 0 443 06245 5

British Library Cataloguing in Publication Data
A catalogue record for this book is available from the British
Library

Library of Congress Cataloging in Publication Data
A catalog record for this book is available from the Library of
Congress

Note
Medical knowledge is constantly changing. As new information
becomes available, changes in treatment, procedures, equipment
and the use of drugs become necessary. The authors and the
publishers have taken care to ensure that the information given in
this text is accurate and up to date. However, readers are strongly
advised to confirm that the information, especially with regard to
drug usage, complies with the latest legislation and standards of
practice.

The
Publisher's
policy is to use
**paper manufactured
from sustainable forests**

Many medical schools in the UK and other countries are designing and implementing new courses which are systems-based. In addition many are taking a problem-based learning approach to the systems. It is hoped that this approach will encourage the student to think rather than just learn didactically. This book is intended to meet the textbook needs of such courses in the digestive system. It provides the basic science needed and places it in a clinical context. This approach is intended to emphasise the importance of a knowledge of basic science for the understanding of medicine. It should help to motivate the students at a very early stage in their course.

In this book the subject matter of each chapter is illustrated by the problems encountered in a carefully selected clinical situation. The clinical cases chosen are those which demonstrate the relevance of many aspects of the basic science to the understanding of the specific clinical problem and by inference, to the understanding of medicine as a whole. This case-based approach should therefore help to motivate students to learn basic science. It should be emphasised that the clinical problems have been chosen because they illustrate a number of different aspects of each area of the digestive system, not because they are common diseases. Indeed some of them are uncommon, or even rare. However, common, relevant diseases are described in the text, and the last chapter draws together information on the common diseases of the digestive system.

A further clinical problem is used for self-assessment at the end of each chapter. Additional self-assessment questions are also included. The self-assessment problem is chosen to illustrate and re-inforce material in the text. With a knowledge of the material covered in the chapter, the student should be able to tackle most of the questions, although in some cases they may need to visit the library and delve a little further in order to provide full answers. Indeed it is hoped that this approach will stimulate the student to wish to learn more about the system and its diseases.

The book has a further purpose: to demonstrate the importance of integration of knowledge of the digestive system with that of the other systems of the body, for the understanding and treatment of disease. With this in mind, many of the cases and problems used address relevant aspects of other systems.

Many of the problems have been tried out in the digestive system course at the University of Birmingham where the authors are based.

ACKNOWLEDGEMENTS

We are grateful for the help given by various people in the preparation of this book. Mr John Hamburger of Birmingham University Dental School read the Mouth chapter, and he and Dr Linda Shaw made some useful general suggestions. Mr Hamburger and Dr J. Rippin kindly provided the photographs for the Mouth chapter. Dr Cliff J. Bailey of the Department of Pharmaceutical Sciences at the University of Aston made useful comments on the Absorptive and Post-absorptive States chapter. Professor R. Coleman and Dr R. Waring of the Department of Biochemistry at Birmingham University provided some useful information for the Liver chapter. Dr Peter Guest, consultant radiologist at the University Hospital, Birmingham provided many of the X-rays and clinical photographs. The encouragement of Dexter W. Smith was very much appreciated.

CONTENTS

OVERVIEW OF THE DIGESTIVE SYSTEM

1

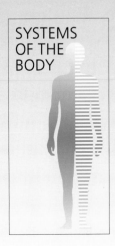

Chapter objectives

After studying this chapter you should be able to:

① Understand the key mechanisms of secretion, absorption, and motility in the gastrointestinal system.

② Understand the coordinated and integrated functioning of the digestive system.

③ Understand how function of the digestive system depends on other systems, such as the cardiovascular system.

Introduction

The cells of the body require adequate amounts of raw materials for their energy-requiring and synthetic processes. The raw materials are obtained from the external environment through ingestion of food. The overall function of the digestive system is to transfer the nutrients in food from the external environment to the internal environment where they can be distributed to the cells of the body via the circulation. In this chapter the general principles and basic mechanisms involved in the functioning of the digestive system will be discussed in the context of the system as a whole. The importance of the integration of the digestive system with the other body systems will be illustrated by the problems encountered in non-occlusive ischaemic disease of the gut, a condition in which the defect originates in the vascular system, but serious consequences result from abnormal absorption in the small intestine.

Ischaemic gut Box 1

Non-occlusive ischaemic disease of the gut

An elderly patient, who was being treated with digitalis for congestive heart failure, suddenly developed severe, constant, abdominal pain. The consultant physician examined him and found that he was in circulatory shock. Thus his systemic arterial blood pressure and cardiac output were severely diminished. The physician suspected from the patient's abdominal symptoms that he was suffering from non-occlusive ischaemic disease of the gut. In this condition the decreased cardiac output results in decreased intestinal perfusion and this, together with other mechanisms, results in the flow of blood to the gastrointestinal tissues being cut off. This disease is often fatal.

Upon consideration of the details of this case we can ask the following questions:

① What are the main causes of the sudden development of this condition in patients with cardiac failure?

② What are the physiological consequences of reduced flow of blood for the functioning of the small intestine?

③ What is the origin of the patient's pain?

④ How are the normal homeostatic mechanisms which control the flow of blood to the gastrointestinal tract perturbed in this condition?

⑤ How can this patient be treated?

Components of the digestive system

Figure 1.1 illustrates the component organs of the gastrointestinal tract, and the associated organs that are essential for the functioning of the digestive system. The gastrointestinal tract consists of the mouth, oesophagus, stomach, small intestine, and large intestine. The food is taken into the mouth and moved into the pharynx by the activity of skeletal muscle, then along the rest of the tract by the activity of smooth muscle. The food material is brought to an appropriate semi-fluid consistency, and the nutrients in it are dissolved and degraded by secretions which enter the tract at different locations. These processes are aided by the contractions of the muscles, which serve to mix the secretions with the food.

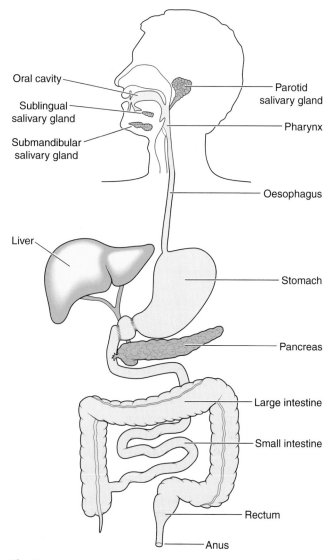

Fig. 1.1
The digestive system and associated exocrine glands.

The associated organs situated outside the gastro-intestinal tract, which are essential for the digestive process, are exocrine glands which secrete important digestive juices. These are:

1. the three pairs of salivary glands producing saliva, which has a range of functions, but most importantly provides lubrication of the upper gastrointestinal tract to allow the food to be moved along it
2. the exocrine pancreas, which secretes pancreatic juice that contains most of the important digestive enzymes required to degrade the food into molecules which can be absorbed
3. the exocrine liver which produces bile, a secretion important for fat digestion and absorption. The liver also provides a medium for the excretion of waste metabolites and drugs.

Saliva is released into the mouth. Pancreatic juice and bile enter the duodenum in the upper small intestine (Fig. 1.1). Their release is stimulated when a meal is present in the gastrointestinal tract.

Physiological processes of the digestive system

The physiological processes that are important for the functioning of the digestive system are digestion, absorption, motility, secretion and excretion. Digestion is the process whereby large molecules are broken down to smaller ones. Food is ingested as large pieces of matter, containing high molecular weight substances such as protein and starch which are unable to cross the cell membranes of the gut epithelium. Before these complex molecules can be utilised they are degraded to smaller molecules, such as glucose and amino acids.

The mixture of ingested material and secretions in the gastrointestinal tract contains water, minerals and vitamins as well as complex nutrients. The products of digestion and other small dissolved molecules, and ions and water are transported across the epithelial cell membranes, mainly in the small intestine. This is the process of absorption. The transported molecules enter the blood or lymph for circulation to the tissues. This process is central to the digestive system, and the other physiological processes of the gastrointestinal tract subserve it.

The gastrointestinal tract is a tube of variable diameter, approximately 15 feet long in living human adults. It extends through the body from the mouth to the anus. The food must be moved along it to reach the appropriate sites for mixing, digestion, and absorption. Two layers of smooth muscle line the gastro-intestinal tract, and contractions of this muscle mix the contents of the lumen and move them through the tract. The process of motility is under the control of nerves and hormones (see below).

Exocrine glands secrete enzymes, ions, water, mucins, and other substances into the digestive tract. The glands are situated within the gastrointestinal tract, in the walls of the stomach and intestines, or outside it (salivary glands, pancreas and liver, see above). Secretion is under the control of nerves and hormones (see below). Some substances are excreted by the liver into the gastrointestinal tract, as components of bile. The gut lumen is continuous with the external environment and its contents are therefore technically outside the body. The faeces eliminated by the intestinal tract are composed mainly of bacteria which have proliferated in the tract, and undigested material such as cellulose, a component of plant cell membranes which cannot be absorbed. Undigested residues largely comprise material that was never actually inside the body, and is therefore not excreted but eliminated from the body. However, a small portion of the faecal material consists of excreted substances such as bile pigments (breakdown products of haemoglobin) which impart the characteristic colour to the faeces.

Quantities of material processed by the gastrointestinal tract

During the course of the day an adult usually consumes about 800 g of food and 1.5 L of water. However, the ingested material is a small part of the material that enters the gastrointestinal tract because secretion into the tract may amount to 7 or 8 L of fluid, the exact amount depending on the frequency and composition of the meals eaten. Figure 1.2 indicates the approximate volumes of fluid entering or leaving the gastrointestinal tract during the average day, and the locations where the processes occur.

Thus 9–10 L of fluid may enter the tract per day. Most of this has been processed when the chyme reaches the large intestine and only 5–10% of it is left to pass on into the colon. Most of this is absorbed in the colon and only approximately 150 g are eliminated from the body as faeces. The latter contain about 30–40% solids which are undigested residues and a few excreted substances (see above).

Regulation of ingestion

Intake of food should be adequate to meet the metabolic needs of the individual, but it should not be so much that it causes obesity. Food ingestion is determined by the sensation of hunger. Hunger includes

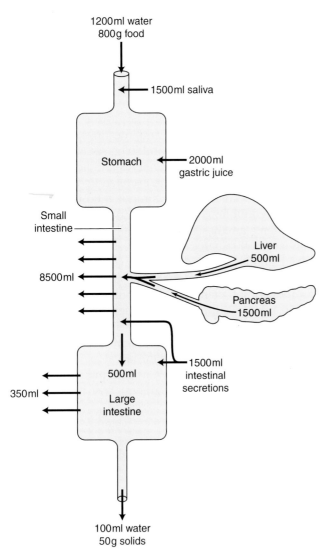

Fig. 1.2
Volumes of material handled by the gastrointestinal tract. The food and fluid ingested, may amount to 2 L or so per day. In addition to the material ingested, large volumes of secretions enter the tract. Most of the nutrients and water are normally absorbed in the small intestine but a small proportion is absorbed in the colon. The volumes indicated are approximate daily amounts.

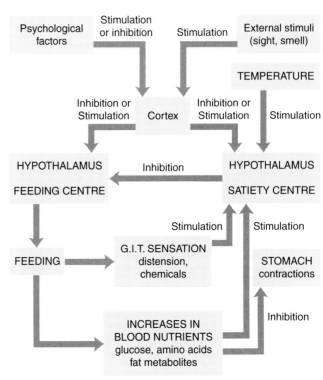

Fig. 1.3
Schematic representation of the role of some factors involved in the regulation of food intake.

individual. The amount of food which causes satiety depends to some extent on whether the individual's energy stores are full (see Chapter 9), but other factors also have a role.

The regulation of food intake can be considered under two headings:

1. 'alimentary' regulation concerned with the immediate effects of feeding on the gastrointestinal tract
2. 'nutritional' regulation, concerned with the maintenance of normal stores of fat and glycogen in the body.

The regulation of food intake is coordinated by neurones in two areas of the brain, known as the feeding centre and the satiety centre. Figure 1.3 indicates some of the factors involved in the regulation of food intake, and the areas of the brain upon which they act. The feeding centre is located in the lateral hypothalamus. Stimulation of neurones in this area causes an animal to eat voraciously (hyperphagia). On the other hand, lesions of this area can cause a lack of desire for food and progressive inanition (loss of weight). In summary, this area excites the emotional drive to search for food. It controls the amount of food eaten

two categories of sensations; sensations from the stomach known as hunger contractions or hunger pangs, and more subjective sensations associated with low levels of nutrients in the blood. Hunger induces an individual to search for an adequate supply of food. A desire for specific foods is known as appetite. Satiety is the opposite of hunger. It is a sensation which usually results from the ingestion of a meal in a normal and also excites the various centres in the brain stem which control chewing, salivation, and swallowing (see Chapter 2).

The satiety centre is situated in the ventromedial nuclei of the hypothalamus. Stimulation of neurones in this area results in complete satiety, and the animal refuses to eat (aphagia), whereas lesions in this area can cause voracious eating and obesity. The satiety centre operates primarily by inhibiting the feeding centre.

The control of appetite appears to be via higher centres than the hypothalamus, including areas in the amygdala, where sensations of smell have an important role in this control, and cortical areas of the limbic system. These areas are closely coupled to the feeding and satiety centres in the hypothalamus.

Alimentary regulation of feeding

The regulation of feeding by sensation from the alimentary tract is short-term regulation. The feeling of hunger when the stomach is empty is due to stimulation of nerve fibres in the vagus nerve which causes the stomach to contract. These contractions are known as hunger contractions, or hunger 'pains'. They are triggered by low blood sugar, which stimulates the vagus nerve fibres. However, feelings of hunger or satiety at different times of the day depend to a large extent on habit. Individuals who are in the habit of eating three meals a day at regular times, but miss a meal on an occasion are likely to feel hungry, even if adequate nutritional stores are present in the tissues. The mechanisms responsible for this are not understood.

Other factors are also important in the alimentary control of hunger, such as distension of the stomach or duodenum. This causes inhibition of the feeding centre and reduces the desire for food. It depends mainly on the activation of mechanoreceptors in these areas of the tract, which results in signals being transmitted in sensory fibres in the vagus nerves. The chemical composition of the food in the duodenum is also important. Thus fat in the duodenum stimulates satiety via release of the hormone cholecystokinin (CCK) into the blood, from the walls of the duodenum (see Chapter 8).

Functional activity of the oral cavity, such as taste, salivation, chewing, swallowing is also important in monitoring the amount of food that passes through the mouth. Thus the degree of hunger is reduced after a certain amount of food has passed through the mouth. However, the inhibition of hunger by this mechanism is short-lived, lasting only 30 minutes or so. The functional significance of this is probably that the individual is stimulated to eat only when the gastrointestinal tract can cope efficiently with food, so that digestion, absorption, and metabolism can work at an appropriate pace.

Nutritional regulation of feeding

The regulation of feeding via nutrient levels in the blood serves to help maintain body energy stores. An individual who has been starving for some time tends to eat more when presented with food than one who has been eating regular meals. Conversely if an animal is force fed for some time, it eats very little when the force-feeding ceases but food is made available. The activity of the feeding centre is therefore geared to the nutritional status of the body. The factors that reflect this and control the feeding and satiety centres are the levels of glucose, amino acids, and fat metabolites available to them. Glucose is very important in this respect. When blood glucose levels fall, an animal increases its feeding. This returns its blood glucose concentration to normal. Furthermore, an increase in blood glucose concentration increases the electrical activity in neurones in the satiety centre. Neurones in the satiety centre, but not other areas of the hypothalamus, concentrate glucose, and this may be related to its role in the control of hunger. The control of feeding by blood glucose levels is known as the 'glucostatic' theory of hunger. To a lesser extent an increase in the concentration of amino acids in the blood can also reduce feeding, and a decrease enhances feeding.

The extent of feeding in an animal depends on the amount of adipose tissue in the body, indicating a role for fat metabolites in the control of feeding behaviour. If adipose tissue mass is low, feeding is increased. It seems likely that lipid metabolites exert a negative feedback control of feeding. This is known as the 'lipostatic' theory of hunger. The nature of the metabolites responsible for this effect is unknown. However, the average concentration of unesterified fatty acid in the blood is approximately proportional to the quantity of adipose tissue fat in the body. Thus free fatty acids or their metabolites probably also regulate long-term feeding habits, and so enable the individual's nutritional stores to remain constant.

Obesity can be due to an abnormality of the feeding mechanism, resulting from either psychogenic factors or from an abnormality of the hypothalamic feeding centres. These can be genetic or environmental factors; overeating in childhood is probably one environmental determinant of obesity. Excessive feeding results in increased energy input over energy output. However, this may occur only during the phase when obesity is developing. Once the fat has been deposited the obesity will be maintained by normal food intake. It can only be reduced if energy input is lower than energy output. This can be achieved only by reducing food intake, or by increasing energy output via exer-

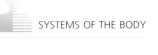
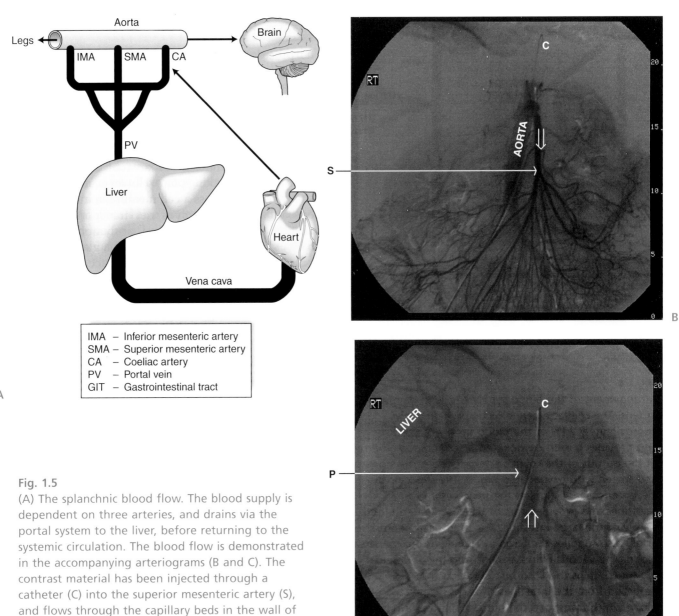

Fig. 1.5
(A) The splanchnic blood flow. The blood supply is dependent on three arteries, and drains via the portal system to the liver, before returning to the systemic circulation. The blood flow is demonstrated in the accompanying arteriograms (B and C). The contrast material has been injected through a catheter (C) into the superior mesenteric artery (S), and flows through the capillary beds in the wall of the small bowel, before collecting in the portal vein (P) and draining into the liver.

concentrations of the ion (in this case a cation) on the two sides of the membrane.

The potential difference across the membranes of secretory cells and absorptive cells (enterocytes) varies from region to region in the digestive system (see Chapter 8).

Mechanisms of transport

Some substances are transported solely by passive diffusion. Others are transported slowly by passive diffusion and more rapidly by special mechanisms.

The special mechanisms include active transport and facilitated diffusion.

Active transport

Table 1.1 on page 10 shows the criteria used to distinguish active and passive processes. A source of energy is required for active transport to take place. This source can be in the form of ATP, glucose, oxygen, or other substances. Passive transport requires no measurable amount of energy. If an active transport mechanism exists for the absorption of a substance it can be transported against a concentration gradient. If the substance is an ion, it may be transported against an

---

Ischaemic gut Box 2

Defect, diagnosis, and treatment

Decreased cardiac output results in decreased intestinal perfusion with blood. As the velocity of flow decreases, the viscosity of the blood increases and the blood tends to stagnate in the small vessels. Then microthrombi develop and disseminate in the blood vessels of the mesenteric circulation. There is also a generalised vaso-constriction of the blood vessels (see Case history on page 18), which causes small vessels to collapse. The consequent increase in resistance to flow in the splanchnic circulation, together with the decreased cardiac output and reduced arterial blood pressure, results in severely reduced blood flow to the intestines, which eventually become ischaemic.

Reduced blood flow to the gastrointestinal tract results in lack of oxygen (hypoxia) and reduced energy substrate supply to the tissues. The result is widespread necrosis of the gastrointestinal mucosa, which is extremely sensitive to hypoxia. This quickly leads to disruption of its functions (see Case history on page 11). The necrosis starts at the tips of the villi, which become hypoxic first. It seems probable also that disruption of the brush border of the enterocytes exposes the underlying tissue to the actions of the digestive proteolytic enzymes in the lumen. The intestines become permeable to toxic substances from the contents of the gut lumen, such as bacteria and bacterial toxins, and toxic substances from the necrotic cells. These substances enter the portal circulation. In summary, the barrier function of the gut is lost. There is a profound toxaemia and impairment of the normal body defences, resulting in septic shock. Loss of fluid, electrolytes, and blood from the gut will also occur. This effect mirrors loss in the skin in burns. The loss of the external barrier allows penetration of bacteria into the body as well as fluid loss from it.

The abdominal pain is due to the inflammatory response to ischaemia that accompanies the necrosis, and also due to inflammation of the parietal peritoneum. Differentiation of this condition from occlusive arterial disease is difficult. Selective angiography, a technique involving the introduction of a radio-opaque substance into the blood, followed by x-radiography, may show narrowed and irregular branches of the superior mesenteric artery, and impaired filling of intramural vessels.

Management of this condition requires measures to maintain the cardiac output, blood pressure and tissue oxygenation, treatment of infection, and replacement of fluid and electrolytes lost from the gastrointestinal tract. Surgery for heart failure may be required but the operation is not safe in the presence of gut infarction. If peritonitis is present, abdominal surgery is required to remove the necrotic intestinal tissue.

---

electrical gradient. In the small intestine the serosal surface of the absorptive cell membrane is positive with respect to the luminal surface. Thus net absorption of cations into the blood must be accomplished by means of active transport. Active transport of an ion may involve exchange for another ion of the same charge, or it may be accompanied by transport of an ion of the opposite charge. These arrangements preserve the electrical status of the cell. Furthermore, in secretory tissues the rate of transport for an actively-transported fluid (for example saliva, bile) can be constant until a pressure above the systolic arterial pressure of the blood serving the secreting tissue is reached.

Passive diffusion is transport down a concentration gradient and the rate of transport is proportional to the concentration difference of the substance across the membrane, over a wide range of concentration differences. However, for active transport the rate is only proportional to the concentration gradient at low concentration differences. This is because at high concentrations the process becomes saturated and a transport maximum (T_m) is reached (Fig. 1.6, page 10). Active transport of a substance is much faster than passive transport of that substance.

Active transport processes, but not passive ones, can be inhibited by metabolic inhibitors such as dinitrophenol (DNP) or iodoacetate. In addition they are temperature-dependent, whilst passive ones are not. A 10°C rise in temperature can result in a 3- to 5-fold increase in the rate of an active transport process. Finally, an active transport process is unidirectional. Thus glucose, for example is actively transported from the lumen of the small intestine into the blood but it is not actively transported in the opposite direction.

Facilitated diffusion

Transport via facilitated diffusion does not occur against a concentration gradient. However, for the transport of a given substance, it is more rapid than passive diffusion. Like active transport, it is proportional to the concentration difference across the membrane only at low favourable concentration gradients.

1

Table 1.1
Comparison between active and passive transport

Criterion	Passive	Active
a) Effect of opposing concentration or electrical gradient	No net transport against gradient	Transport against a gradient
b) Variation with concentration difference	Transport proportional to concentration difference over a wide range	Transport proportional only at low concentrations, saturation at high concentrations
c) Energy supply	Not required	Required, glucose, O_2, ATP etc.
d) Inhibitors	Not inhibited by metabolic or competitive inhibitors	Inhibited by metabolic inhibitors (F^-, DNP etc.)
e) Temperature change	No appreciable effect	Sensitive to temperature change (Q_{10} is high)
f) Direction	Bidirectional	Unidirectional

DNP, dinitrophenol. Q10 Effect of a 10°C increase in temperature.

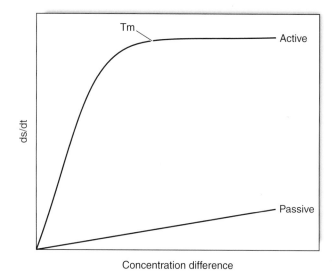

Fig. 1.6
The effect of concentration gradient on active and passive transport processes. Tm, transport maximum.

At high concentration differences the mechanism becomes saturated. This is usually because it depends on the binding of the substance to a carrier protein in the membrane. Facilitated diffusion can be inhibited competitively by substances that bind to the same sites on the carrier protein.

Pinocytosis

Some particles or large macromolecules, such as some proteins, may be absorbed in the small intestine via pinocytosis (endocytosis). This process involves the molecule becoming surrounded by the cell membrane and engulfed into the cell. It resembles phagocytosis but pinocytotic vesicles are small (usually 100–200 nM in diameter) whilst phagocytosed particles are larger (e.g. bacteria). The macromolecules usually attach to specific receptors which are concentrated in small coated pits in the membrane. The cytoplasmic surface of the pit is coated with a dense material containing contractile filaments. After the protein molecule has attached to its receptors the entire pit invaginates into the cell and its borders close over the attached macromolecules together with a small amount of fluid. The invaginated portion of the membrane breaks away from the rest of the membrane. Thus the endocytosed particle is surrounded by the plasma membrane of the cell and engulfed. It is then a membrane-bound particle within the cytoplasm of the cell.

Ischaemic gut Box 3

Effects on membrane transport

Under hypoxic conditions, cellular metabolism becomes anaerobic. Adenosine, a metabolite of ATP is degraded to hypoxanthine. The enzyme hypoxanthine oxidase then catalyses the conversion of hypoxanthine to superoxide and hydroxyl-free radicals, which are cytotoxic. These compounds oxidise cell membrane lipids, and this in turn causes irreversible changes in the permeability of cell membranes and disruption of active transport systems in the cell plasma membranes. As a consequence the cells can no longer maintain their normal intracellular composition and the cells die. Because of its high metabolic activity the mucosa has the highest requirement for oxygen of all layers of the gastrointestinal tract, and consequently it is the most sensitive to anoxia. Necrosis of the absorptive cells reduces the surface area for absorption and disrupts the specialised transport mechanisms for the absorption of nutrients. In addition, because the normal barrier to diffusion has been removed as the mucosal cells die, toxic metabolites and other substances diffuse into the blood. Under normal conditions mucosal cell loss would result in rapid cell proliferation and replacement. As this process requires oxygen, it will not take place unless the blood supply is restored. Thus aggressive treatment of the heart failure is central to the survival of these patients.

The process is active, requiring energy in the form of ATP within the cell, and Ca^{2+} ions in the extracellular fluid. Inside the cell the Ca^{2+} may activate the contractile microfilaments to pinch the vesicles off the cell membrane.

Motility

Smooth muscle in the gastrointestinal tract

The muscle of the gastrointestinal tract is arranged mainly in two layers, an outer longitudinal coat, and an inner circular coat (Fig. 1.7A). In most regions of the gastrointestinal tract the muscular coat is composed entirely of smooth muscle. However, skeletal muscle is present in the pharynx, the upper third of the oesophagus, and the external anal sphincter.

The smooth muscle of the gastrointestinal tract is of two types: phasic and tonic. Phasic muscle contracts and relaxes in a matter of seconds (i.e. phasically). This type of smooth muscle is present in the main body of the oesophagus, the gastric antrum and the small intestine. Tonic muscle contracts in a slow and sustained manner (i.e. tonically). The duration of tonic muscle contractions can be minutes or hours. This type of smooth muscle is present in the lower oesophageal sphincter, the ileocaecal sphincter and the internal anal sphincter. These differences between phasic and tonic muscle reflect the different functions they perform. Thus contraction of the antrum muscle empties food rapidly into the intestines, whereas the tonic contractions of the muscle of the ileocaecal sphincter keeps the junction between the ileum and the colon closed for long periods of time and enables the entry of chyme into the colon to be carefully controlled. Whether the muscle is phasic or tonic depends on properties intrinsic to the muscle cells. Neurotransmitters and hormones alter the amplitude of phasic contractions, and the tone of tonic muscle. These differences relate to the electrical properties of the cells but the basic mechanisms underlying the contractile activity are similar in all smooth muscle cells.

The smooth muscle coats are composed of small spindle-shaped cells. Unlike skeletal muscle cells, these cells are not arranged in orderly sarcomeres. There are no striations, although thick and thin myofilaments are present. Actin and tropomyosin are the contractile proteins that constitute the thin filaments, and myosin is the contractile protein of the thick filaments. Troponin is present only in negligible amounts, if at all. There are many more actin than myosin filaments. The ratio of thin to thick filaments is between

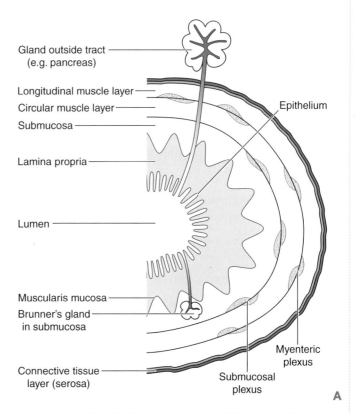

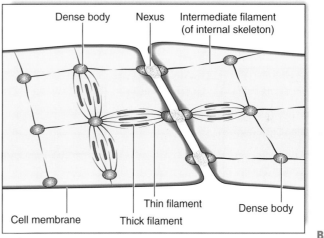

Fig. 1.7
(A) Layers of the gastrointestinal tract showing the locations of glands, the smooth muscle coats, and the enteric nerve plexi. (B) Structural features of visceral smooth muscle.

12:1 and 18:1. This can be contrasted with skeletal muscle where the ratio is 2:1. The thin filaments are anchored either to the plasma membrane or to structures known as dense bodies which are attached to a network of another type of filament of intermediate thickness between the thick and thin filaments. These intermediate filaments form an internal skeleton on which the contractile filaments are anchored. Figure

1.7 shows the organisation of the structures in smooth muscle. The dense bodies correspond to the Z lines in skeletal muscle. Contraction of smooth muscle occurs by a sliding filament mechanism similar to that in skeletal and cardiac muscle, with cross-bridge formation occurring between the overlapping thick and thin filaments. The muscle cells are organised as sheets which behave as effector units because the individual cells are functionally coupled to one another. Opposing membranes of the cells are fused to form gap junctions or nexuses. These are low-resistance junctions that allow the spread of excitation from one cell to another. Contractions of the bundles of cells are therefore synchronous.

Initiation of smooth muscle contraction

Contraction of smooth muscle cells is triggered by Ca^{2+} influx into the muscle cells. Neurotransmitters, hormones and other factors can promote Ca^{2+} influx. In resting muscle the Ca^{2+} concentration is low (approximately $10^{-7}M$) and there is no interaction between actin and myosin. The extracellular Ca^{2+} concentration is approximately 2mM. In phasic muscle cells the Ca^{2+} enters via voltage-determined Ca^{2+} channels (VDCCs). When the cell membrane is depolarised to threshold, an action potential is generated and the VDCCs open. Ca^{2+} enters down its concentration gradient causing the cell to contract. The resulting influx of Ca^{2+} initiates the contractile response of the non-pacemaker cells. The intracellular events that trigger muscle contraction are outlined in Figure 1.8. Inside the cell, the Ca^{2+} binds to calmodulin, a Ca^{2+} binding protein. This complex activates a kinase enzyme on the light chain of the myosin molecules in the thick filaments. The activated myosin light-chain kinase catalyses the phosphorylation of myosin utilising ATP, which is dephosphorylated to form ADP. The phosphorylated myosin can then interact with actin to split ATP, causing the movement of the cross-bridges. The myofilaments slide past each other and the muscle contracts. The myosin is inactivated by dephosphorylation and the ADP formed is converted back to ATP. The process of contraction requires energy, so the ischaemic bowel quickly becomes atonic and passively dilates, resulting in abdominal distension (Fig. 1.9).

Control

Action potentials are triggered in only a few cells by nervous and hormonal influences. These are known as

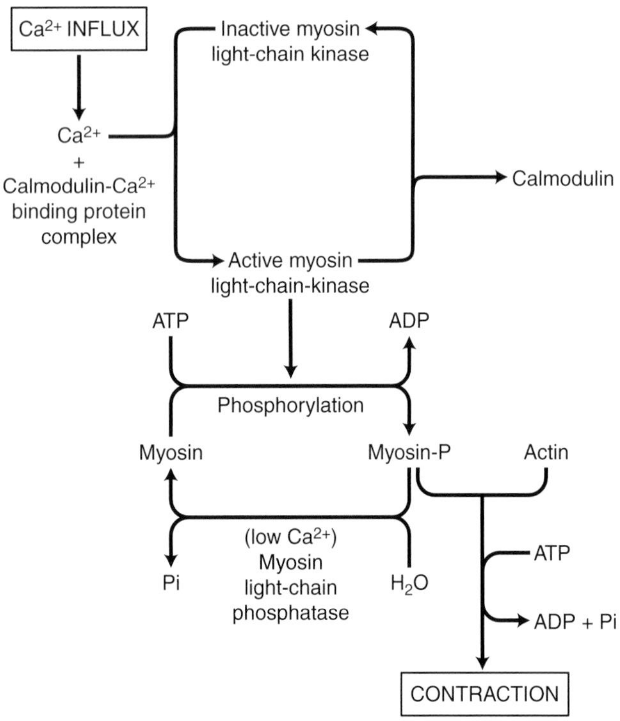

Fig. 1.8
Role of Ca^{2+} in the contraction of smooth muscle. Based on a diagram from Johnson L. J., 'Gastrointestinal Pathology' 4e London: Mosby 1991.

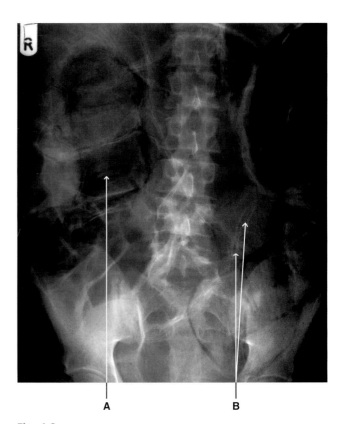

Fig. 1.9
A plain X-ray of large bowel ischaemia, showing dilated large bowel (A), with gas in the oedematous bowel wall, underneath the ischaemic mucosa (B).

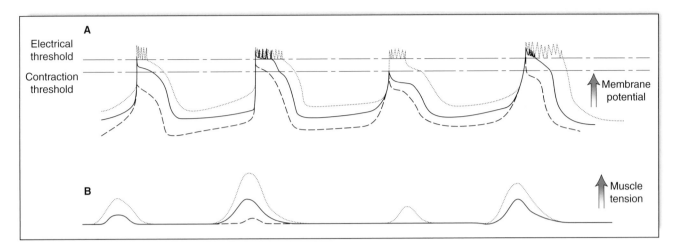

Fig. 1.10

Control of pacemaker cells in gastrointestinal smooth muscle. The generation of action potentials by the cell and their frequency depends on the amplitude of the oscillations in the membrane potential. (A) Oscillating membrane potential. The solid line represents a recording from a cell which is not under the influence of hormones or transmitters. Stimulation shifts the resting membrane potential towards the threshold for electrical excitation (depolarisation), resulting in the generation of action potentials (dotted line). When the membrane potential exceeds the threshold level, muscle tension is developed. Inhibition shifts the resting membrane potential further away from the threshold (hyperpolarisation, dashed line). (B) Development of muscle tension. An increased frequency of action potentials causes the development of increased muscle tension via summation of the contractile response. The contraction threshold of the membrane potential may be slightly lower than the action potential threshold (see A). Solid line, tension developed in the absence of external stimulation. Dotted line, tension developed in response to stimulation.

pacemaker cells. The action potentials set up in these cells are then transmitted throughout the muscle sheet. The pacemaker cells are most numerous in the longitudinal muscle layer. In these cells the resting membrane potential (RMP) is continuously oscillating. This activity is known as the basal electrical rhythm. The control of tension development in smooth muscle is exerted via changing the offset of this basal electrical rhythm (Fig. 1.10). If the amplitude of the depolarisation phase of the oscillation reaches the threshold level, an action potential is triggered. The action potential is conducted via nexuses from cell to cell causing Ca^{2+} influx, and contraction of the smooth muscle cells. With increased frequency of action potentials there is summation of the contractile response and the muscle contracts with increased force. The force generated is related to the intracellular Ca^{2+} concentration.

Action potentials occur spontaneously in pacemaker cells as the amplitude of the oscillations occasionally reaches the threshold potential in the absence of external stimulation. The muscle is therefore under a certain amount of tension even in the resting state. This property of spontaneous contraction is known as tone.

Increased Ca^{2+} influx leads to increased force of contraction. Conversely, because there is normally always a degree of tone present, a decrease in Ca^{2+} influx leads to a decrease in the force of contraction, i.e. relative

relaxation. Control is exerted largely by shifts in the mean RMP (Fig. 1.10). If the membrane potential is shifted closer to threshold (depolarisation), more oscillations reach threshold and more action potentials are generated and the force of contraction will be increased. If the membrane potential is shifted further from the threshold (hyperpolarisation), fewer of the oscillations reach the threshold, the frequency of action potentials decreases, and the force of contraction decreases.

Smooth muscle contracts in response to stretch. This is known as the myogenic reflex. It is an intrinsic property of smooth muscle and does not occur in skeletal muscle. Figure 1.11 shows the relationship between the degree of stretch and the force of contraction in visceral smooth muscle. Stretching the membrane opens Ca^{2+} channels in the membrane and Ca^{2+} flows into the cell. However, whereas moderate stretch results in depolarisation of the membrane and muscle contraction, excessive stretch inhibits the force of contraction.

The membrane potential of the pacemaker cells can be controlled by neurotransmitters and hormones. These act on receptors to cause either depolarisation or hyperpolarisation of the cells. The nerve axons that enter smooth muscle release neurotransmitter from swellings, known as varicosities, along their length. No discrete neuromuscular junctions exist between the

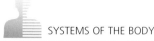

muscle cells and the nerve release sites. Indeed the varicosities are usually some distance from the muscle cells.

Control of secretion and motility

The control of secretion and motility in the gastrointestinal tract is by neural, hormonal, and paracrine mechanisms. The neural control is via both extrinsic nerves of the autonomic nervous system and nerves in the intrinsic enteric nerve plexi of the gastrointestinal tract. In many instances the mediators of neural or hormonal control are peptides. In some cases a given peptide acts as both a neurotransmitter and a hormone. Table 1.2 shows some of the neuropeptides involved in control of the gastrointestinal tract.

Neural control

The gastrointestinal tract is innervated by both autonomic nerves and by nerves in the enteric plexi in the walls of the tract (Fig. 1.7A, page 11). The enteric nervous system controls motility, secretion, and blood flow. However, signals from the central nervous system, travelling in both sympathetic and parasympathetic nerves can alter the activity of the nerves in the intrinsic plexi.

Enteric nervous system

The enteric nervous system may be regarded as a third division of the autonomic nervous system, after the sympathetic and parasympathetic divisions. However, in contrast to the sympathetic and parasympathetic nerves, the enteric nerves can perform many functions independently of the central nervous system.

Anatomy

The enteric nervous system consists of two major plexi (Fig. 1.7A), together with lesser plexi, in the wall of the gastrointestinal tract. Figure 1.12 shows the anatomical arrangement of the enteric nervous system in the tract. The major plexi are the myenteric plexus (Auerbach's plexus), which is situated between the layers of longitudinal and circular smooth muscle, and the submucous plexus (Meissner's plexus), which lies in the

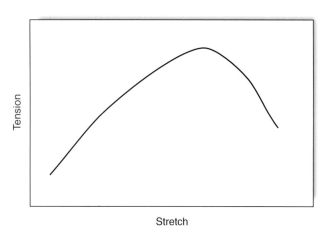

Fig. 1.11
Effect of stretch on tension development in smooth muscle. Tension development is proportional to stretch at low or moderate levels of stretch, but excessive stretch results in reduced tension.

Table 1.2
Some biologically active peptides of the digestive system, their cellular sites of origin in the gastrointestinal tract, and their sites of action

Peptide	Main site of origin	Site of action
Gastrin	APUD cells (stomach antrum)	Secretory cells of stomach, pancreas Smooth muscle of gallbladder, small intestine
GRP	Intrinsic neurones (stomach)	Secretory and smooth muscle cells of stomach
Somatostatin	APUD cells (stomach)	Secretory cells of stomach
Secretin	APUD cells (duodenum)	Secretory cells of stomach, pancreas, liver, small intestine
Cholecystokinin	APUD cells (duodenum)	Secretory cells of stomach, pancreas Smooth muscle of gallbladder, blood vessels
Motilin	APUD cells (duodenum, jejunum)	Smooth muscle of small intestine
GIP	APUD cells (duodenum, jejunum)	Secretory cells of stomach
Enteroglucagon	APUD cells (ileum and colon)	Secretory cells of stomach Smooth muscle cells of stomach, intestines
VIP	Intrinsic neurones (throughout the GIT)	Secretory cells of salivary glands, small intestines, pancreas Smooth muscle of stomach and large intestine, sphincters, blood vessels

GRP, gastrin releasing peptide, GIP, gastric inhibitory peptide, VIP, vasoactive intestinal peptide. APUD cells are the enterocrine cells of the gastrointestinal tract.

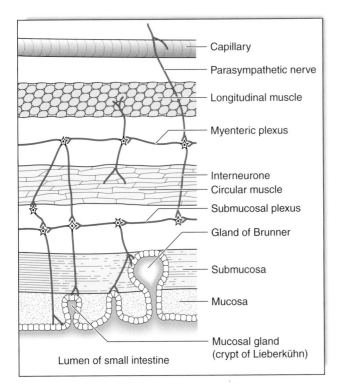

Fig. 1.12
The arrangement of neurones in the enteric nerve plexi.

Capillary
Parasympathetic nerve
Longitudinal muscle
Myenteric plexus
Interneurone
Circular muscle
Submucosal plexus
Gland of Brunner
Submucosa
Mucosa
Mucosal gland (crypt of Lieberkühn)
Lumen of small intestine

mucosa. The myenteric plexus is involved mainly in the control of gastrointestinal motility. This is exemplified in Hirschsprung's disease where ganglion cells are missing from a region of the myenteric plexus (see Chapter 10), resulting in severe constipation, which in the neonate can be life-threatening (muconium ileus). The submucous plexus is more important in the control of secretion and blood flow. It is also important in receiving sensory information from the gut epithelium and from stretch receptors in the wall of the tract. Smaller plexi reside within the smooth muscle layers and within the mucosa.

Within each plexus the neuronal cell bodies are arranged in ganglia. Intrinsic nerves of the enteric nervous system connect the plexi together by synapsing with the ganglion cells. They also innervate smooth muscle, secretory glands, and blood vessels of the tract. In addition many of them synapse with postganglionic sympathetic and parasympathetic nerves, or sensory nerves. These arrangements are shown schematically in Figure 1.12. The enteric nervous system is therefore composed of four categories of nerves:

- extrinsic fibres
- intrinsic motoneurones
- intrinsic interneurones
- sensory neurones.

Extrinsic fibres

If the extrinsic nerves are sectioned there is little impairment of gastrointestinal function, except in the mouth, oesophagus, and anal regions, where control by extrinsic nerves is more important than in the rest of the gastrointestinal tract. Such extrinsic control is clearly required in these regions for the ingestion of food and the expulsion of faeces.

Both excitatory and inhibitory nerves innervate the smooth muscle, blood vessels and glands of the gastrointestinal tract. In addition there are both excitatory and inhibitory interneurones in the plexi. Furthermore, enteric neurones (as well as gastrointestinal smooth muscle cells, see below) exhibit spontaneous rhythmic activity.

In general, stimulation of the myenteric plexus increases the motor activity of the gut, by increasing tonic contractions (tone), the intensity and rate of rhythmic contractions of the smooth muscle, and the velocity of waves of contraction (peristalsis) along the tract. However, some fibres in the myenteric plexus are inhibitory. Many different excitatory and inhibitory neurotransmitters are involved.

Intrinsic motoneurones

Intrinsic motor nerves are predominantly excitatory. Some of the excitatory neurones are cholinergic and their effects can be blocked with atropine, indicating that the receptors involved are muscarinic. However, other excitatory neurones release other transmitters such as substance P. Stimulation of excitatory motor nerves can cause contraction of both circular and longitudinal smooth muscle, relaxation of sphincter muscle, or glandular secretion. Stimulation of inhibitory motor fibres in the enteric nervous system causes smooth muscle relaxation. The inhibitory transmitter involved may be ATP or vasoactive intestinal peptide (VIP).

Intrinsic interneurones

Intrinsic interneurones can also be excitatory or inhibitory. The transmitter released by excitatory neurones is probably acetylcholine, which acts on nicotinic receptors on postsynaptic neurones. The transmitters released by the inhibitory interneurones are largely unknown.

Sensory neurones

Many afferent sensory neurones are present in the gastrointestinal tract. Some of these have their cell bodies in the enteric nervous system. They are stimulated by distension or irritation of the gut wall which activates mechanoreceptors and by substances in the food, which activate chemoreceptors. They form part of reflex pathways, which may or may not be influenced by control via extrinsic nerves. Some of these sensory fibres also terminate on interneurones which in turn can activate excitatory or inhibitory motor neurones.

Some afferent sensory fibres that have their cell bodies in the enteric nerve plexi, terminate in the sympathetic ganglia. Other sensory fibres from the gastrointestinal tract have their cell bodies in the dorsal root ganglia of the spinal cord or in the cranial nerve ganglia. These nerve fibres travel in the same nerve trunks as the autonomic nerves. They transmit information to the medulla, which in turn transmits efferent signals back to the gastrointestinal tract to influence its functions. Specific reflexes are described in the appropriate chapters in this book.

Control by autonomic nerves

At any one time activity in autonomic nerves can alter the activity of the entire gastrointestinal tract, or of a discrete part of it, via its influences on the enteric nervous system. In addition, autonomic nerves may synapse directly on smooth muscle and secretory cells to influence their activity directly, although they synapse principally with enteric interneurones to influence function indirectly.

Parasympathetic nerves

Preganglionic nerves from both the cranial and sacral divisions of the parasympathetic nervous system supply the gastrointestinal tract. The cranial parasympathetic preganglionic nerve fibres travel in the vagus nerve except for a few which innervate the mouth and pharyngeal regions. The vagal fibres innervate the oesophagus, stomach, pancreas, liver, small intestine, and the ascending and transverse colon (Fig. 1.13). The preganglionic nerves of the sacral division of the parasympathetic nervous system, which innervate the tract originate in the second, third and fourth segments of the sacral spinal cord and travel in the pelvic nerves to the distal part of the large intestine. The parasympathetic innervation of the tract is more extensive in the upper (orad) region and the distal (rectal and anal) regions than elsewhere. The preganglionic parasympathetic nerve fibres form excitatory synapses with postganglionic neurones in both the myenteric and submucosal plexi. These are mainly excitatory interneurones of the enteric nerve plexi. Stimulation of the parasympathetic nerves can have a diffuse, far-reaching effect to activate the entire enteric nervous system via these interneurones. In general, the effect of activity in the parasympathetic nerves is to stimulate secretion and motility in the gastrointestinal

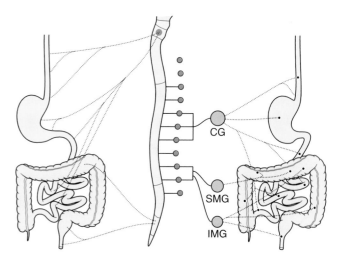

Fig. 1.13

The autonomic innervation of the gastrointestinal tract. LHS, dashed lines indicate the preganglionic parasympathetic innervation by the vagus nerve (cranial nerve 10) from the brain stem, and nerves of the sacral outflow of the spinal cord. RHS, the dashed lines indicate the postganglionic sympathetic innervation arising from the cervical ganglion (CG), the superior mesenteric ganglion (SMG) and the inferior mesenteric ganglion (IMG). The preganglionic sympathetic nerves arise in the thoracic and upper lumbar regions of the spinal cord, and pass through the paravertebral chains to ganglia.

tract. The transmitter released by the preganglionic parasympathetic nerves is acetylcholine and it acts on nicotinic receptors on interneurones in the enteric nerve plexi.

Sympathetic nerves

The preganglionic sympathetic nerves that supply the gastrointestinal tract arise from segments T8 to L2 in the thoracic spinal cord (Fig. 1.13). This is why pain from the gastrointestinal tract is referred to the corresponding somatic dermatomes (areas of the skin innervated by neurones that enter the spinal cord at the same level). The fibres pass through the sympathetic chains and synapse with postganglionic neurones in the coeliac ganglion and various mesenteric ganglia. The postganglionic fibres travel together with blood vessels to innervate all regions of the tract. They terminate mainly on neurones in the enteric nerve plexi, although a few terminate directly on smooth muscle cells or secretory cells. In general, activity in the sympathetic nerves inhibits activity in the gastrointestinal tract, having opposite effects to stimulation of the parasympathetic nerves. Stimulation of postganglionic sympathetic nerve fibres can inhibit the release of acetylcholine from excitatory motoneurones, to cause relaxation of the smooth muscle indirectly. They can also cause constriction of sphincter muscle, or inhibit glandular secretion, and importantly, cause vasoconstriction of arterioles of the gastrointestinal tract, redirecting blood flow away from the splanchnic bed. Most effects of activation of sympathetic nerves are exerted indirectly via its connections in the enteric nervous system. Movement of food through the gastrointestinal tract can be completely blocked by strong activation of the sympathetic nervous system. The transmitter released by sympathetic postganglionic nerve fibres is noradrenaline.

Endocrine control

The gastrointestinal tract is the largest endocrine organ in the body, but the hormone-secreting cells are diffusely distributed in the mucosa, scattered amongst numerous other types of cell. This is in contrast to other endocrine organs such as the pituitary, thyroid, and adrenals, where the cells are organised 'en masse'. The endocrine cells of the gastrointestinal tract are APUD cells. This acronym stands for amine precursor uptake and decarboxylation, after the classical function of the cells, which may relate to their role in hormone synthesis. The APUD cells in different regions of the tract secrete different hormones. Table 1.2 (page 14) indicates some of the peptides secreted, and the locations in the gastrointestinal tract where they are secreted.

The APUD cells that contain peptide hormones can be stained with silver. They contain dense-core vesicles in which the peptide hormones are packaged. These cells are of two types: 'open' and 'closed' (Fig. 1.14).

The open cells in the gastrointestinal mucosa extend to the lumen of the tract, and their luminal surface is covered with microvilli, an indication of their specialisation for secretion. In some cases only a thin neck of cytoplasm exists between the luminal margin and the basilar side of the cell. The secretory vesicles are at the base of the cell. The open APUD cell is the most common type of endocrine cell in the gastrointestinal tract. It is found in areas extending from the pyloric antrum to the rectum. These cells sense chemical substances in the food. Thus they behave as chemoreceptors or 'taste' cells. In addition they may respond to mechanical stimulation.

The closed APUD cells are numerous in the oxyntic area of the stomach mucosa. They sometimes have horizontal processes. They usually make synaptic contacts with intrinsic nerve cells as well as with other APUD cells. Cells of both types release hormones into the interstitial spaces from where they are transported

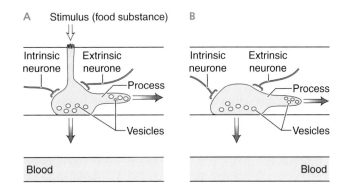

Fig. 1.14
Schematic representation of open and closed APUD cells. (A) Open cell, (B) closed cell. The peptide hormones are stored in secretory vesicles, and released by exocytosis into the blood. They may also be secreted from extensions or processes. They can also act in a paracrine manner on other cells, including other APUD cells, in the mucosa. Open cells can be stimulated by substances in the gastrointestinal lumen. Both open and closed cells can be stimulated by peptides released from other APUD cells, or by transmitters released from intrinsic or extrinsic nerves.

by diffusion or vesicular transport (cytopempsis) into the blood capillaries.

Upon stimulation both the open and the closed type of APUD cells release hormones. The hormones circulate in the blood to act at sites which may be distant from the location where they are secreted. Gastrin, for example, is a hormone secreted by the stomach antrum, but it acts on the liver and pancreas as well as the stomach. However, the hormones are secreted first into the interstitial spaces where they can regulate cells in close proximity to the hormone release sites. They therefore have local and distant influences. The local influences are known as paracrine control.

Control of blood flow

The blood flow to the digestive organs is relatively low in the fasting state but it increases several-fold when a meal is present in the tract and the tissues are actively secreting digestive juices or absorbing nutrients. Blood flow to the gut is controlled by many factors, including haemodynamic factors such as cardiac output, systemic arterial pressure, blood viscosity, and blood volume, which regulate the flow to all tissues in the body. Other factors include increased activity in sympathetic nerves which causes vasoconstriction and reduced blood flow, via release of noradrenaline which activates α-adrenergic receptors. However, this effect is short-lived for several reasons,

OVERVIEW OF THE DIGESTIVE SYSTEM

one of these being changes in local factors. Thus there is a reduction in oxygen tension (hypoxia), when the blood flow is reduced, and this induces vasodilatation. In addition, sympathetic nerve stimulation relaxes gut smooth muscle which results in reduced mechanical resistance to blood flow to the gastrointestinal tract. Other substances constricting the splanchnic vessels are circulating adrenaline, angiotensin II, and vasopressin.

Stimulation of the parasympathetic nerves to the gastrointestinal tract causes an increase in blood flow by various indirect mechanisms. These are a result of the increased secretory activity of the tissues induced by parasympathetic nerve stimulation. Secretion requires an increased metabolism of the actively secreting tissues, which results in an increased production of metabolites such as K^+, amines and polypeptides, and CO_2, as well as reduced O_2 tension, all of which may cause localised vasodilatation, with a consequent increase in blood flow. The transmitter released from these parasympathetic nerves may be VIP.

Stimulation of tissues to secrete can also result in the release of proteolytic enzymes, known as kallikreins, which activate precursors of the vasodilator bradykinin, in the intercellular spaces, to form the active vasodilator (see Chapter 2). These local responses are feedback mechanisms whereby the consumption of energy metabolites results in a greater supply of metabolites via increased blood flow. Other substances that dilate the blood vessels of the gastrointestinal tract are the hormones gastrin and cholecystokinin (CCK), which are released into the blood when food is present in the stomach and duodenum respectively. These have a more localised effect, with gastrin increasing the blood flow to the stomach and CCK increasing blood flow to the pancreas and intestines.

During a meal, the different organs of the digestive system are activated in sequence to secrete, absorb or contract, and their demand for energy substrates and oxygen increases accordingly. These requirements are met by an increased blood supply to the individual component organs and tissues as they require them. Neural activity in efferents from higher centres in the brain, autonomic nerves and enteric nerves, and hormones and local metabolites all interact to mediate the increased regional blood flow (hyperaemia) as each region requires it. In addition, during a meal there is also a generalised increase in blood flow due to an increased cardiac output. Thus when food enters the stomach, the release of gastrin and local metabolites in the stomach stimulates its blood flow. When the food enters the small intestine, the release of CCK and local metabolites results in increased blood flow to the small intestine.

The splanchnic circulation can be compromised in a number of pathological conditions that may arise in other organs of the body, such as haemorrhage and congestive heart failure, or by diseases of the digestive organs. Such diseases include non-occlusive ischaemic disease of the intestines, and cirrhosis of the liver.

Control of gastrointestinal functions during a meal

In general, the presence of food in the gastrointestinal tract stimulates smooth muscle in the main body of the tract and the gallbladder, relaxes the smooth muscle of the sphincters, and stimulates secretion and blood flow in the salivary glands, pancreas and liver. The control can be considered in three phases, depending on the location of the food. The cephalic phase is due to the approach of food and the presence of food in the mouth, the gastric phase is due to the presence of food in the stomach, and the intestinal phase to the presence of food is present in the small intestines. The sequential effects of food or chyme in these various locations enables synchronisation and coordination of activity of the smooth muscle, secretory tissues, and vascular system of the different regions and organs.

Food in the mouth stimulates pressure receptors and chemo- (taste) receptors, and this results in increased blood flow to the salivary glands and secretion of saliva which starts the digestion of starch. It also initiates the secretions of the stomach, pancreas, and liver to prepare the gastrointestinal tract to perform its digestive and absorptive functions. At this time the motility of the stomach is transiently inhibited.

Food in the stomach causes increased blood flow to the stomach and secretion of gastric juice, and stimulates the smooth muscle of the stomach. This enables the stomach to churn the food present within it and start the digestion of the food. However, food in the stomach also stimulates the secretion of pancreatic juice, bile, and intestinal juices in preparation for the chyme when it arrives in the small intestine where most digestion and absorption occurs. In addition it stimulates motility in the ileum and colon. This moves the chyme present in those regions into the next region and makes way for the arrival of more chyme.

Chyme in the duodenum exerts the major control over gastrointestinal function. It inhibits gastric secretion and motility, which transiently prevents further emptying of the stomach, allowing time for the processing of the food material already present in the small intestine. Food in the small intestine also stimulates secretion of intestinal juice, pancreatic juice and alkaline bile, and the blood flow to the intestines, pancreas and liver. It stimulates contraction of the gallbladder and relaxation of the sphincter of Oddi to allow the pancreatic juice and bile to enter the duodenum. These digestive juices can then perform the digestion of the complex nutrients, enabling absorption to take place in the small intestine.

Self-assessment case study: obesity

An excessively overweight middle-aged man visited his general practitioner to seek advice on how to lose weight. The doctor noticed that the man became breathless on slight exertion. The man was weighed at the surgery and found to be five stones overweight for his height. He was also found to have some sugar in his urine, indicating the possibility that he was suffering from type II diabetes mellitus, which is associated with obesity. The doctor examined the patient and found that his blood pressure was abnormally high, also a common finding in obese individuals. The patient was told that it was very important to lose weight and he was given a diet sheet.

Having read this chapter you should be able to attempt to answer the following questions:

① What sort of diet would the patient's diet sheet indicate? Can you explain why?

② Which other measures could the patient adopt to help him lose weight?

③ What do you understand by the 'alimentary' regulation of hunger?

④ Which nutrients are involved in the 'nutritional' regulation of food intake?

⑤ What defects in the hypothalamus could lead to hyperphagia (overeating), albeit in rare cases?

⑥ What is the function of the satiety centre?

⑦ What do you understand by appetite? Which areas of the central nervous system are involved in its control?

⑧ Can you give an example of a drug that could be prescribed for this patient if other measures prove unsuccessful?

Self-assessment questions

After reading this chapter you should be able to answer the following questions:

① Which structures outside the gastrointestinal tract provide important digestive juices?

② Which of the physiological processes is central to the functioning of the digestive system (give reasons)?

③ What are the major components of the faeces?

④ What are the major functions of the splanchnic circulation?

⑤ What are the main determinants of the rate of transport of a substance by passive diffusion?

⑥ How does active transport differ from passive transport?

⑦ How does Ca^{2+} trigger the contraction of smooth muscle?

⑧ What are 'pacemaker' cells in the gastrointestinal tract?

⑨ Which regions of the gastrointestinal tract are innervated by the vagus nerve?

⑩ Which types of neurone are present in the enteric nervous system?

⑪ Which regions of the gastrointestinal tract are innervated by somatic motoneurones?

⑫ What is the difference between 'open' and 'closed' APUD cells?

⑬ What is meant by the cephalic phase of control of the digestive system?

⑭ What is meant by the intestinal phase of control of the digestive system? Which hormones are involved in the control of pancreatic and gastric secretions during this phase? What are the major stimuli for their release? In what ways do they affect the release of gastric juice and pancreatic juice?

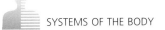
THE MOUTH, SALIVARY GLANDS, AND OESOPHAGUS

Introduction

The functions of the mouth and oesophagus are numerous. They include mastication, taste, swallowing, lubrication, digestion, speech, the signalling of thirst, and protection of the body from harmful ingested substances. The performance of all of these functions depends on the presence of saliva. In this chapter the functional importance of saliva is illustrated by the problems encountered in individuals with xerostomia (dry mouth), a condition characterised by pathological changes in the salivary and mucous glands, which result in impaired secretion.

The mouth

Anatomical features of the mouth

The oral cavity (the mouth) is closed by the apposition of the lips. The lips and the cheeks are composed mainly of skeletal muscle embedded in elastic fibro-connective tissue. Figure 2.2 shows the anatomical features of the oral cavity and the structures within it, including the tongue and the teeth. It also shows associated structures, such as the olfactory mucosa, which are important for the digestive system.

Xerostomia Box 1

Xerostomia

A 60-year-old woman visited her general practitioner and complained of a persistent dry mouth, difficulties in chewing and swallowing, and sore, gritty eyes. She also said that her food seemed tasteless. The doctor examined the patient's mouth. Her gums and teeth appeared inflamed and infected, and her tongue appeared lobulated. The patient was sent for investigation of salivary function.

The most frequent cause of dry mouth (xerostomia) is hypofunction of the salivary glands (which is often accompanied by hypofunction of the lacrimal glands). Figure 2.1 shows the appearance of the tongue in a patient with xerostomia.

The following questions will be addressed in this chapter:

① What are the major causes of dry mouth? Which oral conditions are associated with xerostomia? Which systemic conditions are associated with xerostomia?

② How can salivary function be assessed?

③ Why is saliva important for oral and dental health?

④ Which functions of the mouth would be impaired in xerostomia?

⑤ Which drugs or other treatments can be used to alleviate xerostomia and what side-effects might be expected from these treatments?

⑥ Why is saliva important for the functioning of the oesophagus?

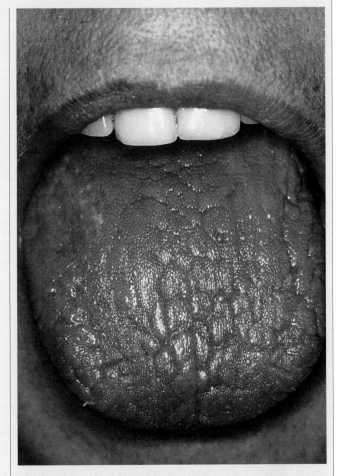

Fig. 2.1
The tongue of a patient with xerostomia, showing a characteristic grooved appearance. (Provided by Mr J. Hamburger, Dental School, University of Birmingham.)

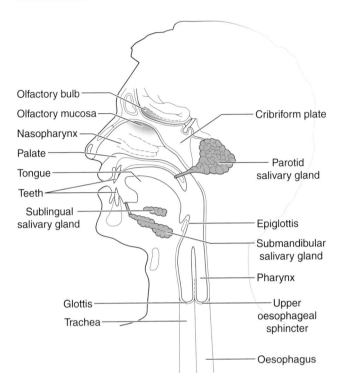

Fig. 2.2
Structures in the mouth, and associated structures.

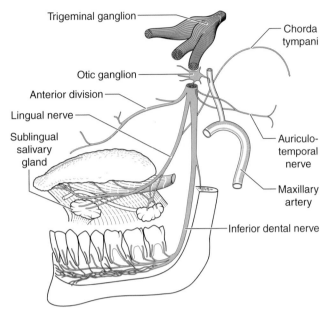

Fig. 2.3
The mandibular division of the trigeminal nerve. The lingual nerve innervates the anterior two-thirds of the tongue and the sublingual and submaxillary salivary glands. The inferior dental nerve innervates the tooth pulp, periodontal ligaments, and gums. The anterior division innervates the muscles of mastication (not shown), and the auriculotemporal nerve innervates structures of the ear (not shown).

Innervation

The innervation of many structures of the mouth is via the four branches of the mandibular division of the trigeminal nerve (Fig. 2.3). These branches are:

1. the anterior division, which innervates the lateral pterygoid, temporal, and masseter muscles which are involved in mastication (see below)
2. the auriculotemporal nerve, which innervates structures of the ear
3. the inferior dental nerve, which innervates the lower lip, tooth pulp, periodontal ligaments and gums
4. the lingual nerve, which innervates the anterior two-thirds of the tongue, the floor of the mouth, and the gum on the lingual side of the lower teeth.

The lingual nerve is joined by the chorda tympani which runs through the lateral pterygoid muscle. The chorda tympani carries sensory taste fibres from the lingual nerve to the facial nerve, and secretomotor (parasympathetic) fibres from the facial nerve to the lingual nerve. These fibres innervate the submandibular and sublingual salivary glands.

Anatomy and histology of the tongue

The tongue has a freely moveable portion known as the body, and a basal or root portion that is attached to the floor of the oral cavity and forms part of the anterior wall of the pharynx. It is divided into anterior and posterior regions by the sulcus terminalis, a V-shaped groove with the apex of the V directed posteriorly. It is composed largely of skeletal muscle fibres and glands, and is covered by a mucous membrane. Some of the muscle fibres are intrinsic and are confined to the tongue. These are arranged vertically, transversely, and longitudinally. There are also extrinsic fibres, which originate outside the tongue, mainly on the mandible and hyoid bone, and pass into the tongue (Fig. 2.4A). The glands are located between the muscle fibres. The glands in the base of the tongue are mainly mucous and their ducts open behind the sulcus terminalis. In the body of the tongue the glands are mainly serous and their ducts open anterior to the sulcus. Near the tip, the glands are mixed and their ducts open on to the inferior surface of the tongue.

On the upper surface of the tongue are numerous small protuberances, or papillae, which give the

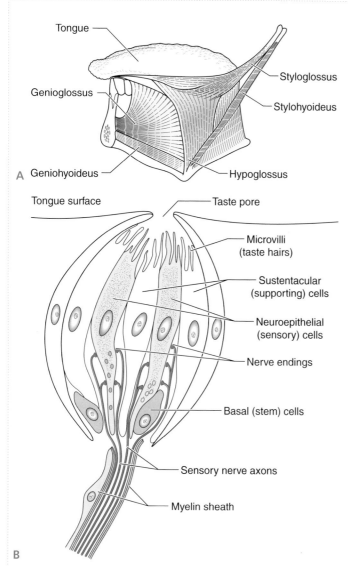

A

B

Fig. 2.4
(A) Locations of the extrinsic muscles of the tongue. (B) Structure of a taste bud. Based on a figure from 'Functional Neuroanatory' Williams P. L. & Warnick R. 1975.

Labels in figure A: Tongue, Styloglossus, Genioglossus, Stylohyoideus, Geniohyoideus, Hypoglossus

Labels in figure B: Tongue surface, Taste pore, Microvilli (taste hairs), Sustentacular (supporting) cells, Neuroepithelial (sensory) cells, Nerve endings, Basal (stem) cells, Sensory nerve axons, Myelin sheath

Taste

Taste buds

There are several thousand taste buds on the human tongue. Each circumvalate papilla contains several hundred taste buds. The taste buds contain the gustatory (taste) receptor cells. Figure 2.4B shows the structure of a taste bud. They are located in the oral (stratified squamous) epithelium, mainly in association with the papillae, but can be situated elsewhere in the oral cavity such as the palate and the epiglottis. They lie within the epithelium. Under the microscope they have a pale, barrel-shaped appearance with a depression, the taste pore, in the surface. This is an aperture that provides communication with the exterior. It contains three types of cell: supporting (sustentacular) cells, neuroepithelial taste cells, and basal cells. The supporting cells lie at the periphery and are arranged like the staves of a barrel. The neuroepithelial cells, which range from 10 to 14 in each taste bud, lie more centrally. Two types of neuroepithelial sensory cell can be distinguished under the electron microscope. One type contains clear vesicles within its cytoplasm and the other contains dense-core vesicles. The presence of different vesicles is consistent with the presence of different transmitter substances. These are stored in the vesicles prior to being released from the cell. Both the sensory cells and the support cells have long apical microvilli, or taste hairs, which project into the taste pore. The taste hairs lie in amorphous polysaccharide material that is secreted by the supporting cells. The basal cell is located peripherally near the basal lamina. These are the stem cells for the other cell types. There are club-shaped endings of sensory nerves lying between the cells. Chemical (taste) stimuli are received by the neuroepithelial cells and transmitted via the release of neurotransmitters from the cells to the nerve endings. The secretions of the serous glands of the papillae wash away food material and permit new taste stimuli to be received by the receptors.

Taste sensation

The solubilisation of food constituents by saliva enables the sense of taste to be experienced. Thus taste depends on the detection of chemicals that are dissolved in the saliva, and for this reason taste is compromised in xerostomia. There are four submodalities: salt, sour, sweet, bitter. Dissolved substances with these properties stimulate the receptors (the taste buds) on the tongue. Acid is the most potent stimulus; in humans, sucking a lemon can lead to the maximum rate of secretion, which can be 7–8 ml of saliva per minute. A taste bud responds to several or all of these submodalities, but each taste bud is most sensitive to

tongue its roughened appearance. Different types of papillae are present and these have different distributions on the tongue: fungiform and foliate papillae are present on the anterior and lateral surface, and circumvalate papillae on the base of the tongue. Papillae contain numerous nerve endings that sense touch. Most papillae have associated taste buds (see below). Lymphatic nodules (the lingual tonsil) protrude from the surface of the posterior one-third of the tongue and give it a nodular, irregular appearance. Between the nodules are crypts where the epithelium is infiltrated with numerous lymphocytes. The inferior surface of the tongue is smooth and is underlain by a submucosa.

one particular taste. However, all taste buds respond to all four stimuli, given high enough concentrations of the appropriate chemicals. The taste buds that respond primarily to sour substances (acids) are situated on the posterior sides of the tongue, whilst salt is detected on the anterior sides. Sweet substances are detected mainly on the front of the tongue, whilst bitter substances are detected on the rear. There are, however, no obvious structural differences in the taste buds in these different regions. It is possible that the differences in sensitivity are partly due to the differences in the projections of the afferent nerves to the central nervous system. The nerves from the taste buds in the anterior of the tongue pass in the chorda tympani (a branch of the facial nerve), and those from the taste buds in the posterior third travel in the glossopharyngeal nerve. These nerves project to the tractus solitarius (Fig. 2.5). The sensory nerves from the taste buds in the palate and epiglottis ascend in the vagus nerve.

Substances dissolved in the saliva diffuse into the taste pore from the fluid layer on the tongue. Appropriate chemicals, such as NaCl, are detected by receptor molecules on the taste hairs, and this results in a depolarisation of the cell membrane of the taste bud cell. The depolarisation response is known as a receptor potential. The amplitude of this response is graded according to the intensity of the stimulus. These receptor potentials give rise to the release of an excitatory transmitter which evokes a generator potential in the endings of the sensory nerve fibres which make contact with the receptor cells. This causes a discharge of impulses in the nerve axon, which is transmitted to the central nervous system. The mechanism involved in the response to salt has been well studied (Fig. 2.6).

Recordings from single afferent sensory fibres show that the intensity of the stimulus (the concentration of the salt solution) is signalled by the frequency of action potentials. The recognition of a particular taste quality by the central nervous system may depend on the patterns of impulses from a population of chemoreceptors.

Smell

Taste as defined by the layman includes smell (olfaction). Activation of olfactory receptors, in conjunction with central nervous system processing of their responses, enable many different types of odour, or flavours, to be distinguished. Smell has more primary qualities than taste. These include floral, ethereal, musky, camphor, putrid, and pungent submodalities. Blockage of the nose by the common cold, or olfactory nerve lesions, renders taste discrimination crude as it then relies only on the taste buds. The sense of smell, like that of taste, is an important stimulant of appetite and digestion. The olfactory mucosa which detects the odours is located in the upper nasopharynx (Fig. 2.2). The odorant molecules are borne to the olfactory mucosa via the inspired air, or from the air in the oral cavity during feeding. The chemical odours are detected by receptors in bipolar cells present in the mucosa (Fig. 2.7). There are about 10 million chemoreceptor cells in the human olfactory mucosa. Immobile cilia on the surface of the cells detect odorants dissolved in the mucous layer that overlies the mucosa. Terminals of unmyelinated nerve fibres

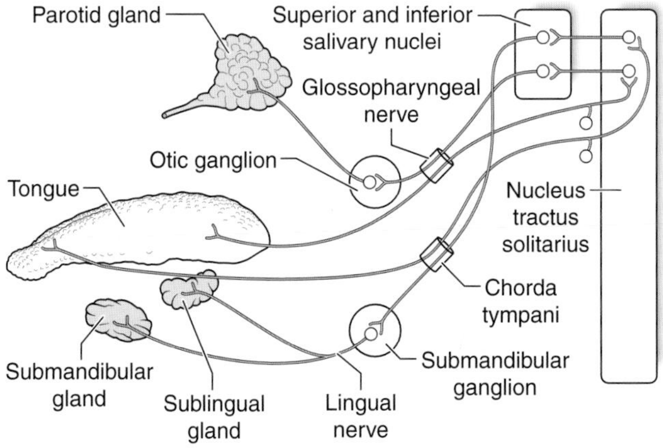

Fig. 2.5
Reflex pathway for the secretion of saliva in response to the stimulation of taste bud receptors.

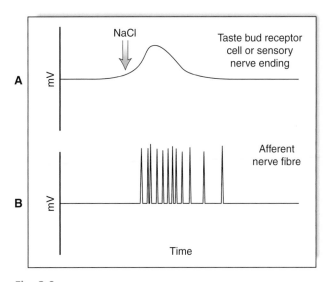

Fig. 2.6
Electrical potentials in (A) taste bud receptors, and (B) primary afferent nerves from the taste receptors.

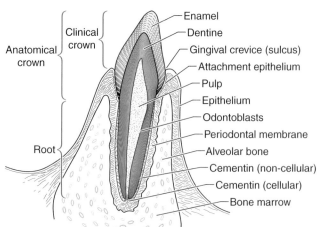

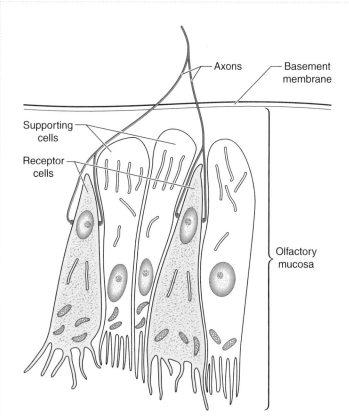

Fig. 2.7
Structure of the olfactory mucosa.

Fig. 2.8
Basic structure of a tooth.

connect with the basal surface of the sensory cells. The chemical odorants depolarise the receptor cell and this triggers a discharge in the sensory nerve. The intensity of the smell is signalled via the frequency of the discharges. The olfactory nerves penetrate the base of the skull via openings in the cribiform plate and make connections in the olfactory bulb, which is located in the cortex. Coding for a particular smell, like coding for taste, depends on the response of a population of receptors. The information is integrated in cortical structures.

Teeth

The teeth are embedded in the bone of the upper and lower jaws. They are arranged in two arcs. The upper arc is larger than the lower arc, and this results in the lower teeth being overlapped by the upper teeth. In the human there are 5 primary, or milk, teeth in each half jaw (20 in total); these erupt between the ages of approximately 6 months and 2 years of age. These teeth are shed between 6 and 13 years of age and are gradually replaced by the permanent adult teeth. The latter number 8 in each half jaw (total 32). The anterior five adult teeth replace the milk teeth.

Teeth of different shapes are present in the mouth. These differences represent modifications that serve different masticatory (chewing) functions. The sharp incisors are specialised for biting, whilst the larger, more flattened molars are specialised for grinding. Figure 2.8 shows the basic structure of a tooth. Each tooth has a basically similar structure: a visible crown projecting above the gingiva (the gum) and a root buried in the alveolus of the maxilla or the mandible. At the junction between the crown and the root is the neck. In the centre of each tooth is the pulp cavity, which is filled by connective tissue. The latter communicates via small pores (apical foramina) with the surrounding connective tissue or periodontal membrane, which holds the tooth in its socket (alveolus). This arrangement forms a peg and socket type of joint which permits slight movement. The hard tissues of the pulp are:

1. dentine, a calcified tissue similar to bone, which surrounds the pulp cavity and forms the bulk of the tooth
2. enamel, the hardest material, which is mainly composed of apatite crystals and covers the dentine of the crown
3. cementin, which like dentine is similar to bone and covers the dentine of the root.

Mastication (chewing)

The sight, smell, and thought of food elicit the secretion of saliva before the food even enters the mouth. However, the palatability of food, and therefore the decision whether or not to ingest it, depends partly on orally sensed properties after food has been taken into the mouth, such as taste, texture, and temperature.

Once it is present in the mouth, food is chewed, a process known as mastication. This involves movements of the jaw and the tongue. It is controlled by sensations from touch and pressure receptors located in the oral mucosa and the periodontum (area around the teeth), as well as from stretch and other receptors in the masticatory muscles, temporomandibular joints, and periosteum.

Mastication process

The vertical (up and down) movements of the mandibles results in biting by the incisor teeth. After a piece of food has been taken into the mouth both vertical movements and horizontal (side to side) movements enable the molars to crush and break the food into fragments of a size suitable for swallowing. These movements also mix the food with the saliva. This serves several functions, including taste and lubrication (see below). Chewing depends on the presence of saliva in the mouth. Saliva contains mucins which give it its lubricant property (see below). It coats the food and makes it slippery and more easily moved about in the mouth. Consequently patients with xerostomia experience difficulty in chewing (see Xerostomia Box 5).

The muscles of mastication are capable of exerting considerable force. The biting forces exerted by the incisors and molars are 110–250 N and 390–900 N respectively. The potential biting force is much greater than the force needed in ordinary chewing. The occlusal contact area between the molars and between the premolars is much more decisive than the biting force in determining the efficiency of mastication in a person with normal dentition. The efficiency of mastication is reduced in people who wear dentures, and they often tend to eat foods that are not difficult to chew; the toughness of the foods chosen seems to be related to the biting force that can be exerted on the dentures. The narrow selection of food by people wearing poorly fitting dentures, for example the omission of meat in the diet, can lead to nutritional deficiency.

Control of mastication

The muscles of mastication are the lateral pterygoids (responsible for jaw opening), and the masseters, the temporalis, and the medial pterygoid muscles (responsible for jaw closing) (Fig. 2.9A). The muscles of closing are more powerful than those involved in opening. There is a reciprocal arrangement between the opening and closing muscles. The control is exerted by neural mechanisms. Two important aspects of the control are:

1. how the movements are generated
2. how the bite is regulated.

Generation of movements

A single bite is a voluntary process involving the cerebral cortex, as are other movements involving skeletal muscles. However, although it was until recently believed that chewing was a reflex (i.e. reflex opening and reflex closing), this is now known not to be the case. Chewing appears to be a programmed pattern of movements organised at a rather low level in the central nervous system. It involves neurones in the nucleus of the fifth cranial nerve. The 'chewing centre' is built into the organisation of this group of neurones. Electrical stimulation of the cortical masticatory area in an anaesthetised animal induces rhythmic jaw movements similar to that observed during chewing. When the electrical changes in the membranes of the neurones are recorded they are seen to exhibit a bursting activity, the bursts being associated with jaw opening and jaw closing (Fig. 2.9B). This pattern is involuntary and seems to be present even if the sensory input is absent. Chewing therefore probably depends on a pattern generator similar to pattern generators seen in other areas of the central nervous system such as the respiratory centres. Such generators are rather primitive basic activities. Figure 2.9C shows the arrangements of the pathways involved in the generation of this chewing activity and its modulation.

Regulation of the bite

As the jaws close, the teeth come into contact with food, or with the opposing set of teeth. Two questions arise:

1. What stops the bite?
2. What regulates the force applied?

Stimulation of mechanoreceptors associated with the teeth is important. Many sensory receptors are present in the tooth pulp and the periodontal ligaments. These are innervated by sensory afferent fibres in the lingual nerve (Fig. 2.3). Activation of these receptors causes information to be transmitted to the brain stem, to inhibit jaw closing when the biting force rises, and therefore to regulate the force applied. This is sometimes described as the jaw opening reflex because if a tooth is tapped, for example an upper incisor, the jaw opens. The lingual nerve afferents ascend via the trigeminal nerve to the brain stem. When these receptors are stimulated, the amplitude of the jaw movement bursting responses changes and activity in the masseter jaw closing muscles increases. These inputs therefore modify the activity of the pattern generator, and contribute to the control of the chewing force. The texture of food is perceived during chewing by excitation of mechanoreceptors in the periodontal ligaments. Slight displacement of a tooth during chewing causes the periodontal ligaments to be stretched and this

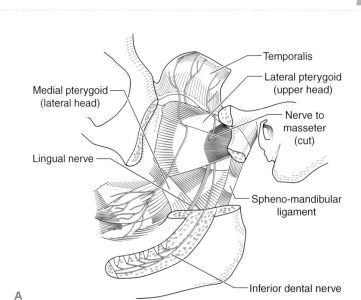

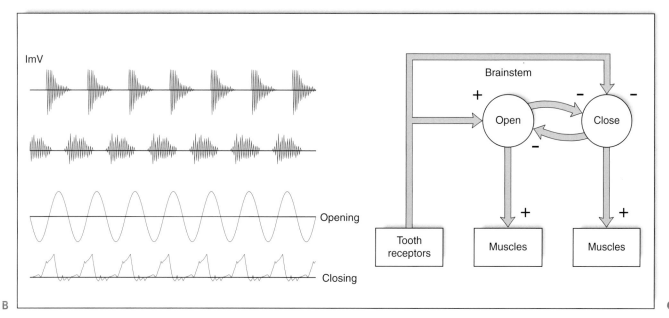

Fig. 2.9

Mastication and its control. (A) Arrangement of the muscles of mastication. The lateral pterygoid is responsible for jaw opening, and the medial pterygoid, the masseters and the temporalis are responsible for jaw closing. (B) Simplified representation of a pattern generator which could control the opening and closing of the jaws. (C) The pattern of electrical activity (EMG) in the muscles of opening and closing.

deforms and excites the receptors. Each afferent responds maximally to one particular direction of applied force. The pressure stimulus threshold for perception of a stimulus applied to a tooth is greater than 10 mN and is higher for the molars than for the incisors or canines. The threshold level is influenced by the velocity of application of the force. The strength of the stimulus is signalled by the frequency of discharge in the afferent nerves. Nevertheless, people who have lost their teeth can control masticatory force, indicat-

ing that tactile sensation in the periodontal ligaments is not the only input controlling the biting force. In fact muscle spindles in the masticatory muscles, temporomandibular joints, and periosteum may also contribute.

Role of tongue movement in mastication

The density of mechanoreceptors is high in the front of the oral cavity and low in the posterior part. The tip of the tongue has the highest density. Two-point discrimination on the tip of the tongue can be less than 1mm. Tactile information from the oral cavity and the tongue is transmitted to the brain via the trigeminal nerve. The tongue is a sophisticated motor organ which moves rhythmically in concert with the lower jaw (usually without being bitten) during chewing. The tongue can perform these movements because of the arrangement of its musculature (Fig. 2.3). The extrinsic muscles enable it to change its overall position. These, together with the intrinsic muscles which terminate on the mucosa or on other muscles of the tongue, enable it to both alter its shape and perform rapid movements. The nerve endings in the papillae transmit the senses of touch, pressure, temperature, and pain. There are also proprioreceptors within the muscles, and abundant muscle spindles in the human tongue, and these are also important for the intricate movements involved in chewing.

Tongue movements during chewing initially involve alteration of the shape of the tongue into a trough-like structure which collects the food bolus on its dorsal surface. The anterior portion is twisted towards the chewing side, the dorsum contracts towards the lateral surface of the teeth, and the food is placed on the occlusal surface of the teeth. The tongue then presses the dorsum against the medial surface of the teeth, whilst twisting to prevent the food from slipping off the occlusal surface. The buccal mucosa is held between the upper and lower teeth and presses the food bolus against the buccal cavity and the tongue. The tongue moves rapidly to select a large food bolus which requires further chewing and places it on the occlusal surface again. The fully ground food is collected on the lateral margin of the tongue. This movement is repeated until the food is completely chewed. The tongue mixes saliva with the crushed food by alternations from one side to the other, coating it with mucus. Then the tongue assumes the posture required for swallowing.

When the mouth is opened passively, the tongue is retracted posteriorly and the root of the tongue is elevated. This is the jaw–tongue reflex. It is evoked by excitation of receptors in the temporal muscle. This movement of the tongue may be important in preventing it from being bitten.

Saliva

Saliva is secreted by three major pairs of salivary glands: the parotids, the submandibular glands (the submaxillary glands in animals), and the sublingual glands. There are also numerous other small glands scattered throughout the oral and buccal mucosa.

The parotids are the largest of the glands. Each parotid is located below and anterior to the ear, between the ramus of the mandible and the mastoid process, with an extension onto the face. Its main duct (Stenson's duct) passes forward to penetrate the cheek and opens into the mouth opposite the second molar tooth.

The submandibular gland lies in the floor of the mouth beneath the body of the mandible, extending below its lower border into the side of the neck. It has a duct (Wharton's duct) which opens beneath the tip of the tongue. In some patients with Sjögren's syndrome (see Xerostomia Box 2, page 31) the ducts of the submandibular glands are obstructed, and the glands become swollen (Fig. 2.10). In such patients the location of the submandibular glands in the neck are clearly indicated.

The sublingual gland is actually a collection of glands that lie near to the duct of the submandibular gland beneath the mucous membrane of the floor of the mouth. Each of these sublingual glands has a separate duct that opens beneath the tongue.

The three pairs of glands differ with respect to the type of acini present, and they secrete saliva that differs in composition with respect to the mucus content. The parotids have acini containing only serous cells. They produce a watery secretion that has a high content of α-amylase but very little mucus. Most acini of the submandibular glands are serous, but some are mucous, and some are mixed and contain mucous

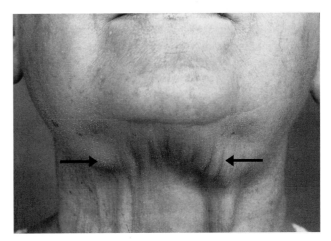

Fig. 2.10
Swollen submandibular glands (arrowed) in a patient with Sjögren's syndrome. The inflammatory process can cause the ducts to become blocked with mucoid saliva. The ducts may also be narrowed (stenosis). As a consequence the glands swell. (Provided by Mr J. Hamburger, Dental School, University of Birmingham.)

THE MOUTH, SALIVARY GLANDS, AND OESOPHAGUS

impart a striated appearance to the cells, under the microscope. These striated ducts drain into larger, excretory ducts, which in turn drain into a large collecting duct that opens into the mouth. The cells lining the striated ducts and the excretory ducts modify the secretion as it flows past them.

Somewhat sparsely distributed myoepithelial cells are present around the ducts and the acini of a salivary gland. These cells support the glandular elements and contract when the glands are stimulated, to assist the extrusion of the saliva from the ducts.

Functions of saliva

The secretion of saliva in response to food has been studied experimentally in animals by surgically making a permanent fistula at the throat, or by inserting a cannula in the appropriate duct under anaesthesia. In humans, a variety of methods are used to assess salivary function. Some of these are discussed in Case history 2, in the box on this page.

Lubrication

The lubricant property of saliva depends on its content of mucins. These glycoproteins form a gel that coats the food and makes it more easily moved about in the mouth. The lubricant property of saliva enables chewing and swallowing to be performed.

Digestion

α-Amylase is the major digestive enzyme in saliva. It hydrolyses α-1,4 glycosidic linkages in starch (see Chapter 8). The efficiency of mastication is important for salivary amylase to infiltrate the food. Despite the short exposure of saliva in the mouth, the salivary digestion of starch is important because it continues even after the food has reached the stomach. Gastric acid in the stomach inactivates α-amylase but the bolus of food does not disintegrate immediately on arrival in the stomach, and so salivary digestion can continue within the bolus for as long as half an hour. When the acid has completely penetrated the food the enzyme is inactivated. α-Amylase works best at a slightly alkaline pH. The starch in potatoes or bread may be digested to the extent of up to 75% before the enzyme is inactivated by the acid in the stomach.

Small amounts of other enzymes are also present in saliva, including lysozyme, sialoperoxidase, lingual lipase, ribonuclease, deoxyribonuclease, and kallikreins. These salivary components are not important for the digestive process, although lysozyme and sialoperoxidase provide important protective functions (see below).

Xerostomia Box 3

Diagnosis

A simple test for xerostomia which can be carried out in the surgery involves swabbing the tongue with 5% citric acid, and measuring the volume of saliva that can be spat out into a graduated tube. Alternatively, a Curby cup can be placed over the opening of Stenson's duct. This creates a vacuum and saliva can be collected. Saliva can also be collected with a pre-weighed sponge. Swallowing difficulty can also be assessed, i.e. whether water has to be taken with dry food for swallowing to be accomplished (for example by the 'cream cracker' test). All of these tests have to be interpreted with care, but on the basis of such tests patients are initially categorised into 'responders' who have functional salivary gland tissue and 'non-responders' who do not. Scintiography (scintioscanning) is a technique involving intravenous administration of a radioisotope, usually technetium pertechnetate, a gamma emitter with a short half-life. This is taken up into the salivary acinar cells. Uptake with time can be measured using a Geiger counter. Responders by definition have functioning $Na^+/K^+/Cl^-$ co-transporters that can move Cl^- ions or technetium pertechnate across the acinar cell membrane. Water moves passively across the membrane as a consequence. Non-responders have no functional epithelium and therefore cannot handle pertechnate correctly. In Sjögren's syndrome there is a slow uptake of the isotope, low peak value and a prolonged excretory phase.

Protective functions of saliva

Saliva has many properties that enable it to promote oral and dental health:

1. The large volume of the fluid produced enables the buccal cavity to be continually rinsed, thereby removing ingested substances and particles from the cavity.
2. It contains mucins that impart a slippery character to the secretion. It coats the mouth, thereby protecting it against abrasion by sharp pieces of food.
3. The alkaline pH of the saliva produced when a meal is being eaten buffers acids present in the food. The copious secretion of saliva prior to vomiting protects the mouth from gastric acid in the vomit by virtue of its mucus content and its pH. Buffering of the acids in food prevents the erosion of tooth enamel.

Xerostomia Box 4

Consequences for oral and dental health

Dental health depends on saliva for many reasons, including its continuous rinsing of the oral and buccal cavities to wash away particles etc. in which micro-organisms grow, its ability to buffer acids (stimulated saliva becomes more alkaline at high rates of flow), its specific and non-specific immune functions due to the presence of immunoglobulins, the anti-microbial constituents sialoperoxidase, thiocyanate and lysozyme, and the presence of calcium phosphate which prevents demineralisation of the teeth. As a consequence of the decreased production of saliva, various oral diseases are associated with xerostomia. These are dental caries, gum disease, mucosal ulceration and atrophy, infections of the mouth (e.g. candida), and ascending infection of the salivary glands.

In addition, in the absence of saliva, retention of dentures is more difficult. Patients who have a dry mouth because they are being treated with tricyclic antidepressants, ganglion-blocking drugs, or para-sympathomimetic drugs (for hypertension), may have a dry mouth and may experience difficulty in oral function if they wear dentures.

---

4. It is bacteriostatic because it contains an antimicrobial substance, thiocyanate, and an enzyme, sialoperoxidase, which catalyses the reaction of metabolic products of bacteria with salivary thiocyanate:

$$H_2O_2 + CNS^- \xrightarrow{\text{sialoperoxidase}} \text{oxidation products, e.g. } OSCN^-$$

Hydrogen peroxide (bacterial activity) — thiocyanate (saliva) — hypothiocyanate (toxic to bacteria)

The oxidised derivatives produced in this reaction are highly toxic to bacterial systems. The oxidation products oxidise -SH groups on many enzymes, including some of those involved in energy metabolism. Saliva also contains the enzyme lysozyme, which acts on the cell walls of certain bacteria, including some streptococci, causing lysis and death. However, most organisms that colonise the mouth resist lysozyme attack by developing protective cell capsules. Infections in the mouth are rare, even after oral or dental surgery when aseptic precautions are difficult to maintain, because of the bacteriostatic properties of saliva.

Control of water intake

Thirst is the desire for increased water intake and it is perceived as a dry mouth. The sensation is signalled by receptors in the oropharynx and upper gastrointestinal tract but the mechanisms involved in the response of the receptors are still poorly understood. However, the relief of thirst sensation via these receptors is short-lived. The desire for increased water intake accompanies an increase in plasma hypertonicity or a reduction in blood volume or pressure (see Chapter 1). The sensation of thirst is initially satisfied by the act of drinking, but this occurs before sufficient water is absorbed from the gastrointestinal tract to correct these disturbances. The desire to drink is completely satisfied only when the plasma osmolarity, volume and pressure are adjusted to within the normal range.

Speech

Speech depends on the movements and positioning of the tongue, lips, and cheeks during controlled expiration. As movements of the tongue are facilitated by the lubricant effect of saliva, speech can be difficult in xerostomia. Speech is a function not directly related to the digestive process and it will not be considered further here.

Absorption in the mouth

Absorption of low molecular weight molecules can occur, to some extent, directly from the oral cavity. This route of absorption can be useful for treatment with certain drugs, especially when a rapid response is required. Such drugs are usually placed under the tongue. One example is glyceryl trinitrate, which is used to treat an angina attack. It can also be a useful route for drugs that are unstable at the pH of the stomach, or which are rapidly metabolised by the liver. Drugs that are absorbed from the oral cavity enter the systemic circulation directly and therefore escape the 'first-pass' metabolism that occurs in the liver, unlike substances that are absorbed into the portal system (see Chapter 7). An example of a drug that is rapidly inactivated in the liver is isoprenaline, which is sometimes used to treat heart block. This drug can be effective if given sublingually. Unfortunately high molecular weight substances are not well absorbed from the mouth.

Mechanisms of secretion

The basal rate of secretion of saliva is very low during sleep, approximately 0.05 ml per minute. In the resting, awake, state it increases to about 0.5 ml per minute, which is just enough to keep the mouth moist. During the course of the day 1–2 L of saliva are secreted. Most

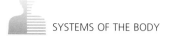

THE MOUTH, SALIVARY GLANDS, AND OESOPHAGUS

2

Xerostomia Box 5

Consequences for the functioning of the mouth

① Lubrication: saliva is necessary to aid chewing, swallowing, and speech because of the lubricant properties conferred on it by its mucin content. Therefore these functions are all compromised in xerostomia.

② Digestion: lack of salivary α-amylase does not result in malabsorption of starch if pancreatic α-amylase secretion is adequate, as the amylases from the two sources have similar catalytic actions in starch digestion, and adequate amounts are secreted by the normal pancreas.

③ Solution: saliva is important for taste as this sense depends on substances dissolved in saliva. It is also important for the solution of substances which are absorbed by mouth. Therefore taste is affected in xerostomia.

④ Protection: saliva is also important for oral and dental health: it washes the mouth, buffers acids in the food, and contains antimicrobial substances. Infections of the mouth and associated structures are common in xerostomia.

⑤ Moistness: control of water intake. Lack of saliva signals thirst. Thirst is therefore a constant sensation in xerostomia.

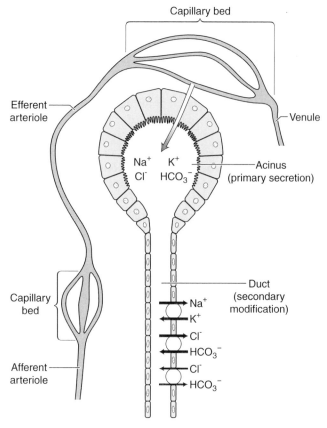

Fig. 2.13
Secretion of primary saliva in the acinus of a salivary gland, and secondary modification in the duct.

of it is swallowed. The proteins in saliva are broken down by the digestive enzymes in the gastrointestinal tract, and the amino acids and peptides produced, together with the water and ions, are reabsorbed across the walls of the intestines.

Figure 2.13 is a simplified representation of a salivary secretory unit (a salivon) which consists of an acinus and a duct. The blood flows first past the ducts and then past the acinus. The blood supply constitutes a portal system, because substances reabsorbed from the duct cells into the blood capillaries surrounding the duct are transported to the capillaries surrounding the acinus via an efferent arteriole, prior to being returned to the heart via the veins. The acinar cells secrete the primary saliva that passes down the ducts. The primary secretion consists of an ultrafiltrate of plasma to which some components synthesised by the acinar cells (such as α-amylase and mucins) are added. It is therefore almost isotonic with plasma. The rate of secretion of the primary juice and the α-amylase concentration vary with the type of stimulation, but the ionic composition of the primary juice is fairly con-

stant. The main ionic constituents of primary saliva are Na^+, K^+, Cl^-, and HCO_3^-.

As the primary juice flows past the duct cells it undergoes secondary modification via transport systems in the membranes of the secretory and striated duct cells. Certain substances are produced by the duct cells and secreted into the saliva and others are extracted from the saliva by the cells. Na^+ and Cl^- are extracted from the saliva and K^+ is added to it. In fact Na^+ and K^+ are exchanged by an active mechanism in the duct cells. However, more Na^+ is extracted than K^+ is added by this mechanism, and the duct epithelium has a very low permeability to water. Consequently secondary saliva becomes more hypotonic as it flows down the ducts and in the human, saliva is always hypotonic compared to plasma. The tonicity is higher at high flow rates.

The HCO_3^- in saliva is produced from CO_2 and water in the duct cells, via the reactions:

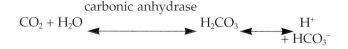

The duct cells are rich in carbonic anhydrase, an enzyme that catalyses the formation of carbonic acid from CO_2 and water. HCO_3^- is secreted across the membranes into the ducts. However, there is also an exchange mechanism whereby HCO_3^- is extracted in exchange for Cl^- (Fig. 2.13). HCO_3^- transport can therefore occur in both directions across the ducts. The rate of secretion determines which process predominates (see below).

The composition of saliva changes with rate of flow because at fast flow rates there is less time for the exchange processes occurring in the ducts to modify the composition. Thus at high flow rates the composition approaches that of the primary juice. Figure 2.14 shows the changes in the concentration of some ions in the saliva flowing from the ducts, with the rate of flow, and compares them with the concentration of those ions in the plasma. The concentrations of Na^+ ions and HCO_3^- ions increase with rate of flow until they reach a plateau, whilst the concentration of K^+ ions decreases to reach a plateau at low flow rates. Na^+ is exchanged for K^+, but the $Na^+:K^+$ exchange ratio is $3:1$. It is only at low flow rates that the active transport processes for these ions in the ducts makes a measurable difference to their concentrations in the saliva. At maximum rates of flow the tonicity of human saliva is approximately 70% of that of plasma. The ducts extract more ions than they deliver to the saliva, and the osmotic gradient is therefore in the direction of the plasma, but the ducts are relatively impermeable to water and so the saliva is always hypotonic to plasma. Table 2.1 compares the ionic composition of primary saliva produced in the acinus, secondary saliva produced at a low flow rate (unstimulated), and secondary saliva produced at a high flow rate (stimulated).

Resting human saliva is slightly acid and its HCO_3^- concentration is lower than that of the primary juice. However, it becomes more alkaline with increasing rate of flow as the concentration of HCO_3^- ions increases. At maximum rates of flow the pH may reach a value of 8.0 and the HCO_3^- concentration is higher than that of the primary juice (Table 2.1). The reasons for these changes are that at low flow rates HCO_3^- is extracted from the saliva in the ducts (in exchange for Cl^-). However, at high rates of flow HCO_3^- is secreted into the ducts (in exchange for Cl^-).

Control of secretion

In the human, the secretion of saliva is mainly in response to nerve stimulation. The efferent control is via autonomic nerves. The glands are innervated by both parasympathetic and sympathetic nerves. The postganglionic sympathetic nerve fibres have their cell bodies in the superior cervical ganglion. The preganglionic parasympathetic nerve fibres travel in branches of the facial (cranial nerve VII) and the glossopharyngeal (cranial nerve XI) nerves, and these synapse with postganglionic fibres in or near the glands. There is a parasympathetic innervation of all acini and most usually also have a sympathetic innervation. Several nerve fibres supply each acinus but

Table 2.1
Concentrations of some important constituents in primary and secondary saliva

Ions (mmol/l)	Primary saliva	Secondary saliva	
		Unstimulated	Stimulated
Na^+	145	2	85
K^+	4	25	18
Cl^-	100	23	55
HCO_3^-	24	4	40
α-amylase (g/l)		<0.1	1.0
Flow rate (ml/min)		0.5	3.5

The ionic composition of the primary juice is similar to that of blood plasma. The differences in ionic compositions of the primary and secondary salivas are due to the modifications that take place as the saliva flows down the ducts. Thus Na^+ is extracted and K^+ is added in the ducts. HCO_3^- is extracted in the ducts (in exchange for Cl^-) but its secretion from the ducts is stimulated at high rates of flow. The fate of Cl^- is complex; it is exchanged for HCO_3^- and it is transported down the electrical gradient created by the transport of Na^+. In stimulated saliva there is less time for such modifications to take place, as the flow rate is faster. The composition of the stimulated secondary juice is therefore intermediate between that of the primary juice and the unstimulated secondary juice. The concentration of α-amylase is higher at high flow rates as its secretion from the acinar cells has been stimulated.

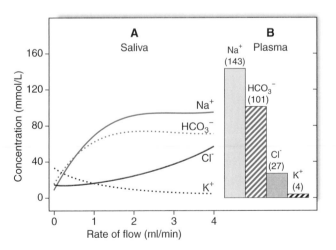

Fig. 2.14
(A) Changes in concentration of some ions in saliva with rate of flow. (B) Concentrations of the same ions in blood plasma. Based on figure from Thaysen J. H. American Journal of Physiology 1954; 178: 155.

not every cell is innervated. However, the acinar cells are electrically coupled so the membrane depolarisation brought about by nerve impulses in the innervated cells is transmitted to the neighbouring cells. Myoepithelial cells in the vicinity of the acini are innervated by the same nerve fibres. The duct cells, myoepithelial cells, and the arterioles of the gland are also controlled by both parasympathetic and sympathetic nerves.

Nerve stimulation produces changes in both the composition and the volume of the secretion. Simulation of either the parasympathetic nerves or the sympathetic nerves increases the rate of secretion. However, the parasympathetic nerves provide a stronger and longer-lasting stimulus. If the parasympathetic supply is interrupted the glands atrophy but interruption of the sympathetic nervous supply causes no major defect in salivary secretion. The parasympathetic nerves release acetylcholine, substance P and vasoactive intestinal peptide (VIP), whilst the sympathetic nerves release noradrenaline.

The processes stimulated by parasympathetic nerve activity include the flow of saliva, the release of α-amylase and mucins from the acinar cells, transport events in the duct cells, the extrusion of the saliva from the ducts, the blood flow, and the metabolism and growth of the acinar and duct cells. Stimulation of the sympathetic nerves is a more transient effect causing the release of saliva rich in α-amylase, mucins, HCO_3^- and K^+, and contraction of the myoepithelial cells. It also causes vasoconstriction, which reduces the blood flow to the glands. This effect may be exaggerated when an individual is frightened and may explain why some people experience a dry mouth when they are afraid. Circulating catecholamines reinforce the effect of sympathetic nerve stimulation. Acinar cell membranes have both α- and β-adrenergic receptors. Other hormones are not a major influence in the control of secretion of saliva, although both vasopressin and aldosterone can stimulate Na^+/K^+ exchange in the duct cells.

Cellular mechanisms of control

The acinar cells of the resting glands contain granules. These can be stained histologically. They are the locus of storage of the zymogen precursor of α-amylase. If the gland is stimulated, the number of granules diminishes as the enzyme is released. The formation of new enzyme occurs rapidly in the acinar cell after stimulation, although it is the release, by exocytosis, not the synthesis, that is directly stimulated by the transmitter. It has been shown that after stimulation of the rat submandibular gland by feeding or by injection of acetylcholine to deplete the enzyme, the content of α-amylase increases 10-fold.

The second messengers involved in the actions of the neurotransmitters on acinar cells are intracellular cAMP and Ca^{2+}. Activation of either β-adrenergic receptors or VIP receptors causes an increase in intracellular cAMP, whilst activation of α-adrenergic receptors, muscarinic acetylcholine receptors or substance P receptors results in increased Ca^{2+} influx into the cell. Substances that increase intracellular cAMP tend to produce a secretion that is richer in α-amylase than those that increase intracellular Ca^{2+} concentration. Those that increase intracellular Ca^{2+} concentration tend to produce a greater increase in the volume of acinar cell secretion. Mucins are also released by exocytosis as a consequence of influx of Ca^{2+} into the cell.

Blood flow

When the parasympathetic nerves are stimulated, there is a rapid vasodilatory effect that can result in up to a 5-fold increase in blood flow. This is followed by a slower vasodilatory effect. The immediate effect is probably due to a direct action of the transmitters acetylcholine and VIP released from parasympathetic nerve fibres which end on the arterioles in the glandular tissue. The two transmitters are probably released from the same nerve terminals. Stimulation of the sympathetics causes vasoconstriction via the release of noradrenaline, which acts on α-adrenergic receptors on the arteriolar smooth muscle.

The slower vasodilatory effect is an indirect consequence of stimulation of the parasympathetics. It is due to the formation of vasodilator metabolites, mainly bradykinin, by processes occurring as a result of the stimulation of the acinar cells. Stimulation of the acinar cells results in the release of proteolytic enzymes known as kallikreins, into the interstitial fluid. These enzymes catalyse the conversion of the vasodilator precursor bradykininogen, to bradykinin, the active vasodilator, and a small peptide:

$$\text{bradykininogen} \xrightarrow{\text{kallikreins}} \text{bradykinin} + \text{peptide}$$

Bradykinin acts on the arteriolar smooth muscle to cause vasodilatation. When the arterioles dilate there is less of a pressure drop across them and the pressure is transferred to the capillaries. The increased hydrostatic pressure and consequent increased transcapillary pressure result in increased filtration in the gland. The consequence is an increased flow of saliva. Furthermore, saliva can actually be secreted at a pressure higher than the arterial pressure to the gland, as the triggering of active processes at the luminal surface of the gland by the parasympathetics causes secondary water transport.

Xerostomia Box 6

Treatment and side-effects

The treatment of xerostomia depends on whether the patient can secrete saliva in response to a stimulus, i.e. whether he or she is a 'responder' who has functioning salivary gland epithelium, or a 'non-responder' who does not. Artificial salivas can be used in non-responders, but these are not wholly satisfactory. Low doses of pilocarpine are often used to treat the condition in individuals with residual salivary function. This drug is a partial agonist of muscarinic acetylcholine receptors. It mimics the effect of stimulation of the parasympathetic nerves, causing the acinar cells to secrete saliva and kallikreins (which in turn cause vasodilatation via bradykinin). However, systemic parasympathetic side-effects can occur, including bradycardia and decreased cardiac output, increased sweating, increased gut motility. If the dry mouth is a consequence of treatment with other medication, it is unwise to prescribe pilocarpine. In these circumstances the possibility of treatment with an alternative drug that does not cause dry mouth should be explored. However, pilocarpine is often prescribed to treat xerostomia that occurs as a consequence of radiotherapy, although side-effects can lead to its use being discontinued.

Control of secretion by food

Saliva is secreted in response to the approach of food, and to the presence of food in the mouth. The effect is mediated via the parasympathetic nerves. Up to 50% of the secretion during a meal comes from the parotid glands. Two reflexes are involved; a conditioned reflex and an unconditioned reflex.

The conditioned reflex is due mainly to the sight and smell of food, although other sensory inputs such as sounds can also trigger this reflex. The reflex was first studied by Pavlov, a Russian physiologist who worked with dogs in St Petersburg. He usually fed the dogs at a time when the bells of the cathedral chimed, and discovered that the dogs salivated when the bells chimed even on occasions when they were not being fed, presumably in anticipation. Thus the conditioned reflex is a learned response because the first time the stimulus is presented it does not elicit a secretion.

The unconditioned reflex is due to the presence of food in the mouth. It occurs in response to activation of touch or taste receptors. Stimulation by food of taste receptors on the tongue, or pressure receptors in the mouth, results in impulses being set up in the afferent nerves to the brainstem. Figure 2.5 (page 25) shows the arrangement of the neural pathways of the secretory reflex that occurs following stimulation of the taste buds. This involves afferent pathways from the tongue to the superior and inferior salivary nuclei. The afferent nerve fibres run in the chorda tympani and the glossopharyngeal nerves (see above). The efferent preganglionic parasympathetic nerves to the salivary glands also run in these nerves. The preganglionic fibres in the glossopharyngeal nerve synapse with postganglionic fibres in the otic ganglion and the postganglionic fibres innervate the parotid glands. The preganglionic fibres in the chorda tympani synapse with postganglionic fibres in the submandibular ganglion, and the postganglionic fibres innervate the submandibular and the sublingual glands.

The precise roles of the sympathetic nerves in stimulating saliva secretion in different physiological states is still unclear.

Oesophagus

Anatomical arrangements of the oesophagus

The structures associated with the oesophagus are shown in Figures 2.2, 2.15 and 2.18. The arrangement of the smooth muscle in the wall of the oesophagus is similar to that of the rest of the gastrointestinal tract in that there is an inner circular layer and an outer longitudinal layer (see Chapter 1). However, only the lower two-thirds of the oesophagus is surrounded by smooth muscle. The top third is surrounded by skeletal muscle. The muscle tissue in an area in the middle of the oesophagus consists of a mixture of skeletal muscle and smooth muscle fibres, the skeletal muscle gradually being replaced by smooth muscle in the caudad direction. Both the skeletal muscle fibres and the smooth muscle fibres are under the control of the vagus nerve. The skeletal muscle is innervated directly by somatic motor neurones from the nucleus ambiguous, whilst the smooth muscle is innervated indirectly by neurones in the vagus nerve which synapse with neurones in the myenteric plexus. The intrinsic nerves are, in effect, postganglionic autonomic nerves. Preganglionic parasympathetic neurones in the vagus nerve from the dorsal motor nucleus synapse with the cell bodies of these neurones.

The upper oesophageal sphincter (the hypopharyngeal sphincter or cricopharyngeus muscle) is composed of skeletal muscle. It is a thickening of the circular muscle layer. The lower sphincter comprises the last 1–2 cm of the oesophagus. It is not anatomically distinguishable as a sphincter but the pressure is normally greater in this region than in the stomach.

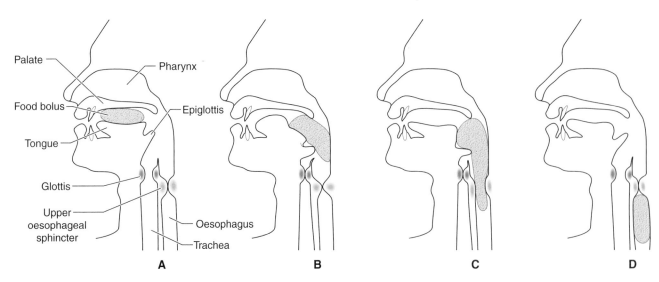

Fig. 2.15
(A,B,C,D) Sequential events involved in swallowing.

Swallowing (deglutition)

The arrangement of the structures associated with swallowing is shown in Figure 2.2 (page 23). The events involved are represented in Figure 2.15. The whole process lasts only a few seconds. It is initiated voluntarily but once initiated it cannot be stopped voluntarily, i.e. it becomes a classical 'all or none' reflex. The process can be divided into three phases:

- voluntary
- pharyngeal
- oesophageal.

Phases of swallowing

Voluntary phase
In the voluntary phase the tongue separates the food into a bolus and then moves it backwards and upwards towards the back of the mouth.

Pharyngeal phase
As the bolus of food moves into the pharynx, it activates pressure receptors in the palate and anterior pharynx. These receptors send impulses in the trigeminal and glossopharyngeal nerves to the brain stem swallowing centre. Each impulse serves as a trigger for the swallowing reflex. This causes the elevation of the soft palate, which seals the nasal cavity and prevents food from entering it. The swallowing centre inhibits respiration, raises the larynx, and closes the glottis (the opening between the vocal chords). This prevents food from getting into the trachea. As the tongue forces the food further back into the pharynx, the bolus tilts the epiglottis backwards to cover the closed glottis. It is closure of the glottis, however, not the tilting of the

epiglottis that is primarily responsible for preventing food from entering the trachea.

The upper oesophageal sphincter is closed at rest. It opens during swallowing, allowing the bolus of food to pass into the oesophagus. Immediately after the bolus has passed, it closes again, resealing the junction. The glottis then opens and breathing resumes. The skeletal muscle of the upper oesophageal sphincter is so arranged that when the sphincter opens it contracts

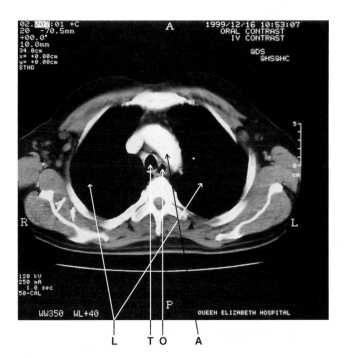

Fig. 2.16
A cross-sectional CT scan of the mid thorax showing the anatomical relationship of the lungs (L), aortic arch (A), overlying the trachea (T), and the oesophagus (O).

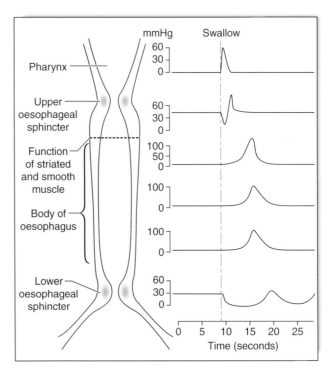

Fig. 2.18
Sequential pressure changes in different regions of the oesophagus during swallowing.

and when it closes it relaxes. This pharyngeal phase of swallowing lasts approximately 1 second. The relationship between the oesophagus and other thoracic structures is shown in Figure 2.16.

Oesophageal phase

The food is moved along the oesophagus by peristalsis. A peristaltic wave consists of a wave of contraction of the circular muscle, followed by a wave of relaxation. The wave of contraction passes along the walls of the oesophagus and moves the food towards the stomach (Fig. 2.17). The wave takes about 9 seconds to travel the length of the oesophagus. The progression of the wave is controlled by autonomic nerves and is coordinated by the swallowing centre in the medulla. Thus it is not primarily gravity, but peristalsis, that moves the food towards the stomach, although gravity assists the process. The importance of peristalsis to the process is seen by the fact that food can be swallowed and will reach the stomach even in someone who is upside down. It is noteworthy that in other parts of the gastrointestinal tract the peristaltic waves are coordinated largely by the internal nerve plexi, the extrinsic nerves being less important, and can be cut without gastrointestinal function being dramatically affected.

As the peristaltic waves begin in the oesophagus, the muscle of the lower oesophageal sphincter relaxes, opening the sphincter and allowing the food bolus

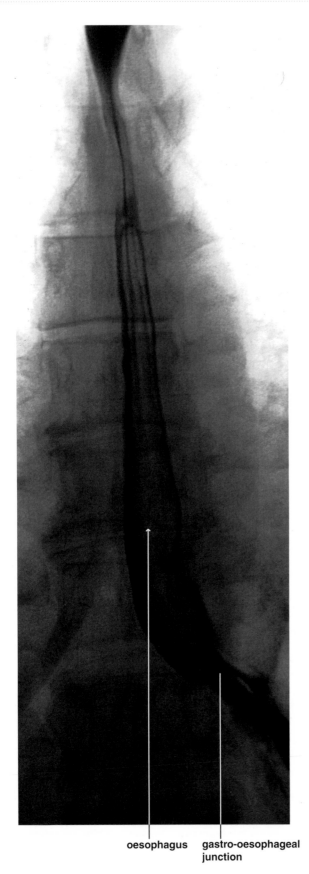

oesophagus   gastro-oesophageal
junction

Fig. 2.17
An X-ray of the oesophagus taken after swallowing barium, showing a normal peristaltic wave.

to enter the stomach. The sphincter muscle then contracts and reseals the junction. It remains closed in the absence of peristalsis, preventing reflux of the stomach's contents. Figure 2.18 shows the pressure changes in different regions of the oesophagus during swallowing.

Control of swallowing

The process of swallowing is coordinated by the swallowing centre in the medulla. It involves efferent impulses from the medulla to 25 different skeletal muscles of the pharynx, the larynx, and the early oesophagus and the smooth muscles in the lower oesophagus.

Control of motility in the oesophagus

The control of peristalsis in the oesophagus is via nerve fibres in the vagus. Impulses in these nerves control both skeletal muscle and smooth muscle in the wall of the oesophagus. The material is propelled to the stomach by the coordinated contraction of the muscle layers in the body of the oesophagus. This wave of contraction is due to a sequential activation of the muscles in the pharynx and oesophagus by neural impulses in the segmental efferent neurones, which utilise acetylcholine as the neurotransmitter (Fig. 2.19).

The sphincter smooth muscle is innervated by both extrinsic and intrinsic nerves. Cholinergic nerve fibres in the vagus are partly responsible for the maintained contraction of the muscle, i.e. its tone, when peristaltic activity is absent in the oesophagus. Stimulation of noradrenergic sympathetic nerves also causes contraction via activation of α-adrenergic receptors. However, if the extrinsic nerves are cut, there is still some tone indicating that the intrinsic nerves are also important. An increase in the blood levels of gastrin released from the gastric antrum can also increase the tone of this sphincter (see Chapter 4). This mechanism may be important in preventing reflux of stomach contents into the oesophagus whilst the stomach is contracting.

Relaxation of the lower oesophageal sphincter is due to impulses in inhibitory nerve fibres that innervate the circular smooth muscle. The transmitters involved may be VIP and nitric oxide. A decrease in cholinergic impulses also promotes relaxation of the sphincter.

Clinical conditions associated with the oesophagus

Motor disease of the oesophagus can be due to disorders of the skeletal muscle or disorders of the smooth muscle.

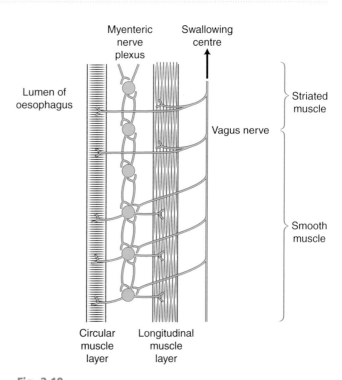

Fig. 2.19
Segmental innervation of the skeletal and smooth muscle of the oesophagus. Somatic motor neurones in the vagus nerve innervate the skeletal muscle directly. Autonomic nerve fibres in the vagus innervate the smooth muscle indirectly via the intrinsic nerves in the myenteric plexus. NB. The transition from skeletal muscle to smooth muscle, in a region approximately one third of the way down the oesophagus, is gradual.

Xerostomia Box 7

Consequences for swallowing

Saliva is necessary for swallowing because it coats the food and lubricates it, making it more easily moved back into the pharynx where it stimulates the pressure receptors that initiate swallowing, enabling food to pass smoothly into the oesophagus. Individuals with xerostomia therefore require fluid intake with food to enable swallowing to take place.

The lubricant properties of saliva assist the passage of the food bolus down the oesophagus and prevent abrasion of the walls by hard material in the swallowed food. The constant rinsing of the oesophagus by saliva, and its buffering and antimicrobial properties, help to protect the oesophagus from damage by acids and to prevent infections.

Disorders affecting skeletal muscle

In primary diseases of skeletal musculature, for example myasthenia gravis or myotonic dystrophy, or primary disease of the nervous system involving the somatic motor nerves, for example amyotrophic lateral sclerosis or poliomyelitis, the striated muscles of the tongue and pharynx, the upper oesophageal sphincter, and the wall of the upper oesophagus are usually affected. Difficulties in swallowing (dysphagia) are experienced and there is loss of propulsive force of the upper oesophagus. Moreover, following a stroke, lesions in the brain stem can interfere with the coordination of the movements of the tongue and pharynx.

Disorders affecting smooth muscle

A condition known as cricopharyngeal spasm, characterised by swallowing difficulty, appears to be due to increased fibrosis of the cricopharyngeal muscle. Achalasia (cardiospasm) is another common oesophageal condition. In this condition there is both defective relaxation of the lower sphincter, which impedes the flow of material into the stomach, and an abnormality of the function of the smooth muscle in the lower two-thirds of the oesophagus whereby the coordinated control of peristalsis is lost. These defects are due to defective innervation of the smooth muscle of the body of the oesophagus and the lower oesophageal sphincter. Chaga's disease, which is prevalent in Latin America, is caused by infection with the parasite *Trypanosoma cruzi*. It can be characterised by similar problems, although defects in the function of the colon are probably more common than defects of the oesophagus in this condition (see Chapter 10). In Chaga's disease there is an absence of ganglion cells in the myenteric plexus.

A common condition in which prolonged contraction of the lower oesophagus occurs after swallowing (instead of a normal peristaltic wave) is known as diffuse oesophageal spasm. The aetiology of this condition is not known, but thickening of the smooth muscle of the oesophagus has been observed in many patients.

If gastric contents are refluxed into the oesophagus (reflux oesophagitis) this causes 'heartburn'. This may or may not be accompanied by inflammation of the oesophagus. In many cases reflux is due to dysfunction of the lower oesophageal sphincter. Raising the head during sleep can prevent episodes of heartburn during the night in susceptible individuals.

Self-assessment case study: denervation following wisdom tooth extraction

An 18-year-old man was admitted to hospital to have an impacted wisdom tooth extracted. The operation involved reflection of a flap of tissue to allow extraction of the tooth. In this patient the inferior dental nerve ran unusually close to the apical part of the tooth root and the nerve was accidentally damaged. (Figure 2.20 on page 42 shows an X-ray from a subject in which the dental nerve is abnormally close to the root of a wisdom tooth.) Unfortunately in the patient the lingual nerve was also damaged during the surgical procedure because it also ran unusually close to the tooth. As a result, after the anaesthetic had worn off, the side of the patient's tongue and the lower lip on the operated side of his mouth were numb. Fortunately for this patient, sensation in the affected areas slowly returned over the course of the following few weeks.

Having read this chapter, you should be able to attempt to answer the following questions relating to the above case:

① Would you expect damage to the inferior dental nerve to affect the patient's ability to chew? Explain your answer, indicting the mechanisms involved in the regulation of the bite.

② Would you expect damage to the lingual nerve to affect the patient's ability to chew? Explain your answer.

③ Would you expect the patient to have difficulty in swallowing? Explain your answer.

④ Would you expect the patient to have a dry mouth? Explain your answer.

⑤ Would you expect the nerve damage to affect the patient's speech?

⑥ Would you expect damage to the lingual nerve to have affected the patient's sense of taste? Explain your answer.

⑦ Would you expect the loss of pain sensation to be a problem for this patient? Explain your answer.

⑧ Why was the patient's lower lip numb?

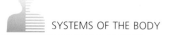
Introduction

The primary function of the stomach is to store the food ingested during a meal and to regulate its release into the duodenum. Another function is to churn and mix the food with the secretions of the stomach, to produce a thick mixture known as 'chyme'. In addition it has a range of exocrine, paracrine, and endocrine functions. The exocrine secretions which are secreted into the stomach lumen are digestive juices, collectively known as gastric juice. The major paracrine secretion is histamine, a substance that stimulates gastric acid secretion. The major endocrine secretion is the hormone gastrin, which acts both locally on the stomach smooth muscle and mucosa to stimulate gastric motility and acid secretion, and distally on the intestines, pancreas, and liver.

In this chapter the secretory and emptying functions of the stomach will be considered in the light of a clinical problem concerning the consequences of gastrectomy, a condition in which these functions are compromised. The process of vomiting and its treatment are also discussed. A second clinical problem relating to the consequences of excessive vomiting is presented at the end of the chapter.

Anatomy of the stomach

The stomach is a storage sac located between the oesophagus and the duodenum. Figure 3.1A indicates the major features of the stomach. Folds, known as rugae, are present on the inner surface of the empty stomach. Figure 3.2 shows an X-ray of a stomach. The rugae flatten out as the stomach fills. The wall of the stomach consists of various layers of tissue (Fig. 3.3). The inner lining is known as the mucosa. It comprises the lamina propria and the gastric glands (or pits). Beneath this lies the submucosa, the muscularis mucosae and the serosa, which is covered by the peritoneum. The wall structure of the stomach is similar to that present throughout the rest of the gastrointestinal tract (see Chapter 1), except that the stomach has an oblique muscle layer in addition to the circular and longitudinal layers in the muscularis mucosa. This facilitates distension of the stomach and the storage of food. The muscle layers are not evenly distributed over the wall of the stomach. The external circular muscle layer is relatively thin in the fundus and body, and thick in the antrum where strong muscular contractions aid the mixing of food. In addition it is highly developed in the pylorus where it becomes a functional sphincter which regulates stomach emptying.

The lining of the stomach is covered with a protective layer of columnar epithelial cells. These have well-developed tight junctions to protect the underlying tissue from acid secretion. In addition the columnar cells secrete mucus and alkaline fluid to further protect the stomach from injury. Numerous gastric pits (approximately 3.5 million in the human) penetrate the surface. These are short ducts into which the more deeply lying gastric glands empty their secretions. The secretions enter the main compartment of the stomach via the necks of these ducts.

The stomach is separated from the duodenal bulb by the pyloric sphincter. Figure 3.1B shows the main structural features of the pylorus. It is not an anatomically discrete sphincter but a development of the circular smooth muscle layer. A ring of connective tissue separates the pylorus from the duodenum,

---

Gastrectomy Box 1

Partial gastrectomy

A 72-year-old man complained to his general practitioner that he had recently started to feel tired and listless. He also complained of longstanding symptoms of dizziness, sweating, and palpitations, after meals. Eight years previously he had undergone a partial gastrectomy and at first had felt reasonably well. In the last two years, however, he had become forgetful and had neglected to attend for his medication, vitamin B_{12} injections. The doctor told him that he should start the medication again and should also try to regulate his food intake more carefully by eating smaller, but more frequent, meals as his symptoms were partly due to the rapid entry of large amounts of material into the small intestine. The doctor also sent him for a blood test. The patient was found to be suffering from megaloblastic anaemia and mild metabolic acidosis. He also exhibited iron-deficiency anaemia. His blood vitamin B_{12} level was low and he was found to be mildly iron deficient.

We can infer from studying the details of this case that a good quality of life can be maintained after partial gastrectomy if:
(1) measures are taken to replace factors which prevent the development of pernicious anaemia, (2) measures are taken to prevent the development of iron-deficiency anaemia, and (3) food intake is carefully regulated.

We can also infer that the digestive functions of the stomach are not essential for life. These issues will be addressed in this chapter.

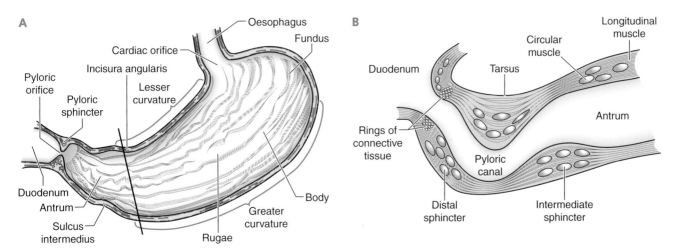

Fig. 3.1

(A) The main anatomical features of the stomach. The diagonal line shows the approximate division of the stomach into the two secretory regions: the oxyntic secretory area consisting of the fundus and the body, and the pyloric secretory area consisting of the pyloric antrum. (B) The structural features of the pylorus.

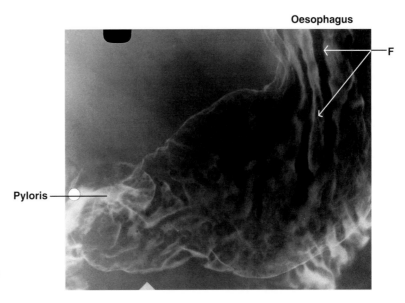

Fig. 3.2

An X-ray of the stomach taken after ingestion of barium. The thick mucosal folds (F) are clearly shown.

enabling the contractions of the two regions to be independent. However, the myenteric nerve plexi of the pylorus and duodenum are continuous (see Chapter 4).

Secretory mucosa of the stomach

The stomach mucosa can be considered as two separate regions (Fig. 3.1): the upper region comprising the fundus and the body of the stomach, known as the oxyntic glandular area, and the lower antral and pyloric region which secretes the hormone gastrin.

The secretory cells of the oxyntic glandular area produce the exocrine digestive juice known as gastric juice. The major secretory cells present in this area are oxyntic (or parietal) cells, which secrete acid and intrinsic factor, and chief (or peptic) cells which secrete pepsinogen, the precursor of the proteolytic enzyme pepsin.

The gastrin-secreting cells, the G cells, are restricted largely to the antral region. The secretions of these cells are involved in the control of many digestive functions including gastric secretion and motility (see Chapter 4). The stomach also contains enterochromaffin-like (ECL) cells which secrete histamine, and D cells which secrete somatostatin.

The consequences of partial surgical resection of the stomach depend on the part being removed. Resection of the lower part of the antrum and pylorus will remove most of the G cells. Lower serum levels of

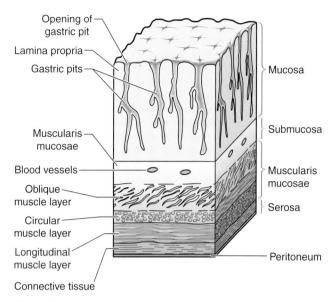

Fig. 3.3
Structure of the gastric mucosa.

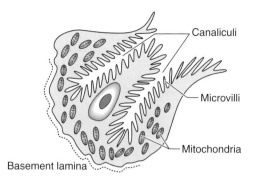

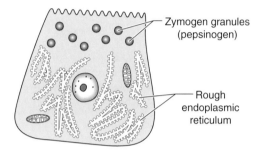

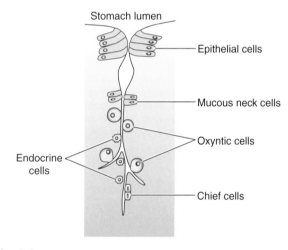

Fig. 3.4
Locations of different cell types in a gastric pit.

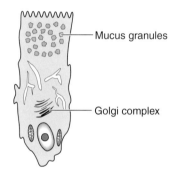

Fig. 3.5
Schematic diagrams of the three major types of exocrine secretory cell in the gastric mucosa. Note that each cell type has characteristic features associated with specialisation for secretion.

gastrin will result in considerably reduced acid secretion in the stomach. Removal of the upper part of the stomach (body and fundus) will remove the majority of the oxyntic cells. This will reduce acid secretion but in addition will result in a more severe lack of intrinsic factor secretion resulting in inadequate absorption of vitamin B_{12}.

Histology

The oxyntic cells and chief cells are located in deeper regions of the pits, as are the endocrine cells. Mucus-secreting cells are located in the neck region

providing a protective barrier to the deeper lying secretory cells. The location of endocrine cells in the deeper aspect of the gastric pits (Fig. 3.4) facilitates uptake of their secreted granules by the underlying capillaries.

Figure 3.5 shows the three major exocrine cell types which produce secretions that enter the lumen of the stomach. These cells are all specialised in various ways to perform their secretory function. The oxyntic cell has a vast surface area enabling it to produce large amounts of secretion. Invaginations of the luminal cell membrane form canaliculi (tubular passages) that penetrate deep into the cell. The canaliculi open on to the cell's free surface. They are lined with finger-like processes, known as microvilli, and these provide a large surface area for transport of secreted substances (see Chapter 1). When the cell is actively secreting, the canaliculi enlarge as they fill with secreted juice. These cells are also rich in mitochondria, which provide the energy in the form of ATP required for the secretory process.

The chief cell is specialised for the secretion of enzyme protein. It contains an extensive network of rough endoplasmic reticulum, the site of protein synthesis. Numerous dense zymogen granules, the loci of storage of the enzyme precursor protein, are located towards the luminal side of the cell.

The mucous cell has a fairly extensive network of endoplasmic reticulum and a prominent Golgi complex, a characteristic of cells specialised for the secretion of glycoproteins, in this case mucins. This cell also contains numerous clear vesicles, which are the sites of storage of mucins.

Composition of gastric juice

The adult human secretes approximately 2 L of gastric juice per day. When a meal is being eaten, the food material stimulates the stomach to secrete gastric juice. The stomach produces two different secretions; an acid secretion known as parietal juice, which is released from the oxyntic (parietal) cells, and an alkaline juice released from the mucous cells. Gastric juice is isotonic with plasma but the concentrations of its various constituents vary with the rate of flow: the higher the rate the greater the acidity. During a meal therefore the chyme becomes more acid, and the acidity can reach pH 2.0. Maximum acid secretion can be induced by injection of histamine. Figure 3.6 shows the changes in concentration of some of the constituent ions in an individual in whom secretion was stimulated by injection of histamine. This procedure is used clinically to assess the secretory function of the stomach. It is known as the Gray and Hollander test after the physicians who first developed it. Absence of HCl secretion is known as achlorhydria. This is seen when the gastric pits are destroyed. As a consequence it is usually associated with lack of intrinsic factor, which results in vitamin B_{12} deficiency and pernicious anaemia (see below). When loss of HCl secretory capacity occurs the first clinical manifestation is usually iron deficiency because lack of acid and gastroferrin result in ingested iron being retained in an unabsorbable form (see below). Vitamin B_{12} deficiency is a later manifestation because total body stores are usually sufficient to maintain normal bone marrow function for several years.

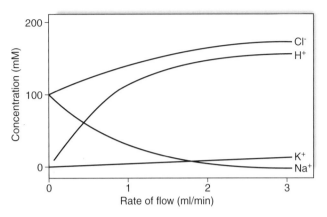

Fig. 3.6
Variation in the ionic composition of gastric juice with rate of flow.

The concentration of H^+ ions increases with rate of flow, as does that of Cl^- ions and K^+ ions, whilst the concentration of Na^+ ions decreases. These changes in composition occur because when food stimulates the stomach to secrete it is only the rate of the acid parietal secretion that increases appreciably. The secretion of alkaline fluid is mainly a passive process and so its rate is relatively unaffected. Thus dilution of the chyme by the alkaline juice is less at high flow rates and the H^+ and Cl^- ion concentrations increase. Both acid and alkaline secretions are isotonic with plasma.

Cellular mechanisms of secretion

Secretions of the oxyntic cell

Hydrochloric acid
The secretion of H^+ and Cl^- ions by the stomach are both active processes. The energy is derived from the hydrolysis of ATP. The H^+ ions are transported against an enormous concentration gradient: the concentration of H^+ ions in the blood is approximately 10^{-8} M, whilst the concentration in the stomach lumen can reach 1.5×10^{-1} M. As in the case of other active transport processes there are mechanisms that regulate the rate of secretion. These are described in the next chapter.

The mechanism whereby the H^+ ions are generated within the cell is outlined in Figure 3.7. Carbon dioxide diffuses into the cell from the plasma. Inside the cell it combines with water to form carbonic acid. This reaction is catalysed by the enzyme carbonic anhydrase. The carbonic acid dissociates to give H^+ and HCO_3^- ions. The HCO_3^- ions are transported into the blood,

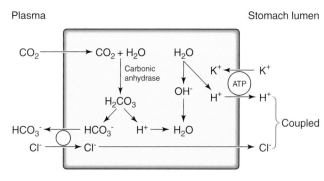

Fig. 3.7
Hydrochloric acid secretion by the oxyntic cell.

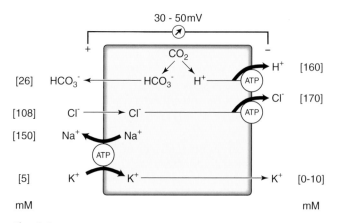

Fig. 3.8
Active and passive transport of ions in the secreting oxyntic cell.

down a concentration gradient, in exchange for Cl^- ions. The secretion of HCO_3^- ions into the blood when the stomach is secreting acid into the lumen results in the plasma becoming transiently alkaline. This phenomenon is known as the 'alkaline tide', and it is this process that is responsible for the development of metabolic alkalosis in patients suffering from persistent vomiting (see below).

Hydrogen ion secretion across the secretory surface of the oxyntic cell is accomplished by proton pumps in the secretory membranes of the canaliculus. The proton pump, which contains an ATPase, secretes H^+ ions in exchange for K^+ ions in a ratio of 1:1. In the resting cell the pumps are located in the intracellular compartment but when the cell is stimulated they are transported along tubulovesicles to the luminal border of the cell and incorporated into the canalicular membrane. When the cell is stimulated to secrete, the tubular vesicle system diminishes and the microvilli become more abundant and cause a substantial increase in the 'secretory' area of the plasma membrane. With inhibition of acid secretion the reverse occurs. Similar changes also occur in the duct cells of the pancreas and these are described in detail in Chapter 5.

Chloride ions are also secreted against a concentration gradient. The concentration of Cl^- ions in the blood is approximately 107 mM, whereas in the lumen of the stomach it can reach 170 mM. However, chloride is also secreted against an electrical gradient as the luminal surface of the resting cell is electronegative (between $-60\,mV$ and $-80\,mV$) with respect to the serosal surface. In the resting cell the potential difference is due to K^+ and Cl^- diffusion potentials. When the cell is stimulated to secrete it becomes less electronegative ($-30\,mV$ to $-50\,mV$, Fig. 3.8). Na^+/K^+ coupled pumps are present at the serosal surface and chloride pumps are present at the mucosal surface. The serosal surface is permeable to chloride and this ion enters the cell bound to a chloride ion transporter

protein, the cystic fibrosis transporter (CFTR). This protein is also present in many other cells, including the pancreatic duct cells. Lack of this transporter results in the clinical condition known as cystic fibrosis, which is a consequence of defective chloride transport (Chapter 5). Passive flow of Cl^- ions into the cell down their concentration gradient occurs in exchange for HCO_3^- ions (Fig. 3.7). The concentration gradient for chloride across the serosal surface of the cell is created by its being actively pumped out of the cell at the mucosal border, thereby keeping the concentration within the cell low. The chloride pump at the mucosal surface is electrogenic, i.e. it produces net transport of negative charges and operates without the exchange of an anion. When the cell is stimulated to secrete, the potential difference falls. The proton and the chloride pumps on the mucosal surface are coupled in the secreting cell so that H^+ and Cl^- ions are secreted in a ratio of 1:1. The coupling mechanism is not yet understood.

Drugs that are powerful inhibitors of the proton pump in the oxyntic cell are used to treat mucosal disorders such as duodenal ulcers, which are potentiated by acid secretion (see Chapter 4). Omeprazole, the most commonly used, is a weak base which acts by blocking the H^+/K^+ ATPase activity of the proton pump. Omeprazole is inactive at neutral pH, but it is activated in acid conditions (pH 3.0). Such conditions exist only in the canaliculi of the oxyntic cell. The action of the drug is therefore restricted to this location in the gastrointestinal tract thereby avoiding the unwanted side-effects of disruption of Cl^- ion transport which could occur in other organs such as the lungs, pancreas, and skin (sweating) with use of other H^+ transport inhibitors that are active in less acid conditions.

Gastrectomy Box 2

Gastrectomy: acid–base disturbance

Secretion of acid by the stomach during a meal is accompanied by transport of HCO_3^- ions into the blood (the alkaline tide). When the food reaches the duodenum it is mixed with the alkaline secretions from the pancreas, liver and walls of the intestines. The cellular mechanisms whereby these alkaline juices are secreted are in some ways the reverse of those whereby acid is secreted in the stomach (Fig. 3.7). Thus transport of HCO_3^- ions into the glandular ducts of these organs occurs simultaneously with the transport of an equal number of H^+ ions into the blood. The consequent increase in blood H^+ concentration is normally neutralised by the HCO_3^- ions of the alkaline tide of the blood from the stomach. In addition the H^+ ions secreted by the stomach into the lumen are neutralised by the HCO_3^- ions present in the digestive juices (bile, pancreatic juice, and intestinal juice) acting in the small intestine (Fig. 3.9). This balance can be upset by the process of vomiting, whereby acid is lost from the body, as well as by gastric resection, which restricts acid production. Feedback control mechanisms normally regulate the secretion of H^+ and HCO_3^- ions to keep the pH values in the gut lumen within appropriate limits (Chapters 4, 5, and 6). Many metabolic functions in the body are extremely sensitive to pH change, and the pH of body fluids such as plasma must therefore be maintained within a very narrow range.

Abnormalities can occur in the acid–base balance of the patient who has undergone partial gastrectomy but the body compensates for these disturbances. After removal of the stomach the 'alkaline tide' obviously does not occur, but during a meal H^+ ions are still transported into the blood from the secreting pancreas, liver and intestines, and the blood tends to become acidic. This 'metabolic' acidosis can be compensated in the short-term by the respiratory system, which responds with an increase in the rate and depth of breathing. This results in CO_2 being blown off from the blood. The reaction:

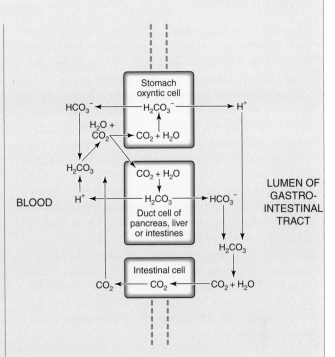

Fig. 3.9
Neutralisation of acid in the blood and in the intestinal lumen.

$$H^+ + HCO_3^- \rightarrow H_2CO_3 \rightarrow CO_2 + H_2O$$

is consequently driven to the right (the law of mass action) and the H^+ ion concentration in the blood falls.

Full compensation of the acidosis takes longer and depends on processes in the renal tubules, which conserve HCO_3^- and secrete acid. In the presence of impaired renal function, the patient's blood tests would show a low pH, low HCO_3^- concentration, and a low pCO_2. In a compensated patient, following a meal, acidotic urine would be excreted. A detailed explanation of the control of acid–base balance can be found in the companion volumes on the Respiratory and Renal systems.

Intrinsic factor

Intrinsic factor is the only substance secreted by the stomach which is essential to life. Intrinsic factor is a 55 000 kDa glycoprotein that complexes with vitamin B_{12} (cobalamin). The glycoprotein dimerises and the dimer binds two molecules of vitamin B_{12}. The complex is resistant to digestion. There are four physiologically important forms of vitamin B_{12}. These cyanocobalamins bind to proteins in the food, and are released from them by the action of acid and pepsin in the stomach. The vitamin is absorbed inefficiently by passive diffusion in the free, uncomplexed state, along the length of the intestine, but a specialised absorption mechanism exists in the distal ileum whereby vitamin B_{12} which is complexed with intrinsic factor can be absorbed at a relatively rapid rate (see Chapter 9). Therefore vitamin B_{12} deficiency can result from disorders of the stomach mucosa which releases intrinsic

> ### Gastrectomy Box 3
>
> #### Pernicious anaemia
>
> We can now understand why the patient who had undergone gastrectomy developed pernicious anaemia, and consider how it was diagnosed and the measures that could be taken to correct it.
>
> After gastrectomy, pernicious anaemia eventually develops as a consequence of Vitamin B_{12} deficiency unless replacement therapy is instigated. In pernicious anaemia, abnormal immature macrocytic red cells are produced by the bone marrow. The results of the patient's blood tests would show a low red cell count and a high mean cell volume (macrocytosis). Treatment could be administration of intrinsic factor by mouth. However, the preferred treatment is intramuscular injections of vitamin B_{12}. The injections are only required every 3 months because the liver has a large storage capacity for this vitamin. Massive doses of the vitamin would be required if it were administered by mouth because of the slow rate of absorption in the absence of intrinsic factor.

> ### Gastrectomy Box 4
>
> #### Iron-deficiency anaemia
>
> We can now consider (1) why iron-deficiency anaemia could be a complication in the gastrectomised patient, (2) how it would have been diagnosed, and (3) how it could be corrected.
>
> After removal of the stomach, iron-deficiency anaemia can eventually develop because of the lack of substances such as gastroferrin which combine with Fe^{2+} and prevent it from forming insoluble complexes in the stomach. In addition the acid in the stomach tends to convert Fe^{3+} in the diet to the ferrous form, the only form that can be absorbed to any appreciable extent. Even if it is only the antrum of the stomach that is removed, iron deficiency can develop because of the reduction in acid secretion.
>
> However, the body's iron stores are more limited than those of vitamin B_{12}, and iron-deficiency anaemia can manifest itself within a few months of partial gastrectomy. The treatment for iron deficiency is daily administration of ferrous sulphate, which is usually effective if given by mouth.

factor, or from disorders affecting the terminal ileum such as Crohn's disease (see Chapter 8).

Pernicious anaemia

In the absence of intrinsic factor, pernicious anaemia develops because vitamin B_{12} deficiency results in impaired maturation of red blood corpuscles. The disease is usually caused by atrophy of the gastric mucosa, which results in destruction of the oxyntic cells. The mucosa is then unable to secrete intrinsic factor, HCl or pepsin. In most individuals with pernicious anaemia, antibodies against oxyntic cell proteins are present in the blood. It is not clear, however, whether the antibodies are the cause of the disease or a secondary response to damage by some other means. Anaemia does not develop until several years after the changes have occurred in the gastric mucosa, when the liver stores of vitamin B_{12} have become depleted. Childhood forms of the disease also exist. These are rare conditions. There is an auto-immune type with similar defects to the more common adult form of the disease, and a type characterised by congenital intrinsic factor deficiency. In the latter type, HCl and pepsin secretion are normal as the oxyntic cells and chief cells are preserved. Another form of the disease is caused by a defect in the mechanism for vitamin B_{12} absorption in the ileum (see Chapter 8).

Gastroferrin and iron absorption

Iron is absorbed mainly as the ferrous (Fe^{2+}) ion, and ferric (Fe^{3+}) iron is absorbed very inefficiently. The body's stores of iron are small and need to be frequently replenished to promote adequate haemoglobin synthesis and red blood cell function. The acid environment in the stomach tends to maintain soluble iron in its absorbable ferrous form.

Gastroferrin is a 350 000 kDa glycoprotein secreted by the oxyntic cells of the stomach. It complexes with Fe^{2+} in the stomach lumen. This complex formation facilitates the absorption of iron in the small intestine (see Chapter 8). This is because there is a tendency for Fe^{2+} ions to form insoluble complexes with OH^-, HCO_3^-, and PO_4^{2-} ions in the duodenum and jejunum. Fe^{2+} ions are not absorbed from these insoluble complexes. However, if Fe^{2+} is complexed with gastroferrin it is kept in an absorbable state. Complex formation with ascorbate (vitamin C) or fructose also tends to keep Fe^{2+} available for absorption.

Secretion of the chief cell

Pepsin, the proteolytic enzyme of the stomach, is normally responsible for less than 20% of the protein digestion that occurs in the gastrointestinal tract. It is an endopeptidase that degrades proteins to peptides. It preferentially hydrolyses peptide linkages where one of the amino acids is aromatic. Pepsin, like other protease enzymes, is formed from an inactive precursor, pepsinogen, which is stored in granules in the stomach chief cells and released by exocytosis. The synthesis and exocytosis of the enzyme protein is essentially similar to that described for pancreatic enzymes in Chapter 6. Pepsinogen is also secreted by other cell types (mucous cells and cells in the glands of Brunner in the duodenum). At least two immunologically distinct pepsinogens are secreted by the stomach, denoted pepsinogens 1 and 2. Pepsinogen 1 is secreted by the chief cells in the oxyntic glandular area, and pepsinogen 2 by cells throughout the stomach as well as in Brunner's glands.

Pepsinogen 1, the precursor of the major pepsin, pepsin 1, is activated in the stomach lumen by hydrolysis, with the removal of a short peptide:

$$\text{Pepsinogen} \atop (42\,500\,\text{kDa}) \quad \xrightarrow[\text{pepsin}]{\text{H}^+} \quad \begin{array}{cc} \text{pepsin} & + & \text{peptide} \\ (35\,000\,\text{kDa}) & & (7\,500\,\text{kDa}) \end{array}$$

Activation of pepsinogen initially requires the presence of acid. The H^+ ions secreted by the stomach perform this function. Then the activated enzyme can act autocatalytically to increase the rate of production of more pepsin. Acid is also important for pepsin action because it provides the appropriate pH for the enzyme to act. The optimum pH for pepsin is approximately pH 3.5. It also denatures ingested protein. Denatured protein is a better substrate for enzymes than native protein.

The presence of pepsin is implicated in acid-induced ulceration. This enzyme can digest damaged mucosa in the oesophagus, stomach, and duodenum, in the presence of acid. Reduction of acid secretion by treatment with proton pump inhibitors such as omeprazole will reduce the activity of pepsin and so protect the mucosa. The mucosa is normally protected by mucus (see below). Disruption of this barrier will provide the opportunity for pepsin to digest the columnar epithelium and create an ulcer. Thus pepsin potentiates (rather than initiates) ulcer formation. The mucosa can be damaged via a number of substances, including prostaglandin inhibitors such as aspirin and other non-steroidal anti-inflammatory drugs (NSAIDS). The mechanism probably involves disruption of the normal body repair mechanisms, preventing healing of small abrasions in the mucosa.

Gastrectomy Box 5

Consequences for digestion

We can assume from the fact that gastrectomy is compatible with life that the role of the stomach in the digestion of food is not indispensable.

If the stomach is removed, the lack of pepsin does not pose a problem as far as the overall digestion of protein is concerned. It is normally responsible for the digestion of only 10–20% of the protein present. In its absence the proteases secreted by the pancreas, which act in the small intestine, can normally cope with the digestion of all the digestible protein present. Chymotrypsin, an enzyme produced by the pancreas (see Chapter 5), has a similar substrate specificity to pepsin. However, pepsin and acid in the stomach have a further role in destroying aerobic bacteria which have been ingested with the food. Thus, in a well-fed normal individual, infections such as cholera, for example, are rare. However, such infections more often affect individuals who have undergone a gastrectomy or who do not secrete acid (achlorhydria).

Secretions of the mucous cell

Mucus is a viscous sticky substance that contains glycoproteins known as mucins, which consist of about 80% carbohydrate, largely galactose and N-acetylglucosamine. The molecules are tetramers with a molecular weight of approximately two million. The carbohydrate chains protect the molecule from digestion by pepsin. It lubricates the pieces of food (in conjunction with salivary mucus) enabling them to be moved about and churned by the contractions of the stomach. The epithelial cells secrete an opaque alkaline mucus which has a high bicarbonate content. This secretion increases when food is eaten. In addition the mucus neck cells secrete a clear mucus in response to food. Mucin tetramers form a dissolved gel when their concentration exceeds approximately 50 mg per ml. This gel forms a layer on the surface of the mucosa. Its stability depends on charged SO_4^-, COO^- groups and H^+ bonds, and dramatic changes in pH can cause precipitation of the mucus. The surface epithelial cells secrete non-parietal alkaline fluid (see above) and this fluid is entrapped in the layer of mucus. The alkaline mucus forms a barrier that lines the stomach and protects it from damage by acid and pepsin.

Mucus is released from the mucous neck cells and surface epithelium by exocytosis. It can also be released by desquamation of the epithelial cells from the surface. Menetrier's disease is a condition characterised by hypertrophy of the gastric epithelium which results in abnormally large amounts of mucus, containing plasma proteins, being secreted. This dangerous loss of protein can lead to reduction in the extracellular fluid volume, shock, and dehydration.

Damage to the mucosal barrier

The stomach normally has a low permeability to acid due to the presence of a protective mucosal barrier. The barrier is partly due to the presence of mucins but other factors such as adequate blood flow and the presence of growth factors which promote the replacement of damaged cells are also important. However, it should be noted that mucus does not form a continuous layer and the protection is due to a great extent to the fact that the rate of acid production keeps pace with the buffering capacity of the food. Peptic ulcers (Fig. 3.10) form in the stomach due to the action of acid and pepsin when the mucosal barrier is damaged and the stomach is unable to protect itself and replace the damaged cells. Thus ulcers in the stomach are not usually due to an increased rate of acid secretion but rather to a defect in the ability of the mucosa to withstand damage (which may be caused by substances such as aspirin, ethanol, and bile salts). In fact in some individuals with peptic ulcers the rate of acid secretion is lower than normal. The decreased rate of acid secretion is caused in part by H^+ ions leaking into the mucosa in exchange for Na^+. The H^+ ions accumulate and the pH of the cells falls. This results in cellular injury and cell death. The H^+ ions also damage mucosal mast cells causing them to release histamine. This exacerbates the condition by acting on the mucosal capillaries causing ischaemia and vascular damage. If the damage is severe, bleeding can occur.

Ulcers form more frequently in the duodenum than in the stomach. In individuals with duodenal ulcers there is often a higher than normal basal secretion of acid and an abnormally high rate of maximum secretion in response to histamine stimulation. Individuals with duodenal ulcer may have twice the average normal number of oxyntic cells in their mucosae. In addition, pepsinogen secretion is also usually high. The sensitivity to gastrin, the hormone that stimulates acid secretion (see Chapter 4), is also usually increased in these individuals. The consequence is that chyme with an abnormally high

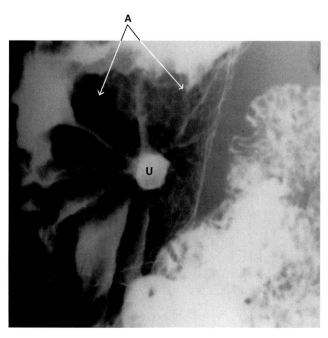

Fig. 3.10

An X-ray of the stomach taken after ingestion of barium. The normal folds of the antrum (A) have been disrupted by the chronic ulceration, giving rise to linear scarring around the ulcer (U).

level of acid and pepsin is passed into the duodenum where the mucosa is not protected, resulting in the formation of ulcers. These occur most frequently in the upper region of the duodenum near the pylorus.

Ulcers can be treated in various ways; including omeprazole treatment to block the proton pump and H_2 receptor blockers to prevent the histamine-mediated stimulation. The various treatments are discussed in detail in Chapter 4.

Absorption in the stomach

Very few substances are absorbed in the stomach and the stomach is virtually impermeable to water. Aspirin and alcohol are the main substances that are absorbed at this location. Alcohol is lipid-soluble and aspirin becomes more lipid-soluble at the acid pH present in the stomach (see Chapter 7). However, ingestion of aspirin can cause ulcers (see above) as it inhibits prostaglandin synthesis, which results in a reduced inflammatory response to injury and reduced cell turnover that inhibits repair mechanisms (see Chapter 4). Interestingly, however, this reduction in cell turnover by aspirin is protective against cancer in the mucosa of the colon (see Chapter 10).

Gastrectomy Box 6

Intestinal absorption

The sensations experienced by the gastrectomised patient after meals indicate activation of the sympathetic nervous system. We can now consider the explanations for these sensations and attempt to understand why the symptoms might be alleviated if the patient changed his eating habits.

If the stomach is removed a normal-sized meal moves rapidly into the small intestine resulting in the absorption of nutrients at an abnormally rapid rate. Furthermore there will be insufficient time for the meal to be completely digested and absorbed before it is moved on along the intestines. If the meal has a high carbohydrate content the absorption of glucose can be so fast that the homeostatic mechanisms for attenuating the increase in blood glucose concentration during absorption are disturbed. Normally the blood glucose rises to a maximum level at 30–60 minutes after the meal. An increase in blood glucose stimulates insulin secretion from the pancreas into the blood. This hormone lowers the blood glucose by promoting glucose uptake into muscle and adipose tissue. The blood glucose therefore returns to normal after 1.6–2 hours (Fig. 3.11). The insulin levels also return to normal. This is normally a finely tuned feedback control system (see Chapter 9). If the blood glucose levels rise too rapidly, however, the blood insulin concentration also rises rapidly to reach an abnormally high level in the plasma (Fig. 3.11). This results in rapid clearance of the blood glucose which can overshoot to an abnormally low level (hypoglycaemia).

Sympathetic nerves are stimulated by low blood glucose and so hypoglycaemia causes symptoms associated with activation of the sympathetic nervous system: palpitations, sweating, vasoconstriction, and pallor.
N.B. The acid in the normal stomach inactivates salivary amylase but obviously not until it penetrates the food bolus. Salivary amylase can therefore act within the food bolus in the stomach. It normally digests up to 70% of the starch in a meal (see Chapter 2). The remainder is digested by pancreatic amylase. After removal of the stomach the concentration of active amylase in the small intestine can be abnormally high. This accelerates the rate of glucose production in the lumen and the rate of increase in blood glucose, and the hypoglycaemia that ensues could be exacerbated.

Another consequence of the rapid entry of material into the small intestine is a rapid loss of fluid into the

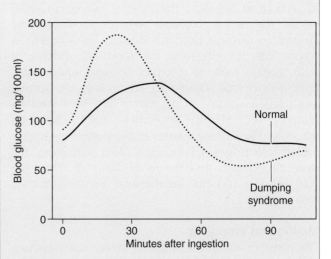

Fig. 3.11
Effect of eating an average-sized, high carbohydrate meal on the concentration of blood glucose in a normal adult and in a patient who has undergone gastrectomy.

gastrointestinal tract, resulting in a reduced intravascular volume. This will exacerbate the fainting sensation produced by the overdrive of the sympathetic nervous system (see below). The contents of the intestinal lumen become hyperosmotic due to large quantities of osmotic particles, resulting from the breakdown of macromolecules in the food, being dissolved in an abnormally low volume of digestive juices. The presence of a hyperosmotic solution in the intestines results in the transport of water from the blood, down its osmotic gradient into the lumen. Other, unknown, factors may also be involved in fluid loss in this condition. The loss of water from the body can result in a dangerous fall in the extracellular fluid volume (ECF). A concomitant fall in the intravascular volume results in hypotension which can be accompanied by fainting etc.

The symptoms that develop when a meal enters the small intestine too rapidly are collectively known as 'dumping syndrome'. The passage of hypertonic chyme through the small intestine into the large intestine will impair water absorption in the colon, causing diarrhoea. All these symptoms can be prevented by reducing the size of meals and so restricting the transit of food into the small intestine.

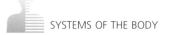
Motility in the stomach

The most important function of the stomach is its action to regulate the rate at which material enters the small intestine where digestion and absorption of most nutrients occurs. The stomach is responsible for churning the food and mixing it with gastric juice to produce a semi-liquid mass known as chyme. The empty stomach in the normal adult has a volume of approximately 50 ml and its lumen is only slightly larger than that of the small intestine. The surface interior of the stomach is highly folded into ridges. Upon being filled with food, the stomach expands and the folds diminish. Thus the wall tension and the intraluminal pressure change only slightly.

Mixing and emptying

The contractions of the stomach, which are responsible for mixing the chyme and emptying it into the small intestine, depend primarily on the activity of the smooth muscle in the wall. The stomach, like the rest of the gastrointestinal tract, is surrounded by layers of smooth muscle (Fig. 3.3, page 46).

During the first half hour after a meal, waves of contraction, known as peristalsis, cause weak ripples which proceed at approximately 1 cm per second over the body of the stomach pushing the food material towards the antrum. The muscle surrounding the antrum region (Fig. 3.1) is much thicker than that surrounding the rest of the stomach. Gradually the contractions become more intense, especially in the antrum. This contractile activity is responsible for churning the food material and mixing it with gastric juice. Eventually a large part of the muscle in the terminal antrum undergoes an intense concerted contraction. This strong contraction is responsible for emptying material into the duodenum. Only a small spurt of material is emptied at any one time. The antral contractions force the rest of the chyme back into the body of the stomach where it undergoes further churning and mixing, becoming more and more fluid.

The pyloric sphincter separates the stomach from the duodenum. Only a small amount of material is ejected through the sphincter each time the antrum contracts but immediately the food has entered the duodenum the back pressure helps to close the sphincter. Thus the function of the sphincter is to allow the carefully regulated emptying of gastric contents, and also to prevent regurgitation of the duodenal contents into the stomach. The latter is important as the gastric mucosa is highly resistant to acid but may be damaged by bile. (The duodenal mucosa on the other hand, is resistant to bile but may be damaged by acid.) Too rapid emptying of gastric contents can lead to duodenal ulcers, whereas regurgitation of duodenal contents can contribute to gastric ulcers.

Vomiting

Vomiting is part of the protective role of the stomach as it protects the body from ingested toxic substances. Thus it augments the other protective mechanisms of the stomach, including acid and pepsin secretion, which inactivate ingested aerobic bacteria, and mucin secretion which protects the columnar epithelium.

Vomiting or emesis is the forceful ejection of gastric contents, and sometimes duodenal contents, through the mouth. It is a reflex usually preceded by a feeling of nausea. This can be accompanied by salivation, sweating, pallor, a fall in blood pressure, pupillodilation, increased heart rate, and irregular breathing. It is usually also preceded by retching in which the gastric contents are forced into the oesophagus without entering the pharynx. A series of retches of increasing strength often precedes vomiting.

The vomiting reflex is controlled by the vomiting centre in the reticular formation in the medulla oblongata and the chemoreceptor trigger zone (CTZ) in the area postrema, which resides in the floor of the fourth ventricle near to the vagal nuclei, which innervate the gastrointestinal tract. The reflex response involves stimulation of the respiratory and abdominal skeletal muscles as well as the smooth muscle of the gastrointestinal tract. A large number of different areas of the body have receptors that provide afferent inputs to the vomiting centres to trigger vomiting. Table 3.1 lists the major stimuli that can trigger vomiting.

Sequence of events

Vomiting starts with a deep inspiration. This is followed by closure of the glottis, which protects the respiratory passages and holds the diaphragm down as the lungs cannot let air out. Air and saliva are drawn into the oesophagus, which becomes distended. The soft palate is elevated to prevent vomit entering the nasopharynx. Then expiration occurs against a closed glottis with simultaneous contraction of the abdominal skeletal muscles. This increases both the intrathoracic and intra-abdominal pressures. The essential component of the vomiting reflex is relaxation of the lower oesophageal sphincter, without which the gastric contents cannot pass into the oesophagus. As the intrathoracic pressure is lower than the intra-abdominal pressure, relaxation of the lower

Table 3.1
Factors that can trigger vomiting

1. Stimulation of sensory nerve endings in the stomach and duodenum (for example by solutions of copper sulphate and hypertonic sodium chloride)
2. Cytotoxic drugs (for example cisplatin used in the treatment of cancer)
3. Endogenous substances produced as a result of radiation damage, infections, or disease
4. Touch receptors at the back of the throat
5. Disturbances of the vestibular apparatus (known as motion sickness)
6. Stimulation of the sensory nerves of the heart and viscera (uterus, renal pelvis, bladder, testicles)
7. A rise in intracranial pressure
8. Nauseating smells, sights, and emotional factors acting through higher central nervous system centres
9. Endocrine factors (for example increase in oestrogen concentration in morning sickness)
10. Migraine
11. Circulatory syncope.

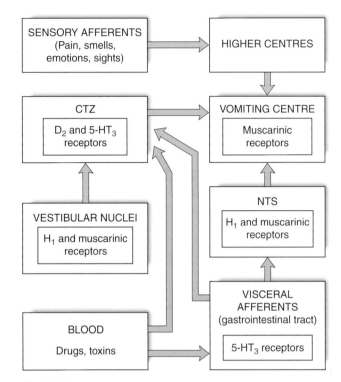

Fig. 3.12
The major peripheral and central areas involved in the control of vomiting, and the receptors utilised.

oesophageal sphincter allows passive flow of gastric contents down the pressure gradient. The importance of the abdominal muscles in vomiting is demonstrated by the fact that vomiting can still be induced in an animal if the stomach has been replaced by a bladder. In the pathological state, the oesophageal sphincter may be incompetent. This allows passive reflux of stomach acid into the oesophagus and results in damage to the unprotected oesophageal mucosa. An incompetent sphincter can be repaired surgically by wrapping the stomach around the lower oesophagus within the abdominal cavity (known as a stomach wrap). This effectively creates a one-way valve thereby preventing reflux of the gastric contents into the oesophagus, but can also prevent the process of vomiting by not allowing opening of the lower oesophageal sphincter.

Prior to vomiting a number of cycles occur whereby the oesophagus is repeatedly filled and emptied but, as the hypopharyngeal sphincter is closed, gastric contents cannot enter the mouth and they flow back into the stomach. Finally a violent expulsive effort forces the material through the upper sphincter into the mouth. If the stomach still contains sufficient material a second cycle can occur. Massive contractions of the duodenum can force intestinal contents into the stomach with the appearance of bile in the vomit. This is not due to reverse peristalsis but to the fact that when the stomach is relaxed, contractions of the duodenum will reverse the normal pressure gradient.

Control of vomiting

Figure 3.12 summarises the major pathways involved in the vomiting reflex. The final common pathway involves impulses from the vomiting centre to the skeletal and visceral smooth muscles. The vomiting centre is a functional rather than an anatomical entity. The vomiting centre receives impulses from the CTZ and the nucleus tractus solitarius (NTS) as well as from higher centres (which respond to repulsive sights, smells, and emotional factors). The CTZ is 'functionally' outside the blood–brain barrier and it is affected directly by substances in the bloodstream such as the opioid analgesics morphine and apomorphine, and glycosides such as digitalis, used in the treatment of cardiac conditions, and by high concentrations of urea (uraemia) associated with renal failure. It is also probably involved in motion sickness, as removal of the area postrema in dogs has been shown to prevent motion sickness from being induced. Both the CTZ and the NTS also receive inputs from the visceral afferents (via the vagal nerves).

Transmitters involved in vomiting

The neurotransmitters in the areas of the brain which control vomiting are numerous. They include γ-aminobutyric acid, acetylcholine, noradrenaline, dopamine, 5-hydroxytryptamine, histamine, glutamate, substance P, endorphins, and neurophysins, but their precise roles are still unknown. The main stimulatory factors and their pathways of action are indicated in Figure 3.12. In some clinical circumstances, for example after ingestion of a toxic substance, it is necessary to stimulate vomiting. The drug used is usually ipecacuanha. Its active ingredients are emetine and cephaeline which act locally on receptors in the stomach and stimulate vomiting via the NTS.

Table 3.2 lists the major anti-emetic drugs and their uses against vomiting induced by different stimuli. All of these drugs can cause unwanted side-effects, especially drowsiness, as they all have an inhibitory effect on the central nervous system.

Table 3.2
Anti-emetic drugs and their actions

Receptor involved	Drug(s)	Used against vomiting induced by
Histamine H_1 receptor	Piperazine derivatives	Motion, morphine
Muscarinic receptor	Hyoscine	Motion, copper sulphate
Dopamine receptor	Phenothiazines	Apomorphine, radiation gastrointestinal infections, cancer chemotherapy (cisplatin), oestrogen (morning sickness), narcotics
5-hydroxytryptamine ($5-HT_3$) receptor	Ondansetron	Cancer chemotherapy (cisplatin)
Cannabinoids	Nabilone	Cancer chemotherapy (cisplatin)

Self-assessment case study: excessive vomiting

A 55-year-old woman is being treated with a course of chemotherapy using cisplatin, an anti-cancer drug. Unfortunately she becomes nauseous and cannot stop vomiting. This is a side-effect of the drug treatment. It can become a chronic condition if the therapy has to be continued. A sample of the patient's blood was tested to assess her acid–base status and electrolyte concentrations.

Using your knowledge of the physiological consequences of gastrectomy you should be able to predict some of the consequences of persistent vomiting. You can now try to work out the answers to the following questions.

① What blood measurements would be made to determine the patient's acid–base status?

② What would you expect the patient's acid–base status to be?

③ Can you outline the cellular mechanisms in the gastrointestinal tract involved in causing the disturbance in acid–base balance?

④ How would the patient's body attempt to compensate for the disturbance?

⑤ Would you expect the patient's blood to show a low K^+ concentration (hypokalaemia)? If so, what would be the mechanisms involved?

⑥ What steps could be taken to correct the disturbances?

⑦ Where are the chemoreceptors that are involved in the response to cisplatin probably located?

⑧ What drugs could be used to treat cisplatin-induced vomiting? Why would you expect these drugs to be effective?

Self-assessment questions

① What are the most important functions of the stomach?

② Which functions of the stomach can be dispensed with?

③ How does the composition of gastric juice vary with the rate of flow and what are the reasons for this variation?

④ How is the oxyntic cell specialised for secretion?

⑤ What is the alkaline tide and when does it occur?

⑥ How does omeprazole relieve ulcer formation in the gastrointestinal tract?

⑦ Can you state three ways in which acid promotes the digestion of protein in the stomach?

⑧ What part does pepsin play in ulcer formation?

⑨ What are the functions of mucus?

⑩ Why is there little change in the wall tension and intraluminal pressure of the stomach when it is distended with food?

THE STOMACH
CONTROL

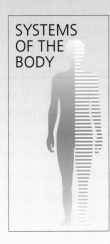

SYSTEMS
OF THE
BODY

Chapter objectives

After studying this chapter you should be able to understand:

① The interplay of nervous and hormonal control of gastric function, and how this is coordinated by food in the gastrointestinal tract.

② How these control mechanisms result in coordinated function of the digestive system.

③ How dysfunction can result in mucosal ulceration and how this can be diagnosed and treated.

④ How dysfunction can result in secondary effects on the gastrointestinal tract and on systemic acid–base balance.

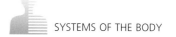
Introduction

Food in the gastrointestinal tract stimulates the release of chemical substances and exerts a mechanical pressure on the walls of the tract, to stimulate or inhibit gastric secretion and motility. Nervous, paracrine, and endocrine signals are involved.

A leading role in the coordination of gastrointestinal functions is played by the hormone gastrin, which is released from the stomach into the bloodstream during a meal. It stimulates both secretion and motility in the stomach. It also stimulates the blood supply to the gastric mucosa. In addition it controls many other functions of the gastrointestinal tract and its associated organs. Gastrin is released from G cells, which are located mainly in the mucosa of the pyloric antrum and so are ideally placed to respond to the presence of ingested material in the stomach. Tumours of ectopic G cells, known as gastrinomas, can give rise to the Zollinger–Ellison syndrome. This rare disease is characterised by oversecretion of gastrin, which results in excessive secretion of acid, and hypermotility of the gastrointestinal tract. In this chapter the physiological and clinical importance of the hormone is illustrated by discussion of the functional abnormalities that arise in Zollinger–Ellison syndrome.

Control of gastric secretion

The control of secretion of gastric juice involves extrinsic and intrinsic nerves, hormones such as gastrin, and paracrine mediators such as histamine.

Gastrinomas Box 1

Gastrinomas (Zollinger–Ellison syndrome)

A 40-year-old woman who had been suffering for several years from intermittent abdominal pain, diarrhoea, and steatorrhoea (the elimination of pale, greasy stools), visited her general practitioner. She had previously been diagnosed as having peptic ulcer disease, and had been prescribed omeprazole and a short course of antibiotics, but with no long-term relief of her symptoms. Consequently she had undergone surgical resection of the distal stomach (a partial gastrectomy). Surprisingly, her symptoms persisted following the surgery. Further tests were initiated to investigate the possibility that they were due to a gastrinoma. Her basal acid secretion and her acid secretion in response to an injection of pentagastrin were investigated. This involved aspiration of gastric juice. A radioimmunoassay for gastrin was performed on a blood serum sample. She was maintained on a high dose of omeprazole to protect against further ulceration, and arrangements were made for her to have an endoscopy. Hypertrophy of the gastric rugae, and ulceration in the second part of the duodenum, were seen. In the light of these observations, and the abnormal plasma gastrin level found, a computerised tomogram (CT scan) of her upper abdomen was performed. This demonstrated a mass in the pancreas. A laparotomy (opening of the abdomen) was performed and the surgeon discovered a tumour in the pancreas, which was identified from a biopsy specimen as a gastrinoma. Removal of the tumour cured the patient's symptoms and her serum gastrin concentration declined to within the normal range.

After studying the details of this case we can consider the following:

① What abnormalities in blood gastrin levels, gastric acid secretion, and pepsinogen secretion might we expect to see in this patient? What changes might we expect following distal gastrectomy?

② Why was hypertrophy of the gastric mucosa present?

③ Why was ulceration seen in the second part of the duodenum? Which other sites in the gastrointestinal tract are likely to be ulcerated in this condition?

④ Which of the diagnostic tests used would have given indications that the condition was Zollinger–Ellison syndrome and not simple gastric or duodenal ulceration?

⑤ What is the rationale for treating this condition with a high dose of omeprazole?

⑥ What are the explanations for the patient's diarrhoea?

⑦ What are the physiological consequences of excessive gastrin and acid production?

⑧ What is the reason for the presence of steatorrhoea?

Hormonal control

Gastrin

Gastrin is a hormone that is secreted from the G cells in the stomach. It stimulates gastric juice secretion, and has a general role in the preparation of the gastrointestinal tract for the digestion and absorption of food.

The existence of a substance that is released into the blood in response to food in the stomach, and that circulates in the bloodstream to stimulate acid secretion, was first proposed by Edkins in 1905. However, when it was realised that histamine, a substance present in abundance in gastric mucosa, stimulated acid secretion, it was assumed that this was the mediator. It was not until 30 years later that Grossman and his colleagues showed that material placed in the gastric antrum of a dog stimulated acid secretion in a gastric pouch (made from the body of the stomach) which had been transplanted in the neck region. Increased secretion occurred even if the antrum was denervated. This indicated that the stimulus was a blood-borne factor released from the gastric antrum; that is, a hormone. In 1964, Gregory and Tracey isolated the pure peptide hormone (subsequently called gastrin) from hog stomach.

Biologically active forms of gastrin

In the normal human, gastrin is produced mainly in the gastric antrum, although smaller amounts are produced in the proximal small intestine. Two major forms of gastrin exist: gastrin-34 (G34, composed of 34 amino acids) and gastrin-17 (G17, composed of 17 amino acids). In humans, over 90% of the gastrin present in the antral mucosa is G17. Gastrin-17 has a half-life in the circulation of approximately 6 minutes, and G34 approximately 36 minutes. Both peptides stimulate gastric acid secretion. The short half-life of the G17 form indicates that its main influence is probably via local receptors in the stomach. The active part of the molecule is the carboxy-terminal tetrapeptide sequence. This sequence is contained in the pentapeptide drug pentagastrin (see below).

G cells and gastrin secretion

Gastrin is secreted from G cells (Fig. 4.1A), which are 'open' APUD (amine precursor uptake and decarboxylation) endocrine cells (see Chapter 1). Microvilli are present along their apical surface, which is in contact with the lumen of the stomach. This structural feature of the cell enables it to sample the gastric contents. Receptors present on the luminal surface membrane sense chemical substances in food, known collectively as 'secretogogues', to regulate the release of gastrin (see below). In normal individuals most of

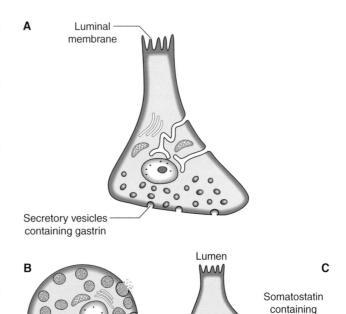

Fig. 4.1
Cell types in the gastric mucosa that release factors which control secretion. (A) Gastrin-secreting G cell, (B) histamine-secreting ECL cell, (C) somatostatin-secreting D cell.

the G cells are found in the mucosa of the gastric antrum, although some (less than 20%) are present in the duodenal mucosa. The G cells comprise less than 1% of the mucosal cells. In the human, these, together with other endocrine cells, are found between the basal and neck regions of the gastric glands (see Chapter 3). The mature cells are replaced from immature precursor cells located in the isthmus of the antral glands. The turnover of the G cells is slow (unlike the epithelial cells). It is stimulated by gastrin. Acid is a potent inhibitor of G cell proliferation, and because of this, the chronic administration of omeprazole, which blocks acid secretion, results in proliferation of G cells. For this reason, if omeprazole treatment is suddenly discontinued, rebound hyperacidity can result.

Gastrin is stored in secretory granules present along the basolateral border of the cell which lies in close proximity to the blood vessels. It is released into the circulation at the basolateral membrane in response to neural, endocrine, or paracrine stimuli, and by local factors in the lumen of the stomach.

Cellular actions of gastrin on acid secretion

Gastrin receptors

Gastrin acts on a variety of cell types that possess specific surface receptors. The oxyntic cell is the type that has been most studied. Interestingly gastrin and cholecystokinin (CCK, a hormone secreted by the duodenal mucosa) have the same carboxy-terminal tetrapeptide and act on the same receptors. There are two such receptors, the CCK-A receptor, present in the pancreas and the gallbladder, and the gastrin-CCK-B receptor, present on the enterochromaffin (ECL) cell and the oxyntic cell. The two hormones exhibit different potencies at these receptors. CCK has a 10-fold higher potency than gastrin at the CCK-A receptor. This difference in binding affinities between gastrin and CCK at the two CCK receptors is the main reason for their different patterns of biological activity. CCK exerts its main physiological effects on the biliary tree and the pancreas where CCK-A receptors predominate.

Oxyntic cell

The secretion of acid and the secretion of intrinsic factor by the oxyntic cell are normally regulated in parallel, so that stimulation of acid is accompanied by increased secretion of intrinsic factor. Gastrin stimulates acid secretion by two mechanisms: it stimulates the oxyntic cell directly, and it stimulates it indirectly through stimulation of the ECL cell to release histamine, which in turn stimulates the oxyntic cell (Fig. 4.2). It binds to CCK-B receptors on the cell membranes in both types of cell. The result of this stimulation is the incorporation of proton pumps into the canalicular membrane of the oxyntic cell (see Chapter 3). Gastrin also stimulates the expression of the gene for the proton pump in the oxyntic cell, thereby increasing its synthesis. Omeprazole, a drug used to reduce gastric acid secretion and so allow mucosal damage to heal, inhibits the activity of the pump. This causes an increase in serum gastrin concentration, because the production of acid (which inhibits gastrin release, see below) is inhibited.

ECL cell

Gastrin binds with a high affinity to CCK-B receptors on ECL cells (Fig. 4.1B), to cause the release of histamine (Fig. 4.2). Histamine acts in a paracrine manner on the oxyntic cell to release acid. The binding of gastrin to the ECL cell also stimulates histamine production (from histidine, see below).

D cell

D cell (Fig. 4.1C) releases somatostatin, which inhibits gastrin secretion. These cells exhibit gastrin-binding

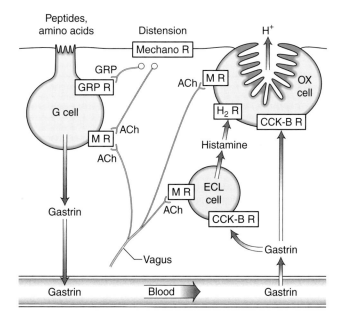

Fig. 4.2
Mechanisms of stimulation of acid secretion from the oxyntic cell by gastrin, histamine, and neurotransmitters.
Abbreviations: ACh, acetylcholine; GRP, gastrin releasing peptide; CCK-BR, cholecystokinin B receptor; H$_2$R, histamine H$_2$ receptor; MR, muscarinic receptor; OX, oxyntic.

sites, and gastrin can therefore stimulate somatostatin release from these cells. However, these binding sites are probably CCK-A receptors, which are more sensitive to CCK than to gastrin. Inhibition of somatostatin release via these receptors is therefore probably normally due mainly to circulating CCK.

Pharmacological stimulation of gastric acid secretion

Pentagastrin is a synthetic drug that consists of the C-terminal tetrapeptide of gastrin to which a substituted β-alanine has been added to stabilise the molecule. It exhibits all the physiological actions of gastrin. It stimulates acid and pepsinogen secretion, gastric blood flow, and contraction of the circular smooth muscle of the stomach. It can be administered to test gastric secretion.

Histamine actions

Histamine acts on H$_2$ receptors on the oxyntic cells to release acid (Fig. 4.2) via a cyclic AMP-mediated mechanism. It is produced in large amounts by the gastric mucosa. It is synthesised by decarboxylation of histidine:

$$\text{Histidine} \xrightarrow{\text{histidine decarboxylase}} \text{histamine} + CO_2$$

If histamine is injected it causes the release of a secretion that is rich in acid. Its presence is necessary for the secretion of normal amounts of acid. Thus inhibition of the enzyme histidine decarboxylase reduces acid secretion.

Neural control of gastric secretion

The stomach is controlled by intrinsic nerves in the internal nerve plexi of the enteric nervous system and by extrinsic nerve fibres in the vagus nerve and sympathetic nerves (see Chapter 1). Axons of nerve fibres (in the intramural plexi) innervate both secretory cells and smooth muscle cells. In general, cholinergic fibres stimulate gastric secretion and motility. Figure 4.3 shows the arrangement of the vagal cholinergic nerve trunks which innervate the stomach. Adrenergic fibres generally inhibit secretion and motility.

It should also be noted that a number of sensory nerves leave the stomach and travel in the vagus nerve and the sympathetic nerves. Sensory nerves in the stomach also provide afferent paths of intrinsic reflex arcs which travel in the intramural plexi of

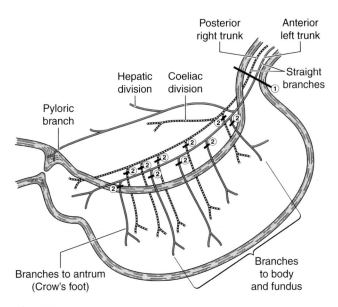

Fig. 4.3
Arrangement of the vagal innervation of the stomach. (1) Site of vagus nerve secretion in a vagotomy, (2) sites of nerve section in a highly selective vagotomy.

the stomach. This provides some intrinsic control of smooth muscle contractions and gastric juice secretion.

Acetylcholine and gastrin-releasing peptide
Acetylcholine released from cholinergic nerve fibres in local nerves can stimulate oxyntic cells to release acid, or G cells to secrete gastrin (Fig. 4.2). Some fibres in the vagus nerve also contain gastrin-releasing peptide (GRP), which exists as two major forms, both containing the nonapeptide active site. The structurally similar peptide bombesin, which has been extracted from the skin of the frog *Bombina bombina,* has similar actions. GRP released from nerves in the stomach stimulates gastrin release from the G cells (Fig. 4.2). It probably also stimulates acid release by a gastrin-independent mechanism. This interaction of the neural and gastrin mechanisms facilitates a rapid response to food ingestion.

Inhibitory control of acid secretion

Feedback control via acid
Gastric acid secretion is blocked if the contents of the stomach become too acid (pH 3.0, or lower). This inhibition is indirect and is exerted via inhibition of gastrin release. It is a negative feedback mechanism that prevents the gastric contents (and probably more importantly the duodenal contents) from becoming too acid. When the acidity of the stomach reaches pH 2.0 it is virtually impossible to stimulate gastrin release by any means. In conditions where achlorhydria (lack of acid secretion) is present (such as pernicious anaemia), there are usually high levels of gastrin in the blood because this feedback mechanism cannot operate. The inhibitory action of acid on the G cell is exerted via stimulation of somatostatin release from D cells in the antral mucosa, which inhibits gastrin and histamine release. Somatostatin acts both locally in a paracrine manner and via the systemic bloodstream in an endocrine manner, to inhibit gastrin release from the G cells in the antrum and histamine release from ECL cells. These interactions are outlined for the antrum region in Figure 4.4.

Somatostatin
Somatostatin is a potent inhibitor of acid secretion from the oxyntic cell. It exists predominantly as the 14 amino acid peptide somatostatin-14 (ST-14) in D cells in the fundic and antral mucosa. It is released from cytoplasmic processes in the vicinity of its

target cell, the G cell (Fig. 4.4). This hormone acts on somatostatin-2 (ST-2) receptors on the G cells. It acts primarily in a paracrine manner via local diffusion in the intercellular spaces, but it also acts systemically through its release into the local mucosal circulation. It also acts upon the oxyntic cells in the fundus to inhibit the release of acid directly. Fundic D cells are 'closed' APUD cells (see Chapter 1) and do not respond to luminal acidity, but antral D cells are 'open' APUD cells and they respond to changes in H⁺ concentration in the stomach lumen. Somatostatin appears to exert a tonic inhibition of acid release in the fundus. During a meal, as the contents of the stomach become increasingly acid, secretion from the oxyntic cell declines, due to the action of somatostatin. The release of somatostatin can be inhibited by neutralisation of luminal acid.

Other inhibitory factors

Numerous peptides inhibit acid secretion. Some of these peptides are released from APUD cells by the presence of chyme in the duodenum (see below). Importantly, CCK, which is secreted in response to fat, competitively inhibits gastrin-mediated stimulation of acid release by binding to CCK-B receptors on the oxyntic cell and the ECL cell. Inhibition of acid and histamine secretion can be produced in two ways:

1. A high level of CCK in the blood (if gastrin levels are high) results in displacement of gastrin from its receptors, but as it is less potent than gastrin this results in reduced acid secretion, when gastrin is present in the circulation.
2. It is also a potent antagonist of gastrin-stimulated acid secretion in humans, by its action on CCK-B receptors on D cells, to release somatostatin, which in turn inhibits acid secretion.

The hormone secretin also produces a profound inhibition of gastrin release and gastric acid secretion. It is released from the duodenum in response to the presence of food at that location. It is a 27 amino acid peptide which has structural similarities to the pancreatic hormone glucagon. The most potent stimulus for secretin release is acid in the duodenum. Secretin inhibits the secretion of gastrin from G cells and the secretion of acid from the oxyntic cells. Other peptides which inhibit gastric acid release, include the 43 amino acid peptide gastric inhibitory peptide (GIP) released in response to fat in the duodenum or ileum, and the 28 amino acid peptide vasoactive intestinal peptide (VIP), which is released into the circulation from nerve endings in the enteric nerves of the submucosal and myenteric plexi. VIP and GIP have considerable sequence homology (14 amino acids) with secretin and glucagon, and they act on the same receptors as secretin on oxyntic cells and G cells to inhibit acid release. The receptors for all these hormones are denoted VIP receptors. Although the primary effect of these peptides is to reduce gastric juice secretion, tumours of APUD cells, such as VIPomas, cause increased motility and consequently diarrhoea. Table 4.1 summarises the actions of

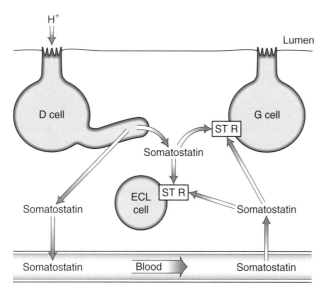

Fig. 4.4
Paracrine and endocrine mechanisms of feedback inhibition of acid secretion by somatostatin released in response to low pH in the antrum. STR, somatostatin receptor.

Table 4.1
Gastrointestinal peptides that inhibit acid production in the stomach

Peptides	Main stimulus	Location	Mechanism of action
CCK	Fat	APUD cells, (duodenum) enteric nerves	Somatostatin release (CCK-B receptors). Competes with gastrin (CCK-A receptors)
Secretin	Acid	APUD cells, (duodenum)	Inhibition of gastrin, and acid release
GIP	Fat	APUD cells, nerves	Inhibition of gastrin and acid release
VIP	Distension of stomach	Enteric nerves	Somatostatin release

CCK, cholecystokinin; GIP, gastric inhibitory peptide; VIP, vasoactive intestinal peptide; ACh, acetylcholine.

some of the endogenous peptides that inhibit acid production, and indicates their sites of release and the likely mechanisms involved.

Finally, prostaglandins synthesised in the gastric mucosa inhibit acid secretion. They function to protect the deeper mucosal layers from damage by acid.

Control of pepsinogen secretion

Pepsin is a cofactor in the acid-induced ulceration of the stomach and duodenum. Its precursor, pepsinogen, is released from the chief cell in response to acetylcholine, as well as by a number of gastrointestinal hormones. Figure 4.5 illustrates the various secretogogues and their receptors and the second messenger systems involved in their actions. Acetylcholine released upon stimulation of the vagus nerve and local nerves is probably the most potent stimulus. It acts on muscarinic receptors on the chief cell membrane. H^+ ions trigger the local cholinergic reflex that stimulates the chief cells. They also enhance the effects of other stimuli on the chief cell. In addition, H^+ ions stimulate the release of secretin in the duodenum (see below) and secretin also stimulates pepsinogen secretion. The effects of H^+ may account in part for the correlation between acid and pepsin secretion. Gastrin stimulates pepsinogen secretion directly via CCK receptors, but the most potent effect of gastrin on pepsinogen secretion is its indirect action via acid secretion.

Activation of muscarinic receptors, and CCK (CCK-A and CCK-B receptors) on the chief cells results in the generation of inositol trisphosphate and diacylglycerol. The relative importance of these two intracellular messengers has not yet been elucidated. The receptors for secretin, VIP, cholera toxin, and prostaglandins are linked to the adenyl cyclase-cAMP second messenger system. Pepsinogen secretion is decreased by somatostatin, which inhibits adenylcyclase in the chief cell.

Control of mucus secretion

Surface mucous cells secrete mucus in response to chemicals such as alcohol, and in response to contact with roughage in the food. Mucus neck cells are also stimulated by gastrin to secrete mucus.

Trophic actions of gastrin

Gastrin may be responsible for controlling the growth and proliferation of a variety of cell types in the gastric mucosa, including ECL cells and the precursors of oxyntic cells. Hyperplasia of ECL cells and oxyntic cells occurs in conditions where hypergastrinaemia is

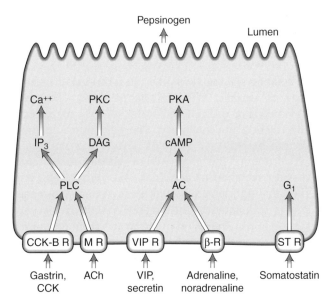

Fig. 4.5
Mechanisms of secretion of pepsinogen from the chief cell. CCK-B R, cholecystokinin-B receptor; ACh, acetylcholine; VIP R, vasoactive intestinal peptide receptor; PKC, protein kinase A; DAG, diacylglycerol; AC, adenylcyclase; IP_3, inositol trisphosphate; β-R, β-adrenergic receptor.

present. Patients with gastrin-secreting tumours exhibit oxyntic cell hyperplasia due to overstimulation by gastrin. Lifelong administration in animals of drugs, such as omeprazole or H_2 receptor blockers, that reduce acid secretion, or resection of the acid-secreting mucosa, all of which can result in consequent hypergastrinaemia due to the reduced feedback inhibition by H^+ ions, can cause ECL cell hyperplasia due to uncontrolled stimulation by gastrin. Moreover, patients who have undergone resection of the antrum and therefore have low circulating gastrin concentrations, display atrophy of the oxyntic glandular mucosa.

Peptic ulcer disease

The duodenum is the most frequent site for ulcer formation. Excessive secretion of acid and pepsinogen are directly implicated in chronic ulceration of the duodenum. High H^+ concentration can lead to the breakdown of the protective mechanisms of the mucosal barrier (see Chapter 3). Patients with simple duodenal ulcer usually have a high basal acid output with normal levels of serum gastrin. In contrast, patients with gastric ulcer usually have normal or slightly low acid secretion. In gastric ulcer the primary defect may be a reduced ability of the mucosa to withstand damage by acid and pepsin.

Gastrinomas Box 2

Causes and diagnosis

In Zollinger–Ellison syndrome the gastrinomas present may be ectopic, often in the pancreas. They may be small and difficult to locate. In 60% of patients the tumours are malignant. The gastrinoma tumours secrete excessive amounts of gastrin into the portal bloodstream. The high serum gastrin levels elicit massive secretion of acid from the oxyntic cells. It is the basal acid secretion (which occurs between meals) that is stimulated to the greatest extent by the high gastrin levels. The secretion of gastrin from the gastrinomas (as with any other secretory tumour) is independent of secretogogues such as peptides in the stomach. Thus secretion of acid during a meal is not abnormally affected. Table 4.2 shows typical values for the basal and maximum acid secretion (induced by injection of pentagastrin), and serum gastrin levels in normal individuals and in patients with gastric ulcer, duodenal ulcer, or Zollinger–Ellison syndrome. The

basal acid output is usually considerably elevated in Zollinger–Ellison syndrome. However, the maximum acid output measured after pentagastrin injection is not increased proportionately to that in normal individuals or patients with peptic ulcer disease. The basal acid output is usually not less than 60% of the maximum output, and is often the same as the maximum output.

In normal individuals a low pH in the stomach lumen inhibits acid secretion by inhibiting gastrin secretion from the antral G cells (see below) but secretion by gastrinomas is independent of this feedback control.

Pepsinogen secretion is also stimulated by gastrin, so its secretion also, is usually abnormally high in Zollinger–Ellison syndrome.

Diagnosis

The diagnosis of Zollinger–Ellison syndrome requires consideration of the results of a number of different

Table 4.2
Acid and gastrin secretion in Zollinger–Ellison syndrome

	Acid secretion rate Basal		Maximum (mmol/h)	Blood gastrin (pmol/l)
	Day (mmol/h)	Night (mmol/12h)		
Normal	1–5	18	25	30
Gastric ulcer	1–5	8	25	30
Duodenal ulcer	4–10	60	40	30
ZES	45	120	55	650

Typical mean values are given for acid secretion and blood gastrin levels in normal subjects, and patients with simple gastric ulcer, duodenal ulcer or Zollinger–Ellison syndrome. Maximal acid output is elicited by injection of pentagastrin (6 μg/kg). ZES, Zollinger–Ellison syndrome.

Table 4.3
The secretin test for Zollinger–Ellison syndrome

	Basal acid secretion rate (mmol/h)		Blood gastrin (pg/ml)	
	Basal	After secretin	Basal	After secretin
Normal	1–5	<5	<80	<80
Duodenal ulcer	4–10	<5	<80	<80
ZES	45	62	650	770

Typical values are given for basal and maximum acid secretion and blood gastrin levels in healthy individuals, in patients with duodenal ulcer, and patients with Zollinger–Ellison syndrome. Maximum values are obtained during a secretin infusion test. ZES, Zollinger–Ellison syndrome.

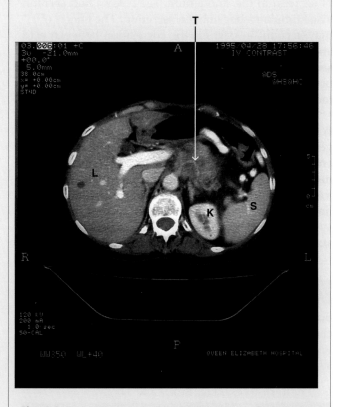

Fig. 4.6
A CT scan showing a cross section of the upper abdomen. A large swelling in the head of the pancreas can be seen, suggestive of a tumour (T). The normal liver (L), spleen (S), and left kidney (K) are seen on the same image.

procedures. Basal acid secretion is dramatically elevated, and serum gastrin levels are often elevated ten times above the normal range, as a consequence of the uncontrolled secretion (Table 4.2). However, high basal acid production by the stomach and high levels of gastrin in the blood are merely suggestive of the condition.

The 'secretin test' has been used in the past to assist the diagnosis of Zollinger–Ellison syndrome, but now that gastrin levels can be measured directly and accurately by radioimmunoassay, it is no longer often employed. The basis of the test depends on the fact that, whereas secretin normally inhibits acid secretion during the intestinal phase of digestion (by acting on the oxyntic cell directly and on the G cell) and normally has little effect on basal acid secretion between meals, it stimulates secretion of gastrin from ectopic gastrinomas; the so-called 'paradoxical' effect of secretin in Zollinger–Ellison syndrome. (It also stimulates the secretion of alkaline pancreatic juice and alkaline bile, Chapters 5 and 6.)

The test involves the intravenous injection or infusion of secretin and investigation of its effect on basal acid and gastrin secretion. In normal individuals and individuals with duodenal ulcer, injection of secretin has little effect on basal acid secretion or basal gastrin secretion, but in patients with Zollinger–Ellison syndrome it usually elicits a marked increase in serum gastrin and gastric acid output. Table 4.3 compares gastrin and acid output following secretin infusion in normal individuals, patients with Zollinger–Ellison syndrome, and patients with duodenal ulcer.

Radiological imaging, such as magnetic resonance imaging (MRI) or computerised tomography (CT), can detect lesions as small as 1–2 cm in diameter (Fig. 4.6). When malignant lesions are present, metastases are usually visible in the liver. Exploratory surgery is required to confirm the lesion (and to remove benign tumours). Malignant tumours are usually treated with proton pump inhibitors to simply control the symptoms of excessive acid secretion.

Gastrinomas Box 3

Gastric hypertrophy

Gastrin has trophic actions on the mucosa of the gastrointestinal tract. It is a growth factor for the stomach mucosa, and in Zollinger–Ellison syndrome the high levels can stimulate hypertrophy of the mucosa. The rugal folds may become extremely thick. This can sometimes be seen in medical imaging procedures such as the barium meal test.

Gastrinomas Box 4

Ulceration of the gastrointestinal tract

The massive secretion of acid and pepsinogen in Zollinger–Ellison syndrome (Table 4.2) leads to widespread ulceration of the upper gastrointestinal tract. Ulcers may occur in the stomach, oesophagus, and duodenum. They occur at the same sites in the duodenum where they are seen in simple duodenal ulcer, in which the first part of the duodenum is the typical site, but they may also occur at more distal sites in the duodenum, because of the very low pH and the high pepsin content of the chyme leaving the stomach.

Treatment of peptic ulcer disease

Surgery

Treatment with proton pump inhibitors or H_2 antagonists is highly effective for duodenal or gastric ulcers (see below). Vagotomy results in a reduced secretion of acid, especially during the cephalic phase of control (see below). However, following vagotomy, although the secretion of pepsinogen (which is also involved in ulcer formation) is effectively reduced, acid secretion is less affected. As a consequence, surgery for peptic ulcer disease is usually restricted to patients with complications. Such complications include haemorrhage from a blood vessel at the base of an ulcer (usually the gastroduodenal artery which passes behind the first part of the duodenum), erosion of the stomach wall through to the peritoneal cavity, which results in perforation, and peritonitis due to leakage of duodenal contents into the cavity.

Prior to the development of effective drug treatment, surgery was the main treatment for chronic peptic ulcer disease. It involved either division of the vagus nerve (vagotomy), or antrectomy (resection of the stomach antrum). Vagotomy was performed to reduce vagal stimulation of acid secretion in the stomach, but unfortunately, this also resulted in impairment of gastric motility and emptying. To overcome this problem, division of the pyloric muscle (pyroplasty) was also performed. In the 1970s, highly selective vagotomy which preserved the function of

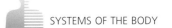

the pyloric muscle was developed (Fig. 4.3, page 61). This circumvented the need for a pyloroplasty. Antrectomy (surgical removal of the antrum) was a more radical approach, which was performed in order to remove the G cells and so reduce gastrin stimulation of acid secretion. Surgical approaches have now been largely superceded by the use of pharmacological treatment, particularly the use of antibiotics (see below).

Pharmacological treatment

At present, the most frequently used treatment for the suppression of gastric acid secretion in peptic ulcer disease is administration of proton pump inhibitors such as omeprazole in combination with antibiotics (see below). Using this treatment the need for long-term therapy is minimised, and it has now largely superceded the use of H_2 antagonists, although these can be very effective. Figure 4.7 shows the sites of action of the different drugs that can inhibit acid secretion in the stomach.

Antibiotics

Over the last few years evidence has accumulated that infection of the gastric mucosa by the bacterium *Helicobacter pylori* is causatively involved in potentiating peptic ulcer disease. These are spiral Gram-negative bacteria present in the stomach of most (over 80%) patients with gastric or duodenal ulcers. The presence of these organisms leads to impairment of the function of the protective mucosal barrier. Combinations of omeprazole (see below) and antibiotics have proved to be extremely effective in the treatment of duodenal ulcers. The bacterium is sensitive to a large number of antibiotics but those penetrating the submucosa where the microorganisms reside, such as clarithomycin and metronidazole, are the most effective. Eradication of *H. pylori* by antibiotic therapy prevents ulcer recurrence and so prevents the need for long-term treatment.

Proton pump inhibitors

The action of omeprazole, and its analogues, has been described in Chapter 3. This powerful drug blocks the H^+/K^+ ATPase proton pump (Fig. 4.7). It markedly inhibits both basal and stimulated secretion of gastric acid, and its use is now the first-line therapy for controlling symptoms in ulcer disease. It has few unwanted side-effects, although there remains concern about lowering acid secretion too drastically, because of the resultant elevation of serum gastrin levels, which in theory could be mitogenic (and therefore tumour-promoting).

Histamine H_2 receptor antagonists

Reduction of acid secretion in peptic ulcer disease can be effected by antagonising the action of histamine (Fig. 4.7). The compounds used include cimetidine and ranitidine. These drugs compete with histamine for H_2 receptors on the oxyntic cell. They can decrease basal- and food-stimulated acid secretion by 90% and can have a very significant effect in promoting the healing of duodenal ulcers. (Secretion of intrinsic factor from the oxyntic cell is also decreased but the doses used clinically are too low to cause pernicious anaemia.) However, if the treatment is withdrawn in patients with duodenal ulcers, the ulcers usually recur within a year. Long-term maintenance with these drugs was widely used until effective treatment with omeprazole and antibiotics became available.

Muscarinic receptor antagonists

Anticholinergic drugs, which bind to muscarinic M_2 receptors on the oxyntic cell and the ECL cell, can antagonise the effects of vagal nerve stimulation and reduce gastric acid secretion (Fig. 4.7). Many muscarinic antagonists are available but most are less effective than H_2 receptor antagonists, although they can have beneficial antispasmodic effects on gut smooth muscle. However, muscarinic receptors are present at many locations within the gastrointestinal tract and outside it, and for this reason parasympathetic side-effects, including effects on the cardiovascular system, are common. Pirenzipine is a relatively specific M_1 receptor antagonist which probably acts on post-

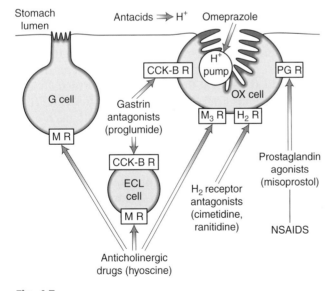

Fig. 4.7
Drugs that inhibit or neutralise acid secretion, and their targets. OX, oxyntic cell; MR, muscarinic receptor; H_2R, histamine H_2 receptor; CCK-B R, cholecystokinin-B receptor; PGR, prostaglandin receptor.

synaptic nerves in parasympathetic ganglia, to block the stimulation of oxyntic cells.

Antacids

Antacids are weak bases that act by neutralising gastric acid (Fig. 4.7). Therefore they can be used to relieve gastric pain caused by excessive acid secretion. Long-term treatment with antacids can produce healing of duodenal ulcers but they are ineffective for healing gastric ulcers. Compounds that are commonly used include magnesium hydroxide, magnesium trisilicate, aluminium hydroxide, and sodium bicarbonate.

Other possible treatments

Gastrin antagonists such as proglumide have been developed (Fig. 4.7) but these compounds are not potent enough for clinical use. Prostaglandins, which are synthesised in the gastric and intestinal mucosa (see Chapter 3), can also be effective in reducing acid secretion. In particular, prostaglandins of the E (PGE) and I (PGI) series can be administered to protect the deeper mucosal cells from damage. Moreover a deficiency of prostaglandins may be a contributing factor in peptic ulcer formation. Ingestion of aspirin, acetylsalicylate, can cause ulceration of the gastric mucosa because it inhibits prostaglandin synthesis. It is a weak acid and at low pH values it tends to exist in the un-ionised form (see Chapter 7). The un-ionised acid is lipid-soluble and it is readily absorbed across the lipid membranes of the stomach. Because prostaglandins inhibit acid secretion, inhibition of prostaglandin synthesis by aspirin results in increased acid secretion. This may result in ulceration in aspirin-sensitive individuals. PGE1 and PGE2 and stable analogues such as misiprostol also inhibit the histamine-mediated stimulation of acid secretion (Fig. 4.7). In practice, their main use is to prevent gastric damage from chronic use of non-steroidal anti-inflammatory drugs (NSAIDS). Finally, agonists of somatostatin and duodenal peptides such as secretin could theoretically be useful in peptic ulcer disease, but at present such drugs are not used clinically to treat gastrointestinal ulcers.

Control of motility in the stomach

In the stomach the pacemaker cells are located in the longitudinal muscle in the greater curvature region of the fundus. The basal electrical rhythm (spontaneously oscillating membrane potential) generates action potentials in the pacemaker cells and these are transmitted through the sheets of smooth muscle. The muscle therefore exhibits contractile activity even in the resting state (see Chapter 1). This contractile activity can be increased or decreased in amplitude and fre-

Gastrinomas Box 5

Treatment

The recognised treatment for Zollinger–Ellison syndrome is, first, to control the overproduction of acid by treatment with a proton pump inhibitor, such as omeprazole. This enables the ulcers to heal and controls the diarrhoea. Patients usually survive for many years with pharmacological treatment alone. When the ulcers are under control, surgery to remove the gastrinoma can be attempted to try to effect a cure. However, many patients with Zollinger–Ellison syndrome (approximately 25%) have multiple endocrine neoplasia type 1 (MEN 1).

In 40% of patients with Zollinger–Ellison syndrome, familial inheritance has been recorded. The syndrome is inherited in an autosomal dominant fashion, and other relatives will usually be affected. For this reason it is important to obtain a family history from patients diagnosed with the disease.

quency by factors that control the electrical activity of the smooth muscle cell membranes.

The electrical changes are of different shape and amplitude in different regions of the stomach. The membrane potential is relatively stable in the fundus region, but a slow wave can be recorded in the rest of the stomach. This slow wave is of relatively small amplitude in the body of the stomach but its amplitude progressively increases in regions closer and closer to the pylorus. The frequency of the slow waves remains the same, approximately 3 per minute, in the different regions because they are driven by the same pacemaker cells (see Chapter 1). In gastric smooth muscle there is a threshold potential for contraction of the muscle. When the membrane potential during the slow wave exceeds the threshold, contraction occurs (Fig. 4.8A). The greater the depolarisation and the longer the membrane potential remains above the threshold, the greater the tension developed.

In the antrum the action potentials exhibit an initial rapid depolarisation phase, followed by a long plateau phase (Fig. 4.8). The rapid depolarisation phase is caused by Ca^{2+} entry through voltage-gated channels, and the plateau phase is due to entry of both Ca^{2+} and Na^+ through slower voltage-gated channels. The influx of Ca^{2+} leads to muscle contraction (see Chapter 1). In the terminal antrum, action potential spikes occur on the plateaux of the slow waves. The trains of action potentials that occur during the plateau phase elicit vigorous contractions in the antrum and these can lead to gastric emptying.

Stretch or distension of the stomach walls increases the tension (the myogenic reflex, see Chapter 1).

Increased levels of circulating gastrin or stimulation of the vagus nerve also lead to a greater force of contraction. This effect is due to an increase in the amplitude and duration of the slow wave depolarisation (Fig. 4.8). The vagus nerve is stimulated by low blood sugar and therefore during fasting, when blood glucose is low, the magnitude of the stomach contractions increases.

Stimulation of the adrenergic sympathetic nerves to the stomach or increasing levels of CCK or secretin (see below) in the blood results in hyperpolarisation of the membrane and relaxation of the muscle (Fig. 4.8C). Sympathetic nerves are activated during exercise and the motility of the gastrointestinal tract is decreased. Stimulation of purinergic fibres in the vagus during the cephalic phase also inhibits muscle contraction.

These nerves release ATP, which hyperpolarises the smooth muscle membranes. Motility of the stomach is slowed during this phase (see below). Table 4.4 summarises the effects of endogenous factors on smooth muscle electrical potential.

After surgical procedures, motility in the stomach is inhibited. This is known as gastric stasis. If severe it can result in acute gastric dilatation (Fig. 4.9). It is a condition that can last for several days. It can be

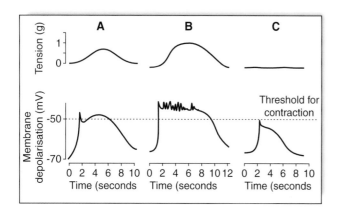

Fig. 4.8
Control of smooth muscle contraction in the stomach. (A). Electrical recordings of the membrane potential in the absence of chemical mediators, (B and C) effects of gastrin and noradrenaline respectively, on the membrane electrical changes and the contractile force in the antrum.

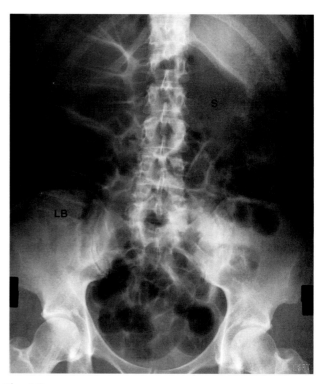

Fig. 4.9
A plain abdominal X-ray showing dilated loops of large bowel (LB) and a massively dilated stomach (S) containing food residue.

Table 4.4
Endogenous factors which control smooth muscle, and their actions on smooth muscle membrane potential

Factor	Location	Stimulus	Action	Receptor
Stretch		Distension	Depolarisation	
ACh	Nerves	Distension, peptides	Depolarisation	Muscarinic
NA, Adrenaline	Nerves	Stress (e.g. exercise)	Hyperpolarisation	β-adrenergic
ATP		Chewing, smells, etc	Hyperpolarisation	Purinergic
Gastrin	Stomach	Peptides, distension	Depolarisation	CCK-B
CCK	Duodenum	Fat	Hyperpolarisation	CCK-A?
Secretin	Duodenum	Acid	Hyperpolarisation	VIP
VIP	Enteric nerves	Distension	Hyperpolarisation	VIP
GIP	Duodenum	Fat	Hyperpolarisation	GIP

ACh, acetylcholine; NA, noradrenaline; VIP, vasoactive intestinal peptide; GIP, gastric inhibitory peptide; CCK, cholecystokinin.

relieved by passing a fine tube into the stomach via the oesophagus (a nasogastric tube), allowing free drainage of the gastric juice and air from the stomach. The condition may be due to activation of the sympathetic nervous system, i.e. excessive release of noradrenaline (Fig. 4.8C). Biopsies of the human antrum of such patients have been investigated electrophysiologically. The action potentials recorded have a shorter plateau phase during repolarisation. This leads to less tension being generated and the stomach dilates. Because the pylorus is closed, the gastric juice accumulates in the stomach (unless nasogastric drainage is instituted).

Control of the pyloric sphincter

The mucosal and muscle layers of the stomach and duodenum are discontinuous due to the presence of a ring of connective tissue on the duodenal side of the pyloric sphincter, but the myenteric plexi of the pylorus and duodenal bulb are continuous (see Chapter 3). The basal electrical rhythm of the duodenum is faster (approximately 10 per minute) than that of the stomach. The duodenal bulb contracts rather irregularly because it is influenced by the basal electrical rhythm of both the stomach and the duodenum. However, the activity in the antrum and duodenum is coordinated, and when the antrum contracts the duodenal bulb is relaxed. The pylorus is densely innervated by both parasympathetic (vagal) and sympathetic nerve fibres. The sympathetic nerves release noradrenaline, which act on adrenergic receptors to increase the constriction of the sphincter. After vagotomy this constriction is unopposed and the outlet of the stomach can be obstructed. The nerve fibres in the vagus are both excitatory and inhibitory. The cholinergic fibres in the vagus increase constriction of the sphincter but the inhibitory fibres release VIP, which relaxes the sphincter. CCK causes constriction of the pyloric sphincter in physiological concentrations that cause gallbladder contraction. Therefore CCK is probably also one of the physiological regulators of the sphincter.

Control of gastric function by food

Motility in the stomach is controlled partly by blood glucose levels. When the blood glucose concentration falls during fasting, gastric smooth muscle is stimulated. Peristaltic contractile activity increases, but not gastric emptying. These contractions can be strong

Gastrinomas Box 6

Diarrhoea

Diarrhoea is usually a prominent symptom in Zollinger–Ellison syndrome. It is present in approximately 65% of cases. There are a number of causes:

① Increased volume of secretions in the gastrointestinal tract. Gastrin increases the secretion of gastric juice, but it also increases the secretion of enzyme-rich juice and alkaline juices from the pancreas (see Chapter 5), alkaline juice from the liver (see Chapter 6) and alkaline juice from the glands of Brunner in the small intestine (see Chapter 7). In Zollinger–Ellison syndrome, elevated gastrin can cause massive volumes of secretion from these organs. The absorptive capacity of the small intestines and colon is consequently overwhelmed, and diarrhoea results. The mechanisms of diarrhoea are discussed in Chapter 7.

② Impaired digestion and malabsorption of nutrients, especially lipids (see above). The chyme becomes highly concentrated with unabsorbed nutrients, and therefore it is hyperosmotic. In the colon, undigested nutrients ferment to produce a further increase in osmotic particles. Water is consequently transported into the lumen of the intestines, down the osmotic gradient, and osmotic diarrhoea results.

③ Increased gastrointestinal motility. As gastrin increases smooth muscle contractility, high levels can result in increased peristalsis and increased force of contraction in the stomach, as well as increased ileal motility. This will cause diarrhoea. It is not clear to what extent these direct effects of gastrin can be exaggerated in the Zollinger–Ellison syndrome. However, they are probably of minor pathological significance compared to the effect of the copious secretions.

enough to cause 'hunger pains'. They are due to impulses in the vagus nerve which is sensitive to low blood glucose.

Acid is secreted at a low rate even when the stomach is empty. The basal rate is approximately 10% of the maximum rate. However, the rate is not constant even when the stomach is empty as it shows a diurnal variation: it is lowest in the morning and highest in the evening.

When a meal is eaten the mechanisms that control the secretion of gastric juice and the motility and emptying of the stomach interact in a complex manner to coordinate the functions of this organ. The control of gastric function during a meal can be conveniently divided into three main phases depending on the location of the food or chyme:

1. The cephalic phase, which occurs before the food reaches the stomach. It is a response to the approach of food (i.e. the smell or sight of food), or food in the mouth.
2. The gastric phase, which occurs in response to food when it reaches the stomach.
3. The intestinal phase, which is due to food material in the intestines, mainly the duodenum and upper jejunum.

In practice of course, for much of the time during a meal, ingested material is present at different locations at the same time.

The cephalic phase

Secretion

During the cephalic phase, gastric acid and pepsinogen secretion is activated by the thought, sight or smell of food, and by food in the mouth. The mechanisms of control of gastric secretion during the cephalic phase are summarised in Figure 4.10. Emotions also influence gastric secretion. The response to the sight and smell of food is a conditioned reflex; a learned response based on previous experiences of food. The release of acid at the sight and smell (approach) of food was first demonstrated by sampling of the gastric contents through a gastrostomy (fistula) in subjects who could not swallow food and had therefore been provided with a permanent fistula so that food could be placed directly in the stomach. Emotions were found to elicit increased or decreased acid secretion. This was shown by Wolff and Wolff, physicians who studied a patient with a closed oesophagus who was provided with a gastrostomy. They showed that hostility and resentment tended to increase gastric secretion whilst depression tended to reduce it.

The taste and the touch of food in the mouth also elicits secretion of gastric juice (before the food reaches the stomach). This is a non-conditioned reflex. It was studied by the physician Janowics, in a patient who had a gastrostomy because she could not swallow food. It was found that if the patient placed some food in her mouth and chewed it, there was an increased secretion of gastric juice. Furthermore, food that the patient enjoyed elicited a more copious secretion than food which she merely tolerated. The secretion in response to palatable food is

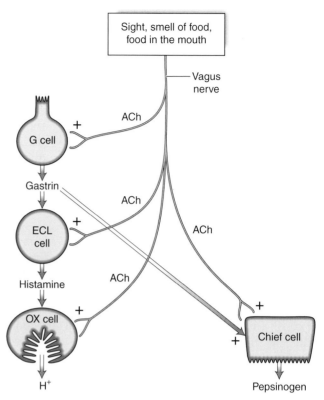

Fig. 4.10
Cephalic phase of control of gastric secretion.

known as 'appetite juice'. This gives some physiological justification for starting a meal with a savoury course (hors d'oeuvre).

The gastric juice secreted during the cephalic phase is rich in pepsinogen, as well as acid. The secretion of both acid and pepsinogen is due to impulses in the vagus nerve. Stimulation of the nerves releases acid both directly from the oxyntic cell and indirectly via the release of gastrin (Fig. 4.10). Less than half the acid produced in response to a meal is secreted during the cephalic phase. Vagotomy reduces the secretion of gastric juice mainly because its effect during the cephalic phase is abolished. When acid is secreted during the cephalic phase whilst the stomach is still empty, there is very little protein present in the stomach to buffer the acid. Therefore a small amount of acid will produce a marked fall in pH. This results in the feedback control mechanism coming into operation, whereby acid secretion is inhibited. The secretion of pepsinogen during the cephalic phase is due to direct stimulation of the chief cells by the vagal impulses, and to the release of gastrin which also stimulates the chief cells.

Motility

Motility in the stomach smooth muscle is reduced during the cephalic phase. The sight, smell, taste, and touch of food in the mouth all inhibit gastric emptying. Pain, depression, fear, and sadness also inhibit it. The mechanism is probably via impulses in inhibitory purinergic fibres in the vagus nerve. The activity in these nerve fibres inhibits gastric emptying and causes relaxation of stomach smooth muscle. At the same time the pyloric sphincter is constricted. The latter effect is probably also due to impulses in cholinergic fibres in the vagus nerve. This delay in the emptying of the stomach permits the stomach initially to store a greater volume when the food enters it, and so allows time for the digestive processes to operate. Interestingly, aggression and anger increase gastric motility but the mechanisms involved have not yet been elucidated.

The gastric phase

Secretion

Food placed directly into the stomach through a gastric fistula (gastrostomy) elicits an increase in both acid and pepsinogen secretion. This is the gastric phase of secretion. The control of secretion during this phase is summarised in Figure 4.11. The amount of secretion depends on the chemical content of the food, and its volume. Secretion of gastric juice is in response to chemicals in the food and to distension of the walls of the stomach by food. The products of protein digestion, especially peptides and amino acids (in particular tryptophan and phenylalanine), caffeine (present in tea, coffee, CocaCola), and alcohol, stimulate gastric secretion. The gastric phase accounts for more than 50% of the acid secreted during a meal. A low pH in the stomach inhibits acid secretion, although it stimulates pepsinogen secretion. These chemical substances, or 'secretogogues', are sensed by APUD cells which behave as chemoreceptors or 'taste' cells. The G cells sense peptides and amino acids whilst the D cells sense pH. Distension is detected by pressure receptors or nerve endings in the mucosa. Distension is not as powerful a stimulant as the chemical constituents of food. The subsequent regulation of gastric secretion is via coordinated neural, hormonal, and paracrine mechanisms. The neural signals are conducted in extrinsic nerves of the vagus nerve and intrinsic nerves of the enteric nerve plexi.

Motility

During the gastric phase of digestion, the stomach empties at a rate proportional to the volume of

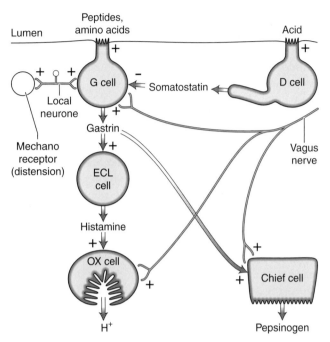

Fig. 4.11
Gastric phase of control of gastric secretion.

material within it. This is due partly to the effect of distension; the chyme stimulates pressure receptors in the wall of the stomach, which trigger impulses in nerves in the internal nerve plexi. It is probably also due to the direct effect of stretching the smooth muscle (the myogenic reflex, see Chapter 1). There is also a vagal mechanism involved in the response to distension, but in the gastric phase (unlike the cephalic phase) impulses in the vagus nerve increase peristalsis and gastric emptying. In this case it is the cholinergic nerve fibres in the vagus that are activated. However, excessive distension inhibits contractility (see Chapter 1) thereby allowing a longer time for the digestive processes to operate. Gastrin release into the blood in response to peptides and amino acids also potentiates peristalsis. Gastric emptying is brought about by strong periodic contractions of the antrum, potentiated by gastrin and acetylcholine in the vagus nerve. The pyloric sphincter relaxes when the antrum contracts and allows a portion of the gastric chyme into the duodenum. The relaxation of the sphincter is probably due to impulses in peptidergic nerve fibres in the vagus nerve, which release VIP.

The intestinal phase

The intestinal phase of gastric function is largely inhibitory. Gastric secretion and motility are both inhibited. In the duodenal phase the food is mixed with the digestive secretions of the pancreas and liver. The inhibition of gastric emptying by food in the duodenum enables the duodenum contents to be processed before more material enters it from the stomach.

Secretion

Although food in the duodenum is largely inhibitory as far as gastric secretion is concerned, there is an early stimulatory phase in response to slight distension of the duodenum, probably due to the release of gastrin from the duodenum. However, appropriate stimulation of the duodenum inhibits gastric secretion. Inhibitory stimuli include distension of the duodenum, fats and peptides in the chyme, increased acidity, and hypertonic solutions. All of these stimuli cause the release of hormones from APUD cells. The duodenal phase of control of secretion is summarised in Figure 4.12.

Acid causes the release of secretin into the blood, and this inhibits secretion of gastric juice. This is a feedback mechanism that prevents the duodenal contents becoming excessively acid. It is important for several reasons:

1. Digestive enzymes that act in the duodenum require neutral or acid pH values for optimum activity.
2. Micelle formation, which is necessary for fat digestion and absorption (see Chapter 8), will only take place at a neutral or slightly alkaline pH.

3. The duodenum is the most common site for ulcer formation in the digestive tract and acid is the prime cause of ulceration in this region. The reduction of acid secretion begins when the pH of the duodenal contents falls to 5.0 and it is complete at a pH value of approximately 2.5.

GIP is also released in the duodenal phase of digestion. This peptide has the same active sequence as secretin, and like secretin, it acts to inhibit acid secretion in the stomach. The mechanisms are discussed above. Both secretin and GIP also inhibit pepsinogen secretion.

Fats in the duodenal contents cause the release of CCK from the walls of the duodenum into the blood. This hormone also inhibits acid and pepsinogen secretion in the stomach. The mechanisms involved are discussed above. It competes with gastrin for CCK-B binding sites. This results in inhibition of acid secretion when gastrin concentrations in the blood are high, as is usually the case when a meal is present in the digestive tract. It also inhibits acid secretion by inhibiting gastrin release via CCK-B receptors.

Motility

Motility in the stomach can be influenced by food in the duodenum, food in the ileum, and food in the colon.

Distension of the duodenum inhibits gastric motility via two mechanisms: a quick enterogastric reflex which employs nerve fibres in the vagus nerve and an unknown neurotransmitter, and a slower humoral mechanism involving the release of hormones from the walls of the duodenum into the blood. These hormones are collectively known as enterogastrones. They include CCK and secretin (Fig. 4.12).

When food material reaches the ileum, the emptying of the stomach is delayed. This is a neural reflex initiated by activation of mechanoreceptors in the walls of the ileum, which triggers impulses in nerve fibres in the internal nerve plexi. Interestingly, when food enters the stomach, the motility of the ileum is increased. Thus ileogastric reflexes operate in both directions.

There is also a neural reflex response when the chyme enters the colon; distension of the colon activates pressure receptors, which triggers impulses in internal nerves to delay gastric emptying.

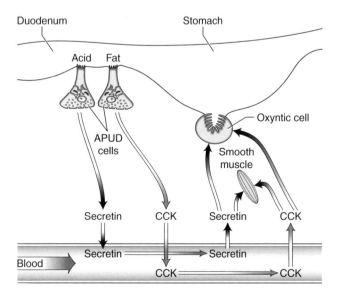

Fig. 4.12
Intestinal phase of gastric control.

Gastrinomas Box 7

Physiological consequences

Acid–base balance

The secretion of H^+ ions into the stomach lumen is accompanied by the secretion of an equal number of HCO_3^- ions into the blood. In Zollinger–Ellison syndrome, excessive secretion of acid, resulting from high levels of gastrin, can therefore lead to a pronounced alkaline tide. This is neutralised in normal individuals by acid secretion into the blood from the pancreas and liver when they secrete alkaline fluids into the ducts. Gastrin not only stimulates acid secretion in the stomach, it also stimulates the production of alkaline juices from the duct cells of the liver and pancreas. Acid in the duodenum stimulates alkaline fluid secretion via secretin, and increased alkaline secretion may also result via this mechanism. However, if these homeostatic mechanisms are overwhelmed by copious acid secretion, as is usually seen in Zollinger–Ellison syndrome, then alkalosis of the blood will occur.

Digestion and absorption

Pale stools indicate steatorrhoea (fat in the faeces). Normally almost all neutral fat ingested is digested and absorbed. Therefore steatorrhoea is an indication of malabsorption and disease. The excessive acid production in Zollinger–Ellison syndrome can lead to malabsorption of fat for two reasons:

① Pancreatic lipase is active at neutral or slightly alkaline pH values and it is reversibly inactivated at acid pH values. Other pancreatic and brush border digestive enzymes also act at neutral or alkaline pH values and malabsorption of other nutrients may also occur.

② Effective absorption of the monoacylglycerol and long-chain fatty acid products of lipid digestion, and lipid-soluble vitamins (A, D, K, and E), depends on them being sequestered in micelles to prevent them separating out of suspension in the chyme (see Chapter 8). The process of micelle formation will only take place at neutral or alkaline pH values. Thus in Zollinger–Ellison syndrome the excessive acid secretion may lead to defective lipid absorption. The consequences are deficiency of essential fatty acids (linoleic, linolenic, and arachidonic) required for healthy nerves and deficiency of vitamins A (required for night vision), D, required for Ca^{2+} absorption (see Chapter 7) and Ca^{2+} homeostasis, and K, required for effective blood clotting.

Vitamin B_{12}

Vitamin B_{12} is poorly absorbed in the ileum at low pH values for reasons not yet understood. Thus pernicious anaemia can develop in Zollinger–Ellison syndrome.

Self-assessment case study: peptic ulcer disease

A 45-year-old man, from a family with a history of peptic ulcer disease, visited his general practitioner and complained of dull, burning pain in his upper abdomen, associated with periodic nausea, vomiting, heartburn, and loss of appetite. He was a heavy drinker and smoker. Upon examination the pain was found to be localised to the epigastrum. The patient said that the pain was worse when his stomach was empty and was eased by eating a meal. He also complained of symptoms of hypersecretion of acid during the night. He often woke in the early hours with a burning sensation behind his lower sternum. He had been taking antacids, which afforded him some relief. The doctor sent him for an endoscopy. This showed the presence of an ulcer in the proximal duodenum. He was advised to stop smoking and not to drink alcohol. He was initially prescribed cimetidine, the preferred treatment for ulcers at the time. However, after 6 weeks the symptoms from the ulcer had not resolved. He was sent for a test to measure his gastric acid output and the results were consistent with chronic duodenal ulcer disease (Table 4.2). He was then prescribed omeprazole, and symptomatic relief was quickly obtained. Unfortunately the patient's symptoms returned after approximately 8 months. Omeprazole treatment was started again, but this time in combination with a course of antibiotics. His symptoms disappeared, and by 2 years later he had suffered no further relapse.

After considering the details of this case you should be able to answer the following questions:

① Why did the general practitioner suspect from what the patient said that he might have a duodenal ulcer rather than a gastric ulcer?

② What findings from the acid secretion tests would have supported the diagnosis of a duodenal ulcer rather than a gastric ulcer?

③ What is the most common location for ulcers in the duodenum? Why do they usually occur at that location?

④ What is the most common site for ulcers in the stomach and why do they occur at that location?

⑤ What is the mechanism of action of H_2 receptor antagonists such as cimetidine? Why are these drugs usually effective in relieving the symptoms of peptic ulcer disease? Why should they be administered at night in this patient?

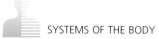

⑥ What is the mechanism of action of omeprazole?

⑦ Why was the patient given a course of antibiotics?

Self-assessment questions

① Which cells in the gastric mucosa are sensitive to gastrin?

② What are the two major receptor subtypes targeted by gastrin?

③ How does acid in the stomach inhibit gastric juice secretion?

④ How does acid in the duodenum inhibit gastric juice secretion?

⑤ What is the effect of (a) gastrin, (b) noradrenaline on the slow wave and contractile force of stomach smooth muscle?

⑥ What is the effect of food in the mouth on gastric secretion and motility?

⑦ How is the secretion of pepsinogen controlled?

⑧ How is the pyloric sphincter affected by stimulation of (a) the sympathetic nerves and (b) the peptidergic vagal nerves that innervate it?

PANCREAS
EXOCRINE FUNCTIONS

5

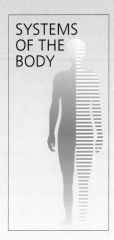

SYSTEMS
OF THE
BODY

Objectives

After studying this chapter you should be able to:

① Describe the macroscopic and microscopic anatomy of the pancreas and relate these to its function.

② Describe the components of exocrine function of the pancreas and apply this knowledge in understanding the pathological conditions of acute and chronic pancreatitis and cystic fibrosis.

Introduction

The pancreas contains exocrine tissue which secretes pancreatic juice, a major digestive secretion, and endocrine tissue which secretes the hormones insulin and glucagon. The hormones are important in the control of metabolism and their roles in the absorptive and postabsorptive metabolic states will be discussed in Chapter 9. This chapter will be mainly concerned with the exocrine secretions of the pancreas, their functions, and the mechanisms whereby the secretory processes are controlled.

Pancreatic juice finds its way into the duodenum via the pancreatic duct which opens into the duodenum at the same location as the common bile duct (see Chapter 1). Entry of both pancreatic juice and bile into the duodenum is controlled by the sphincter of Oddi. The smooth muscle of the sphincter is contracted between meals so that the junction is sealed. When a meal is being processed in the gastrointestinal tract, the sphincter muscle relaxes and allows the pancreatic juice and bile into the small intestine. The control of the sphincter of Oddi is discussed in Chapter 7. Exocrine dysfunction of the pancreas may be due to disorders of the pancreas itself, or to blockage of the main ducts which prevents the exocrine secretions reaching the duodenum. Duct blockage may also result in impaired bile flow from the liver and so cause jaundice.

In the small intestine, pancreatic juice, bile, and the juices secreted by the walls of the intestines, mix with the fluid (chyme) arriving from the stomach. Pancreatic juice provides most of the important digestive enzymes. In addition, by virtue of its HCO_3^- content, it helps to provide the appropriate pH in the intestinal lumen for the enzymes to act on their nutrient substrates. The functional importance of the pancreas to the digestive processes can be illustrated by the problems arising in an individual suffering from chronic pancreatitis, a condition in which pancreatic tissue is destroyed.

Chronic pancreatitis Box 1

Chronic pancreatitis

A forty-year-old man who had been a heavy drinker for many years, went to see his general practitioner. He had made two previous visits over the past year due to his experiencing recurrent episodes of abdominal pain. Although the pain had been intermittent at first, it was now continuous. The patient also said that he had lost a considerable amount of weight since his last visit. Upon enquiry the pain was described to originate in the epigastrum, and to radiate through to the back. In appearance the patient was very thin and the doctor noticed that he was mildly jaundiced. The doctor arranged for the patient to be admitted to hospital for a few days for tests so that his condition could be diagnosed. He was submitted to an X-ray examination, and serum and urine analyses were performed. The patient's stools were collected over three days. These were seen to be pale-coloured and bulky, indicating a high fat content (steatorrhoea). He was told to abstain from food the next morning so that a glucose tolerance test could be performed. The patient's response to secretin was also tested. This involved an injection of secretin (1 CU/kg body weight) and continuous aspiration of the duodenal contents until the water and bicarbonate output had returned to the initial level.

The blood tests showed a reduced serum pancreatic isoamylase, but increased bilirubin and alkaline phosphatase. The glucose tolerance test showed an abnormally high and prolonged rise in serum glucose, and urine analysis confirmed the presence of glycosuria (glucose in the urine), indicating that the patient was diabetic. The secretin test indicated a decreased pancreatic secretory response as manifest by a low level of HCO_3^- secretion. The presumptive diagnosis was chronic pancreatitis. The patient was prescribed pethidine to control the pain. He was advised to abstain completely from alcohol, and to try to eat regular meals.

Examination of the details of this case gives rise to the following questions:

① Is the primary defect in chronic pancreatitis known? What might the X-ray have revealed? What could be the cause of the condition in this patient?

② How are the exocrine and endocrine functions of the pancreas impaired in chronic pancreatitis? How is this condition diagnosed? What did the high faecal fat content indicate? What is the basis of a) the secretin test, b) the glucose tolerance test? Why has diabetes mellitus developed in this patient? Why was the patient jaundiced? Why were the patient's serum bilirubin and alkaline phosphatase abnormally high?

③ What are the main physiological consequences of this disease and how can the condition be treated or managed?

We shall address these questions in this chapter.

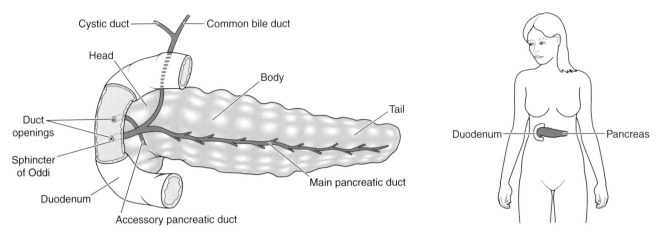

Fig. 5.1
The pancreas and its innervation and blood supply.

Anatomy

The pancreas is an elongated gland which lies in the abdominal cavity. It can be divided into three regions: the head, the body and the tail (Figs 5.1 and 5.2). The head is an expanded portion that lies in the C-shaped region of the duodenum to which it is intimately attached by connective tissue, and which is connected by a common blood supply. The body and tail extend across the midline of the body toward the hilum of the spleen. The pancreatic duct (duct of Wirsung) extends through the long axis of the gland to the duodenum. Pancreatic juice empties from this duct into the duodenum via the ampulla of Vater. In some individuals there is also an accessory pancreatic duct. Bile in the common bile duct from the liver also enters the duodenum at the ampulla of Vater.

Exocrine tissue

The exocrine units of the pancreas are tubuloacinar glands which are organised like bunches of grapes, in a similar manner to the units in the salivary glands (Fig. 5.3). These exocrine units surround the islets of Langerhans, the endocrine units of the pancreas. A thin layer of loose connective tissue surrounds the gland. Septa extend from this layer into the gland, dividing it into lobules, giving it an irregular surface. Larger areas of connective tissue surround the main ducts and the blood vessels and nerve fibres that penetrate the gland. Small mucous glands situated within the connective tissue surrounding the pancreatic duct secrete mucus into the duct.

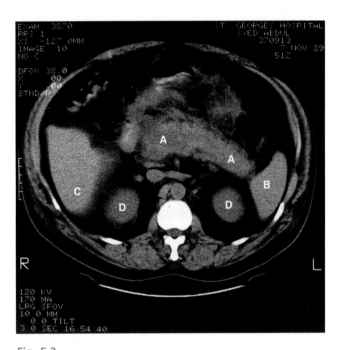

Fig. 5.2
Computerised tomography (CT) scan: cross section of the abdomen showing a swollen pancreas caused by pancreatitis (A) lying posteriorly on the abdominal wall. The spleen (B), lower border of liver (C) and kidneys (D) are also seen.

Endocrine tissue

The endocrine units, or islets of Langerhans, are most numerous in the tail region of the pancreas. They consist of clusters of cells which are surrounded by the pancreatic acini (Fig. 5.3). The islets vary considerably in size. As with all endocrine tissue, the hormones they produce are secreted into the blood. The major endocrine cell types present are α, β, D, and PP cells which secrete glucagon, insulin, somatostatin, and pancreatic polypeptide, respectively (for more information see Chapters 8 and 9). Different types of endocrine cells can be distinguished under the electron microscope by the different appearance of the granules within them. The islet cells have the general features of APUD cells (see Chapter 1). In addition there are a few (less than 5%) small 'clear' cells with as yet no clearly defined function.

Glucagon and insulin, the hormones produced by the α and β cells respectively are taken up by the local blood vessels to act systemically. Somatostatin acts locally in a paracrine manner to inhibit the secretion of the α and β cells, as well as the exocrine secretions of the acinar and duct cells. Pancreatic polypeptide acts in a paracrine manner to inhibit the exocrine secretions of the pancreas.

Oxygenated blood is supplied to the pancreas by branches of the coeliac and superior mesenteric arteries. The blood drains from the pancreas via the portal vein to the liver. The acini and ducts are surrounded by separate capillary beds. Some of the capillaries that supply the islets converge to form efferent arterioles which then enter further capillary networks around the acini. This arrangement is important for the paracrine control of pancreatic exocrine secretion.

Cholinergic preganglionic fibres of the vagus nerve enter the pancreas. These synapse with postganglionic cholinergic nerve fibres which lie within the pancreatic tissue and innervate both acinar and islet cells. Postganglionic sympathetic nerves from the coeliac and superior mesenteric plexi innervate the pancreatic blood vessels as well as the acinar and duct cells.

Histology of the exocrine tissue

Figure 5.3 shows the structure of a pancreatic lobule. The exocrine units of the pancreas, or pancreatons, each consist of a terminal acinar portion and a duct (Fig. 5.4). The duct that drains the acinus is known as an intercalated duct. These empty into larger intralobular ducts. The intralobular ducts in each lobule drain into a larger extralobular duct which empties the secretions of that lobule into still larger ducts, and the latter converge into the main collecting duct, the pancreatic duct.

The acinus is a rounded structure consisting of mainly pyramidal epithelial cells (Fig. 5.4). These cells secrete the digestive enzymes of the pancreatic juice. They display polarised features which are common to secretory cells (Fig. 5.3). The nucleus of the acinar cell is situated at the base of the cell. The cytoplasm in the basal region can be stained with haematoxylin or basic dyes due to the presence of rough endoplasmic reticu-

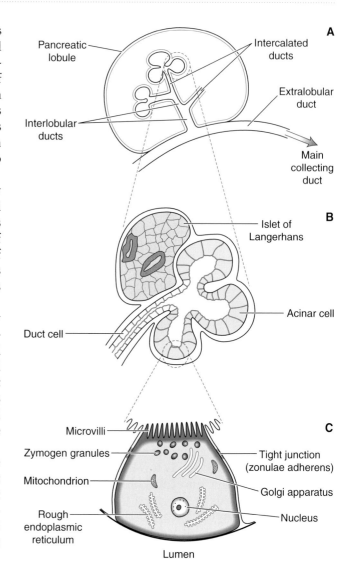

Fig. 5.3
(A) A lobule of the pancreas indicating the duct system, (B) the relationship of an exocrine unit and an islet of Langerhans, (C) an acinar cell.

lum, the site of production of the digestive enzymes. Small mitochondria are situated throughout the cell. The apical portion of the cell contains the Golgi apparatus, and numerous zymogen granules which contain the pancreatic enzymes or enzyme precursors. The apical region therefore stains with acid dyes such as eosin. Microvilli extend from the apical surface of the acinar cell into the lumen. The apical poles of neighbouring cells are joined by tight junctions, known as zonulae adherens. These junctions separate the fluid in the lumen of the acinus from the fluid in the intercellular spaces that bathes the basolateral surfaces of the cells. The tight junctions are impermeable to macromolecules, such as digestive enzymes, in the luminal fluid, but permit the exchange of water and ions between the interstitial spaces and the lumen of the acinus. Disruption of these junctions may be an aetiological factor in the development of chronic pancreatitis (see Case history 5, page 80). Gap junctions between neighbouring cells allow rapid changes in membrane potential to be transmitted between the cells. They also permit the exchange of low molecular weight molecules (less than 1400 kDa mass) between cells.

The intercalated duct begins within the acinus. This is a unique feature of secretory glands. The duct cells within the acinus are known as centroacinar cells (Fig. 5.4). These stain lightly with eosin. They are squamous cells with a centrally placed nucleus. These cells are continuous with those of the short intercalated duct that lies outside the acinus and drains it. The intercalated ducts are lined by flattened squamous epithelial cells. The neighbouring duct cells are joined by tight junctions as in the acinus. These separate the duct lumen from the intercellular spaces and function to exclude large molecules from the spaces. They also have gap junctions which permit the transmission of membrane electrical changes between the cells. These ducts lead into the intralobular ducts which are lined with cuboidal or low columnar epithelium. Larger ducts contain interlobular connective tissue cells and APUD cells.

Pancreatic juice

Composition of pancreatic juice

The pancreatic juice entering the duodenum is a mixture of two types of secretion, an enzyme-rich secretion and an aqueous alkaline secretion. If the ducts are ligated near the acini, which results in acinar cells degeneration, the secretion of the alkaline component of the juice is largely unaltered, but the secretion of enzymes is markedly reduced. This indicates that the enzymes are secreted by the acinar cells, and the alkaline fluid by the duct cells. The alkaline secretion originates largely from the centroacinar cells and the duct cells of the intralobular and small interlobular ducts. These relationships are illustrated in Figure 5.4.

Alkaline secretion

Composition

The cells of the upper ducts secrete an isotonic juice which is rich in bicarbonate but contains only traces of enzymes. There is a continuous resting secretion of this juice, but it can be stimulated up to 14-fold during a meal. It contains Na^+, K^+, HCO_3^-, Mg^{2+}, Ca^{2+}, Cl^- and other ions, present in concentrations similar to those of plasma. It therefore resembles an ultrafiltrate of plasma. It is alkaline by virtue of its high HCO_3^- content.

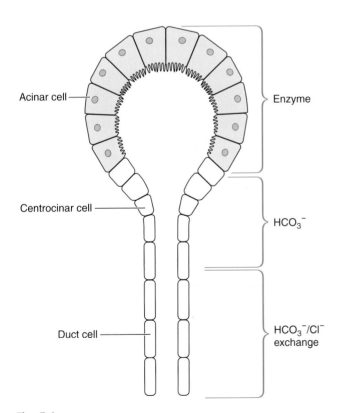

Fig. 5.4
Secretory unit showing the cellular locations of the different secretions.

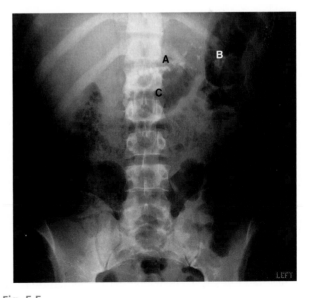

Fig. 5.5
Plain abdominal X-ray showing calcified stones in the pancreatic duct (A), from a patient with chronic pancreatitis secondary to alcoholism. Gas in the left colon (B) and overlying stomach (C) are also seen.

Chronic pancreatitis Box 2

Defect and causes

Now we can ask what the primary defect in chronic pancreatitis might be and how the use of x-rays can reveal it. We can also ask what is the likely cause of the condition in this patient.

The primary malfunction in chronic pancreatitis is probably defective ductal secretion of bicarbonate and water which results in a high protein concentration in the pancreatic juice in the ducts. This results in the precipitation of protein, and the formation of protein plugs, and consequently dilatation of the proximal ducts. The effect of blockage of the ducts is the generation of a high pressure in the ducts which causes pain. Secondary back pressure may lead to disruption of the integrity of the ductal epithelium and result in destruction of the pancreatic tissue. This can lead to an inflammatory and fibrotic process in and around the pancreatic tissue. This in time leads to pancreatic insufficiency. Fibrosis around the autonomic nerves which surround the pancreas may result in back pain, which is a common feature of this condition.

Chronic pancreatitis is characterised by progressive functional damage to the pancreas, with or without evidence of inflammation. There is permanent destruction of pancreatic tissue, and exocrine and endocrine pancreatic insufficiency usually follows. However, owing to the tremendous reserve of pancreatic tissue, the insufficiency may be subclinical and tests of pancreatic function may be necessary to reveal it. The histopathology indicates irregularly distributed fibrosis, reduced number and size of islets of Langerhans, and variable obstruction of pancreatic ducts of all sizes. Protein precipitation initially occurs in the lobular and interlobular ducts, leading to the formation of plugs that calcify by surface accretion. Concentric lamellar protein precipitates appear in the major pancreatic ducts and these subsequently also calcify to form stones. A specific protein, called stone protein, a normal constituent of pancreatic juice, which has a high affinity for Ca^{2+}, appears to be the major protein present in pancreatic stones. The calculi contain calcium bicarbonate or hydroxyapatite (calcium phosphate and calcium bicarbonate). The stones can be seen in x-radiographs (see Fig. 5.5) Foci of acinar ectasia are present, and acinar atrophy, chronic inflammation, and fibrosis, in areas of ductal obstruction. These, together with stricture formation due to periductal fibrosis eventually lead to ductal eclesia. The chronic inflammation may extend to adjacent organs, causing constriction of the duodenum, stomach antrum, common bile duct, or transverse colon. Central epigastric pain is a common feature of chronic pancreatitis and is due to referred pain from the embryological foregut. Fibrosis and inflammation around the pancreas may involve the coeliac plexus of autonomic nerves resulting from the chronic pain that may accompany this condition.

In 90 per cent of patients with chronic pancreatitis there is a history of excessive alcohol intake. However the incidence of the disease is low, being approximately 30 per 100 000 in the United Kingdom. Onset is usually in middle age. The disease is approximately three times more common in males than females. Affected patients are presumably susceptible to pancreatic damage by alcohol, although the genetic mechanism is poorly understood. Rare autosomal dominant inherited forms of the disease have been described. Most alcoholic patients already have sustained permanent structural and functional damage to the pancreas by the time of their first attack of abdominal pain. Moreover the morphological changes seen in chronic pancreatitis are evident at post mortem examination in many alcoholics who had no symptoms of pancreatic disease during life. Asymptomatic alcoholics often exhibit abnormal exocrine function when subjected to the secretin test.

It is not precisely known how alcohol causes chronic pancreatitis. It may promote pancreatic duct obstruction through causing precipitation of proteins that are secreted by the pancreatic tissue.

Functions

The pancreatic juice arriving in the duodenum is mixed with the chyme by contractions of the smooth muscle of the small intestine. The function of the alkaline pancreatic secretion, together with the other alkaline secretions (bile and intestinal juices) that act in the small intestine, is to neutralise the acid chyme arriving from the stomach. This is important for several reasons: i) the pancreatic enzymes require a neutral or slightly alkaline pH for their activity, ii) the absorption of fat depends on the formation in the intestinal lumen of micelles, a process which only takes place at neutral or slightly alkaline pH values, iii) it protects the intestinal mucosa because excess acid in the duodenum can damage the mucosa and lead to the formation of ulcers.

Cellular mechanism of secretion

The mechanisms involved in the production of intracellular HCO_3^- in the centroacinar and upper duct cells are illustrated in Figure 5.6. The initial intracellular step involves the reaction of CO_2 and water. Secreted H^+ ions react with HCO_3^- ions in the blood perfusing the gland and this generates CO_2, some of which diffuses into the duct cell. More than 90% of the HCO_3^- in pancreatic juice is derived from blood CO_2. In the cell the CO_2 combines with intracellular water to generate carbonic acid, in a reaction which is catalysed by carbonic anhydrase II, an enzyme present in the centroacinar and upper duct cells. The carbonic acid dissociates to give HCO_3^- and H^+. Whilst bicarbonate is being secreted the partial pressure of CO_2 (pCO_2) in the cells is lower than in the blood as it is being used up in the production of HCO_3^- ions, and the higher the rate of secretion the greater the downhill gradient for diffusion of CO_2 into the cell. The HCO_3^- ions are

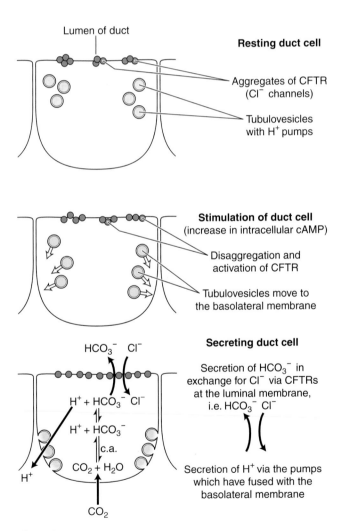

Lumen of duct

Resting duct cell

Aggregates of CFTR (Cl^- channels)

Tubulovesicles with H^+ pumps

Stimulation of duct cell (increase in intracellular cAMP)

Disaggregation and activation of CFTR

Tubulovesicles move to the basolateral membrane

Secreting duct cell

HCO_3^- Cl^-

$H^+ + HCO_3^-$ Cl^-

$H^+ + HCO_3^-$

c.a.

$CO_2 + H_2O$

H^+

CO_2

Secretion of HCO_3^- in exchange for Cl^- via CFTRs at the luminal membrane, i.e. HCO_3^- Cl^-

Secretion of H^+ via the pumps which have fused with the basolateral membrane

Fig. 5.6
Cellular mechanisms involved in the production of HCO_3^- and H^+ in a duct cell. c.a., Carbonic anhydrase. Based on a diagram from 'Gastroenterology', Raeder M. G., London: WB Saunders, 1992.

secreted from the luminal membrane by Cl^- / HCO_3^- exchange, and the H^+ ions are secreted into the blood. Thus for every HCO_3^- ion that is secreted into the duct lumen one H^+ ion is secreted into the blood. Therefore the blood flowing through the pancreas becomes transiently acid when it is secreting HCO_3^-. The H^+ ions in the blood help to neutralise the 'alkaline tide' produced during a meal by the secreting stomach (see Chapter 3), by combining with plasma HCO_3^- to produce CO_2. In post-surgical conditions where the patient has been provided with a draining pancreatic fistula, the pancreatic juice drains to the outside and the patient incurs considerable losses of HCO_3^-. A pancreatic fistula that is in direct communication from the main pancreatic duct to the skin does not contain significant quantities of activated enzymes. However if the fistula communicates from the duodenum to the skin then the digestive enzymes are active and can cause a significant amount of skin excoriation and damage. This will result in considerable management problems until the fistula closes. Loss of HCO_3^- results in a metabolic acidosis. This is usually compensated for by renal and respiratory mechanisms. Fluid and electrolyte losses, however, can be more difficult to manage because the patient may have a restricted oral intake. Replacement via intravenous infusion is necessary.

The exchange mechanism in the centroacinar and upper duct cells, whereby HCO_3^- is secreted in exchange for Cl^-, obviously depends on the presence of Cl^- in the fluid in the lumen. Cl^- ion flux out of the cell into the lumen is via a chloride conductance channel known as the cystic fibrosis transmembrane conductance regulator (CFTR) which is regulated by cyclic AMP. Immunocytochemical studies using fluorescent antibodies against the CFTR have shown that it is localised to the apical region of centroacinar and intralobular duct cells. The CFTR is coupled to the HCO_3^-/Cl^- exchanger. Failure of this secretory mechanism is seen in cystic fibrosis (see below). It results in a high concentration of protein in the pancreatic ducts which can block the lumen. This results in secondary pancreatic damage; a process similar to that which occurs in chronic pancreatitis.

The Cl^- channel is present in clusters in the apical plasma membranes. When the gland is stimulated (by secretin or by an increase in cAMP), the channel clusters disaggregate (see Fig. 5.6) increasing the number of open channels. The channel is regulated in two ways: i) via phosphorylation and dephosphorylation by protein kinase A and a phosphatase respectively, which serves as a molecular switch involved in the gating of the channel, and ii) via activation of the channel by hydrolysis of ATP and other nucleotides.

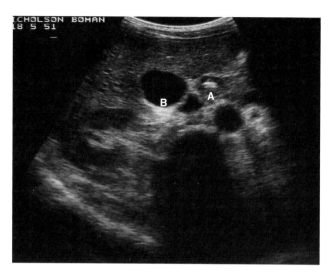

Fig. 5.10
Ultrasound scan of the bilary tree, showing a calcified stone in the common bile duct (A) which is dilated around the stone. The adjacent gallbladder is also seen (B).

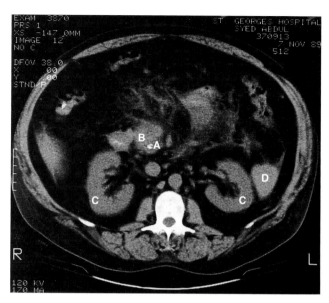

Fig. 5.11
CT scan of the same patient as Fig. 5.10, showing the calcified stone at the lower end of the common bile duct (A) lying within a swollen head of the pancreas (B). The kidneys (C) and spleen (D) are also visible.

vary with respect to its enzyme protein content. It can contain between 1% and 10% protein.

CCK and gastrin compete for the same receptor on the acinar cell. CCK, gastrin and acetylcholine all increase enzyme protein synthesis and secretion via i) increase in phosphatidylinositol turnover and ii) increase in intracellular Ca^{2+} concentration (Fig. 5.12). Secretin and VIP act on the acinar cell to increase the intracellular levels of cAMP. This increase in cAMP by secretin and VIP potentiates the effect of CCK, gastrin and acetylcholine. Thus the enzyme secretion is greater when the two types of secretogogue are acting together.

Somatostatin

Somatostatin, which is present in D cells in the islets of Langerhans of the pancreas, is a powerful inhibitor of pancreatic secretion. It acts in a paracrine manner to inhibit the release of the exocrine alkaline and enzyme secretions, as well as the pancreatic hormones insulin and glucagon. In addition it inhibits the release of a number of gastrointestinal hormones, including CCK, secretin, and gastrin. Circulating somatostatin probably augments the actions of the locally released hormone. It originates from a number of sites in the body, including various locations in the gastrointestinal tract. Pancreatic somatostatin is predominantly the teradecapeptide form, S-14. The release of this hormone is stimulated by CCK, gastrin and secretin.

Analogues of somatostatin such as octreotide are used clinically to inhibit pancreatic enzyme secretion in acute pancreatitis, and following pancreatic surgery.

Octreotide is an octapeptide which contains the tetrapeptide sequence which is known to be essential for somatostatin activity. Somatostatin itself, when injected, has a short half life (less than 4 minutes). However, octreotide injected subcutaneously, has a half life of approximately 100 minutes and its action is therefore relatively long-lasting. This is important in the clinical setting as somatostatin is only effective if given as a continuous infusion, whereas analogues such as octreotide are effective if given as a bolus two or three times per day.

Nervous control

The nervous control of pancreatic secretion is via both parasympathetic and sympathetic nerves. Stimulation of cholinergic fibres in the vagus nerve enhances the rate of secretion of both enzyme and alkaline fluid. Stimulation of the sympathetic nerves inhibits secretion, mainly by reducing the blood flow to the gland (via vasoconstriction of the arterioles) which decreases the volume of juice secreted. However, stimulation of the sympathetic nerves to the pancreas depresses the enzyme content of the secretion as well as the volume of juice secreted.

Control of secretion during a meal

The control of the secretion of pancreatic juice during a meal depends on the volume and composition of the food. Ingested material present at different locations

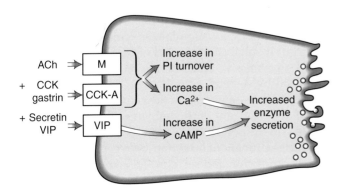

Fig. 5.12
Cellular mechanisms of control in the acinar cell. M, muscarinic receptor; PL, phosphatidylinositol.

within the gastrointestinal tract affects the control of the secretions in different ways. The control during a meal can accordingly be divided into three phases (see Chapter 1) according to the location of the food or chyme; i) the cephalic phase, due to the approach of food or the presence of food in the mouth, ii) the gastric phase, when food is in the stomach, and iii) the intestinal phase when food material is in the duodenum.

Cephalic phase
The sight and smell of food, or other sensory stimuli associated with the impending arrival of food, elicit increased pancreatic secretion via a 'conditioned' reflex. The presence of food in the mouth stimulates secretion via a 'non-conditioned' reflex. The control during this phase is therefore nervous. It is mediated by impulses in cholinergic fibres in the vagus nerve. The juice secreted is mainly the enzyme-rich secretion, containing very little HCO_3^-.

In response to vagal stimulation, the acinar cells also secrete kallikreins, which catalyse the production of bradykinin, a vasodilator. This results in increased blood flow to the pancreas, and increased volume of secretion. The mechanism involved in this effect is similar to that which occurs in the control of salivary secretion which is described in Chapter 2.

Gastric phase
The presence of food in the stomach stimulates the secretion of pancreatic juice via a hormonal mechanism. Activation of chemoreceptors in the walls of the stomach by peptides, and the activation of mechanoreceptors, causes the release of the hormone gastrin from G cells, into the local circulation. Stimulation of cholinergic nerves is also involved in this phase of control. During the gastric phase the secretion of both the enzyme-rich and the alkaline components of pancreatic juice is increased.

Intestinal phase
The intestinal phase of control is probably the most important phase of the response to food. Food material in the duodenum stimulates both the alkaline and the enzyme-rich components of pancreatic juice. The alkaline component of pancreatic juice is secreted in response mainly to acid in the duodenal contents. Acid stimulates the release of secretin from APUD cells in the walls of the intestine and this hormone stimulates the duct cells to secrete the alkaline fluid. This is a feedback control mechanism which helps to control the pH of the duodenal contents.

Chronic pancreatitis Box 4

Physiological consequences, treatment and management

The main consequences of malabsorption and diabetes mellitus are malnutrition and weight loss. Lack of alkaline secretion can lead to alkalosis because the alkaline tide in the blood which results from gastric acid secretion (see Chapter 3) is normally partially neutralised by an 'acid' tide which results from the secretion of alkaline juice. However, in chronic pancreatitis, the alkalosis is normally compensated by respiratory and renal mechanisms.

Complications of chronic pancreatitis include pancreatic necrosis, haemorrhage, acute pseudocysts, and pancreatic abcesses. Treatment is usually non-surgical in uncomplicated chronic pancreatitis. The need for complete abstention from alcohol is emphasised. Pain relief is initially via aspirin treatment, and then, if necessary, via opiates. Nutritional support in the form of simple nutrients (amino acids, glucose, fatty acids) may be advised. Oral pancreatic extract can be prescribed to replace the pancreatic enzymes. Usually the extract is enriched with lipase as the secretion of this enzyme tends to decrease more rapidly than that of proteolytic enzymes. The enzyme preparation can be administered together with antacids or the anti-ulcer drug cimetidine to reduce the acid production by the stomach as this inactivates the enzymes. Alternatively the pancreatic enzyme preparation can be administered in the form of granules within which the enzymes are enclosed in a pH-dependent polymer. The protective coating dissolves only when the pH is more alkaline than 6.0, i.e. not in the stomach but hopefully in the duodenum or upper jejunum.

The metabolic complications of diabetes are discussed in Chapter 9. If diabetes is present it is treated with insulin.

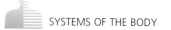

PANCREAS: EXOCRINE FUNCTIONS

5

The enzyme-rich juice is released during the intestinal phase in response to fat and peptides in the food. The fats and peptides cause the release of CCK from the walls of the duodenum into the blood. CCK stimulates the acinar cells to secrete enzymes. Trypsin in the duodenum inhibits the release of enzymes via inhibition of CCK release. This is another feedback control mechanism, which limits the quantity of enzymes present in the intestines, and may have some protective function.

Secretin exerts a permissive effect on the secretion of enzymes; it does not stimulate enzyme secretion on its own, but it enhances the effect of CCK. Likewise CCK exerts a permissive effect on the secretion of the alkaline fluid by secretin. Stimulation of the vagus nerve causes the release of mainly the enzyme-rich secretion, but if the vagi are sectioned, the alkaline secretion elicited in response to secretin is reduced by 50%, indicting a functional overlap between the effects of vagal stimulation and secretin. Thus the vagal mechanism may enhance the effect of secretin.

Self-assessment case study: cystic fibrosis

A twelve-year-boy who was suffering from cystic fibrosis was taken to the outpatient clinic for his regular checkup. His condition had been diagnosed soon after birth and he had both pancreatic and respiratory tract involvement. He had been asked to bring a sample of his stool. This was pale-coloured, poorly formed, and oily in appearance. It was sent to the laboratory for analysis to assess his pancreatic function. His exocrine pancreatic insufficiency was being treated with a pancreatic enzyme preparation and the anti-ulcer drug cimetidine.

After studying this chapter you should be able to suggest the answers to the following questions:

① What is the inherited defect in this condition?

② How is the defect manifest in the pancreas? What abnormalities of pancreatic function result from this pathology?

③ Why is the child being treated with an enzyme preparation? What are the problems with having to give such a preparation by mouth. Why is the boy being treated with cimetidine? Would you expect enteric coated preparations to be more effective than a powder? Would you expect bicarbonate by mouth to be helpful? Would you expect any abnormalities in the acid bases status of this patient?

④ Why was the boy's stool pale-coloured? What tests would be performed on the sample?

Self-assessment questions

① What exocrine cell types are present in the pancreas? What is the composition of each type of juice secreted?

② Can you describe the cellular mechanisms involved in the secretion of alkaline pancreatic juice? How is the CFTR involved in this process?

③ Can you describe the cellular mechanisms of secretion of pancreatic enzymes? What part of this process is under physiological regulation by hormones?

④ How is the secretion of each component of pancreatic juice controlled by food in a) the mouth, b) the stomach, c) the duodenum?

LIVER AND BILIARY SYSTEM

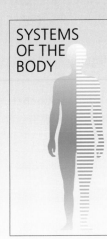

SYSTEMS
OF THE
BODY

Chapter objectives

By studying this chapter you should be able to understand:

① The role of the liver in (a) the digestive process and (b) the excretion of waste metabolites and toxic substances.

② The relationship between the structure of the hepatobiliary tract and its function in the secretion and storage of bile.

③ The mechanisms of secretion of the important components of bile, and their recycling via the enterohepatic circulation.

④ The mechanisms of control of bile secretion and its release into the duodenum.

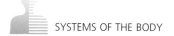
Introduction

The numerous functions of the liver can be divided into two broad categories: one is concerned with the processing of absorbed materials and synthetic reactions, and the other with secretion and excretion. The processing of absorbed nutrients and the role of the liver in the control of energy metabolism are discussed in Chapter 9. This chapter is concerned with the secretory and excretory roles of the liver.

The most important exocrine functions of the liver are:

1. the provision of bile acids and alkaline fluid for the digestion and absorption of fats, and for neutralisation of gastric acid in the intestines
2. the degradation and conjugation of waste products of metabolism
3. the detoxification of poisonous substances
4. the excretion of waste metabolites and detoxified substances in bile.

Detoxified substances and waste metabolites are eliminated from the body either in the bile, via the gastrointestinal tract, or via secretion from the liver into the blood for subsequent excretion by the kidneys. The liver has enormous reserves of function, and normal homeostasis can be maintained even after three-quarters of it have been removed. Clinical manifestation of liver disease therefore implies considerable damage to the organ.

Gallstones form in the gallbladder and biliary tract as a consequence of various derangements of the hepatobiliary system. The problems encountered in gallstone disease are used in this chapter to illustrate many of the roles of the liver in secretion and excretion.

Functioning of the hepatobiliary system

The anatomical arrangement of the liver, gallbladder, and biliary tract is shown in Figure 6.1. The liver is continually secreting substances both into the blood and into the bile. Bile is both a secretory fluid and an excretory medium. In the human it is stored between meals in the gallbladder, where it is concentrated. During a meal it is released from the gallbladder and enters into the cystic duct, which in turn drains into the common bile duct. The bile enters the small intestine at the level of the duodenum. The entry of bile into the duodenum is controlled by a smooth muscle sphincter, the sphincter of Oddi.

The gallbladder is surrounded by smooth muscle. Between meals, when the gallbladder smooth muscle is relaxed, the sphincter of Oddi is closed, preventing

---

Gallstones Box 1

Gallstone disease

An obese middle-aged woman explained to her general practitioner that she had suffered several attacks of severe 'gripping' pain in the upper abdomen, although there were no abnormal physical signs at the time she was seen by the doctor. Upon questioning, she said that the attacks had started after meals. The pain built up gradually to a maximum and lasted for several hours. Her description of the location of the pain indicated that it was epigastric, in the right upper quadrant of the abdomen. She also said that during a recent severe attack a friend had remarked that the 'whites' of the patient's eyes (the sclera) had appeared yellow. In addition, the patient had noticed that her urine became dark in colour, and her stools were pale and greasy-looking and tended to float in the lavatory pan. The doctor suspected that the patient was suffering from gallstones. This was subsequently confirmed by an ultrasound scan, and the patient was referred to a surgeon for a cholecystectomy (surgical removal of the gallbladder).

Examination of the details of this case provokes the following questions:

① What would an ultrasound scan show in gallstone disease? How could the findings explain the cause of the patient's pain?

② How can we explain the abnormal appearance of the patient's stools? What abnormalities of the digestive process does it indicate?

③ How can we explain the yellowing of the sclera (a symptom of jaundice)?

④ Why is the gallbladder important for the digestive process? How would the composition of the bile which enters the duodenum differ from normal after cholecystectomy? Would cholecystectomy have deleterious consequences for the normal functioning of the body?

⑤ What is the composition of gallstones? What causes them to form?

⑥ Can gallstones be treated by oral administration of bile acids? What type of gallstone might be amenable to this treatment?

These issues will be addressed in this chapter.

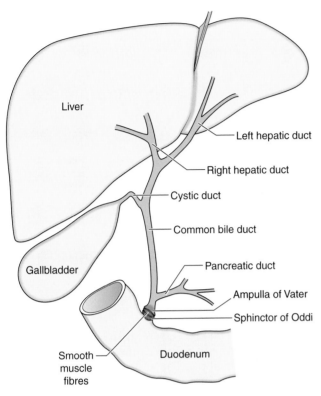

Fig. 6.1
Anatomical arrangement of the liver, gallbladder, and biliary tract.

portal triad) contains a bile duct, a branch of the portal vein, and a branch of the hepatic artery.

The liver has a double blood supply: the hepatic artery supplies the liver with oxygenated blood from the lungs, and the portal vein supplies it with nutrient-rich blood from the intestines (see Chapter 1). The arterial blood comprises approximately 20% of the total blood supply of the liver and the portal venous blood, approximately 80%. The arterial blood and the portal venous blood mix together in the liver sinusoids. The sinusoidal blood drains away via the hepatic veins to the vena cava. This direction of flow is determined by the relatively higher pressure of the blood in the portal vein compared to the central vein.

The liver is covered by a fibroconnective tissue capsule, the capsule of Glisson, from which thin connective tissue septa enter the organ to divide it into lobes and lobules. The capsule is covered by peritoneum, except in an area known as the 'bare area', which is in direct contact with the diaphragm.

The secretory system of the liver begins with minute tubules, the canaliculi. These are formed by oppositely aligned grooves in the contact surfaces of adjacent hepatocytes (Fig. 6.3). The membrane of each liver cell contributes to several bile canaliculi. Bile secreted into the canaliculi flows in the opposite direction to the flow of blood in the sinusoids. The canaliculi drain into terminal bile ductules. The ductules converge to form intralobular ducts, and these converge to form interlobular ducts, which in turn converge to form the right and left hepatic bile ducts. These converge outside the liver to form the common hepatic bile duct.

the bile from entering the small intestine. Consequently the bile passes into the gallbladder, where it is stored and concentrated. Contraction of the gallbladder forces the bile into the common bile duct. At the same time the smooth muscle in the sphincter of Oddi relaxes, and the sphincter opens to allow the bile to enter the duodenum. Food in the duodenum is the main stimulus for gallbladder contraction.

Anatomy and morphology of the liver

The liver is the largest single organ in the body. In the adult it comprises approximately one-fiftieth of the body weight. In the infant it is proportionately even larger. It consists of right and left lobes (Fig. 6.2A), the right lobe being six times the size of the left in the adult.

The liver is composed of lobules (Fig. 6.2B). In the centre of each lobule is the central canal, in which lies a central vein, which is a tributary of the inferior vena cava. Columns of liver cells (hepatocytes) and sinusoids radiate out from the central canal. Several portal tracts lie at the periphery of each lobule. Each tract (or

Histology

The major type of cell in the liver is the hepatocyte, which is an epithelial parenchymal cell. The hepatocytes are arranged in plates that branch and anastomise to form a three-dimensional lattice (Fig. 6.2B). Between the plates are the blood-filled sinusoids. In this respect the liver resembles an endocrine gland. There is usually only one layer of hepatocytes between sinusoids.

The sinusoidal spaces differ from blood capillaries in that they are of greater diameter and their lining cells are not typically endothelial. The basal lamina around the sinusoids is incomplete and this enables direct access of the plasma to the surface of the hepatocyte. This allows active metabolic exchange between the blood and the cells (Fig. 6.2C). The perisinusoidal space is an interstitial space containing reticular and collagenous fibres. A few mesenchymal cells, called lipocytes, produce the fibres. Two main cell types are present in the sinusoidal lining. These are

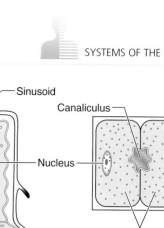
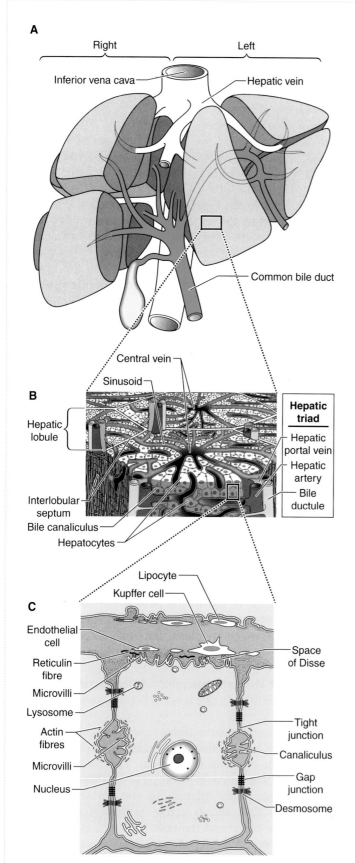

A

Right | Left

Inferior vena cava — Hepatic vein

Common bile duct

B

Central vein
Sinusoid

Hepatic lobule

Hepatic triad
- Hepatic portal vein
- Hepatic artery
- Bile ductule

Interlobular septum
Bile canaliculus
Hepatocytes

C

Lipocyte
Kupffer cell

Endothelial cell
Reticulin fibre
Microvilli
Lysosome
Actin fibres
Microvilli
Nucleus

Space of Disse
Tight junction
Canaliculus
Gap junction
Desmosome

Hepatocyte — Sinusoid
Canaliculus
Nucleus
Hepatocytes
Canaliculus

Fig. 6.3
Early secretory system of the liver. Inset: canaliculus (in cross-section) formed by adjacent hepatocytes.

endothelial cells and Kupffer cells. They lie in a mesh of fine reticular fibres. The endothelial cell has small, elongated nuclei and greatly attenuated cytoplasm. The cytoplasm may interdigitate with cytoplasmic processes from adjacent cells of the same type or another type. They contain few organelles but numerous pinocytotic vesicles. They also contain large fenestrae, which are not closed by a diaphragm. Kupffer cells are phagocytic and often contain degenerating red cells, pigment granules, and iron-containing granules. They have large nuclei and extensive cytoplasm, with processes that extend into, and sometimes across, the sinusoidal space. They increase in number when required for phagocytosis, possibly via differentiation of the endothelial type of cell.

Hepatocytes

The hepatocyte is a polygonal cell with a clearly defined cell membrane, which is closely apposed to the cell membranes of adjacent hepatocytes (Figs 6.2C, 6.3). The membranes of adjacent cells are partially separated to form a bile canaliculus. The plasmalemma of adjacent hepatocytes shows irregularities with tight junctions, spot desmosomes and gap junctions. These

Fig. 6.2
(A) The biliary drainage of the two lobes of the liver. (B) Lobular structure of the liver, illustrating the biliary secretory system and the dual blood supply. (C) Features of the hepatocyte, and its relationship to adjacent cells and the sinusoid.

Gallstones Box 2

Detection and cause of pain

Gallstones (biliary calculi) are hard masses that can be present in the gallbladder or the bile ducts. They are composed largely either of cholesterol or bile pigment. Both types of gallstone may be calcified, although calcification is more frequent in pigment gallstones where calcium bilirubinate is usually a major component. The calcification may be in either a central core or a peripheral 'shell'. Cholesterol stones tend to be large (often in excess of 1 cm in diameter), and several may be present in one individual. The attacks of pain (biliary colic) experienced following meals are due to transient obstruction of the cystic duct when the gallbladder contracts. The pain is due to the pressure of the bile behind the stone. However, most individuals with gallstones are asymptomatic, and require no treatment.

Gallstones that are sufficiently calcified (less than 20% of all gallstones) can be detected by plain abdominal radiography. These may be cholesterol stones that have a calcified shell, or pigment stones composed mainly of calcium bilirubinate. Pure cholesterol stones are radiolucent and cannot be detected using this technique.

Historically, gallstones were detected by oral cholecystography. This involves ingestion of a radio-opaque substance such as an iodinated phthalate, which is absorbed into the blood and secreted into the bile. The substance is concentrated in the gallbladder, and this enables the gallbladder to be visualised by radiography as an opaque mass. Gallstones can then be seen as translucent bodies within it. The gallbladder was then stimulated to contract by intravenous injection of cholecystokinin (CCK) (see below) and further radiographic films were taken. Contraction may cause calculi that were not visible in the filled gallbladder to be seen. The technique was obviously not appropriate for detecting stones in the gallbladder if the cystic duct was blocked as the secreted opaque substance does not enter the gallbladder. The technique is further limited by variable absorption and secretion, making it too unreliable to be used as the examination of first choice. A simpler and more rapid technique employing ultrasonography is now used to reveal gallstones, providing an overall gallstone detection rate of over 90% (Fig. 6.4). It also evaluates the thickness of the gallbladder wall; an abnormally thick wall indicates a diseased gallbladder, usually secondary to chronic inflammation, but occasionally due to a carcinoma of the gallbladder.

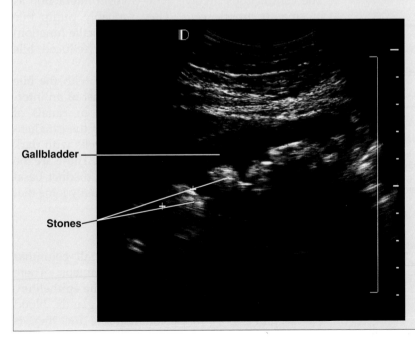

Fig. 6.4
An ultrasound scan showing a distended gallbladder and radio-opaque stones within the lumen.

separate the canaliculus from the rest of the intercellular space (Fig. 6.2C).

The plasma membrane of hepatocytes is specialised in certain regions. Adjacent to a sinusoidal blood space the hepatocyte is separated from the wall of the sinusoid by the perisinusoidal space (the space of Disse) and at this location the plasma membrane of the hepatocyte has numerous long microvilli. Vesicles and

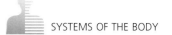
vacuoles are present in the subadjacent cytoplasm. The microvilli provide a large surface area for absorption and secretion.

The nuclei in different hepatocytes show considerable variation in shape and size, and in some cases the cells are binucleate. Clumps of basophilic material are present in all cells. There are numerous small mitochondria throughout the cytoplasm of the hepatocyte. The structure of all hepatocytes is broadly similar but the cytoplasm of the cells shows a gradual variation with the distance of the cell from the periphery. The differences are related to the differences in functional activity of the peripherally and centrally positioned cells. The hepatocytes closest to the afferent blood supply, the 'periportal' cells, are exposed to the highest concentrations of nutrients and oxygen, and those in the central region, the 'perivenous' cells, near to the efferent outflow, are exposed to the lowest concentrations. The periportal cells are the most active in the uptake from the blood of bile salts and in the secretion of bile into the canaliculi as well as in oxidative metabolism and gluconeogenesis (Fig. 6.5). After feeding, glycogen is deposited first in the periportal cells. It is only after a heavy carbohydrate meal that the more centrally located perivenous cells store glycogen. Moreover when the blood sugar concentration falls, glycogen is removed first from the perivenous cells. The perivenous cells, which are exposed to depleted plasma, are the more active in biotransformation reactions and the secretion of potentially toxic xenobiotic and endobiotic substances. They are also more active in glycolytic and ketogenic reactions. Under certain conditions fat is deposited in the hepatocytes and it appears first in the more centrally disposed cells. Thus the cytosol of a given hepatocyte exhibits differences in composition at different times in relation to feeding and whether fat or glycogen has been deposited.

The canaliculus

The lumen of the canaliculus is approximately $0.75\,\mu m$ in diameter. Microvilli project from the canalicular membrane into the lumen, providing a large surface area for secretion. Membranes of adjacent hepatocytes are joined by tight junctions near to the canaliculus (Fig. 6.2C). These junctions are leaky and permit paracellular exchange between the plasma and the canaliculus.

The canaliculus is involved in transport of substances into the lumen, but it is also a contractile structure. Actin filaments are present in the microvilli, and both actin and myosin fibres are present in the cytoplasm surrounding the canaliculus. Contractions of the canaliculi can be stimulated by extracellular ATP. The contractions involve actin–myosin interaction as in smooth muscle cells. They probably pump bile towards the ducts. Atony (lack of contractile function) of the canaliculus causes cholestasis (reduced bile flow).

The junctions of the bile canaliculus with the bile ducts at the periphery of a lobule consist of an intermediate structure called the ductules or canals of Hering. Here the hepatocytes that form the canaliculus are gradually replaced by smaller cells with dark nuclei and poorly developed organelles. These are the ductule cells. They are underlain by a distinct basal lamina. The lumen of the ductule eventually joins that of a bile duct in the portal area.

Extrahepatic ducts

The extrahepatic ducts are lined by tall columnar epithelium (Fig. 6.6) that secretes mucus. There is a layer of connective tissue beneath the epithelium, with numerous elastic fibres, mucous glands, blood vessels, and nerves. In the common bile duct there is also a layer of smooth muscle cells. These cells are sparse in the upper region of the duct but form a thicker layer of oblique and transverse fibres in the regions of the sphincter of Oddi near the duodenum (see below).

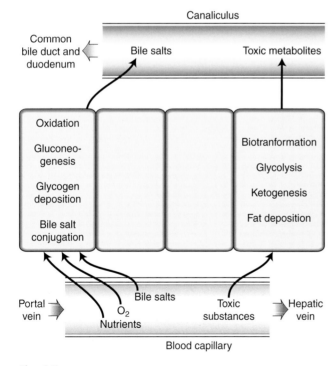

Fig. 6.5
The major functions of periportal and perivenous hepatocytes.

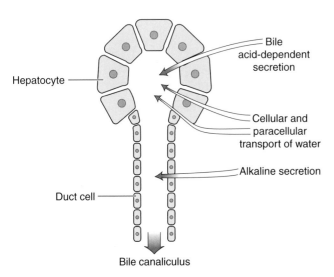

Fig. 6.6
Sites of secretion of the two component secretions of bile.

Table 6.1
Comparison of the concentrations of some substances in hepatic and gallbladder bile. Loss of gallbladder bile via a fistula can quickly deplete K^+ reserves, unless replacement therapy is started

Constituent	Hepatic bile (mM)	Gallbladder bile (mM)
Electrolytes		
HCO_3^-	28	10
Cl^-	100	25
K^+	5	12
Na^+	145	130
Ca^{2+}	5	23
Organic molecules		
Bilirubin	0.7	5.1
Cholesterol	2.6	16.0
Lecithin	0.5	3.9
Bile salts	26.0	145.0

Bile

Composition and functions

Bile is secreted at a rate of 250–1000 ml per day in the adult. It is isosmotic with blood plasma. Bile is a composite of two different secretions: one originating in the hepatocytes, and the other in the cells which line the bile ducts (Fig. 6.6). The two secretions mix together in the ducts.

Secretion of the duct cells

The secretion from the duct cells is a watery, alkaline fluid that is rich in bicarbonate. It comprises approximately 25% of the total bile volume. Its function is, first, to provide an appropriate pH for the process of micelle formation (see below), which requires a neutral or slightly alkaline environment. Second, it contributes (together with pancreatic juice and intestinal secretions) to the neutralisation of stomach acid in the intestinal chyme. This is important both for micelle formation and for digestive enzyme action, in the small intestine (see Chapter 7). In addition the neutralisation of acid in the duodenum protects the mucosa from ulceration. The secretion contains Na^+, K^+, Cl^-, and HCO_3^- ions. Its composition is similar to that of alkaline pancreatic juice. At basal rates of secretion the ionic composition resembles that of plasma. However, as the flow increases upon stimulation by a meal, the Cl^- concentration decreases and the HCO_3^- concentration increases. This is due to the presence of a Cl/HCO_3^- exchange mechanism in the duct cells. HCO_3^- ions are extracted from the bile and Cl^- is added to it, a process similar to that involved in the secretion of

alkaline juice from the pancreatic duct cells (see Chapter 5). At high flow rates the bile is not in contact with the duct cells for sufficient time to allow appreciable modification to take place and there is proportionately less bicarbonate extracted from it, resulting in a more alkaline bile. Thus the secretion becomes more alkaline at flow rates higher than the basal level.

The volume of the alkaline secretion, unlike the secretion produced by the hepatocytes, is not directly determined by the concentration of bile salts in the blood. It has been termed the 'bile acid-independent' component of bile. The control of this secretion during a meal, like that of alkaline pancreatic juice and the alkaline fluid secreted from Brunner's glands in the duodenum, is via the release of the hormone secretin into the blood, from the walls of the duodenum. This occurs mainly in response to the presence of acid in the duodenum (see Chapter 5). The hormone circulates in the blood to stimulate all of these glands. As it is released in response to acid chyme in the duodenum it provides a feedback control of the pH of the intestinal contents.

Secretion from the hepatocytes

The hepatocytes secrete a primary juice into the canaliculi. It contains a number of inorganic monovalent and divalent ions, and various organic substances (Table 6.1). The latter include lipids, bile acids, lecithin, and cholesterol, which are sequestered together in micelles. Bile secretion is a major route whereby cholesterol is lost from the body. The bile acids are essential for the effective digestion and absorption of dietary fats. There are also some proteins in bile, including albumin, polymeric immunoglobulin A (pIgA) which protects the biliary tract and the upper intestines from infection, and some plasma-derived enzymes. Bile also contains bile pigments, chiefly bilirubin, which are conjugated with glucuronic acid. The pigments are breakdown products of haemoglobin. Bile also contains numerous other compounds that are extracted from the blood, metabolised by the liver, and excreted. Many of these substances are potentially toxic endogenous or exogenous substances such as steroid hormones, drugs, and environmental toxins that are detoxified and conjugated by the liver. Conjugation serves to increase the polarity of a substance and therefore its solubility in water (see below). Bile remains isosmotic with plasma at different rates of flow. This implies that an increase in secretion of bile acids and metabolites by the liver results in an increase in bile volume. This is known as the choleretic effect.

Biliary lipids

The structures of the major lipids present in bile are shown in Figure 6.7. The bile acids are derivatives of cholesterol and contain the cyclopentanoperhydrophenanthrene nucleus. One, two or three alcohol groups are attached to this nucleus and there is a short hydrocarbon chain ending in a carboxyl group. Primary bile acids (cholic acid and chenodeoxycholic acid) are synthesised by the liver hepatocytes. Secondary bile acids (deoxycholic acid and lithocholic acid) are formed by dehydroxylation of primary bile acids in the intestines, by bacteria (Fig. 6.7). The bile acids are usually conjugated in the hepatocyte with amino acids, largely glycine or taurine. The ratio of glycocholates to taurocholates is normally approximately 3:1 but the exact proportions depend on the availability of the two amino acids. The conjugated primary and secondary bile acids are reabsorbed actively in the ileum (see Chapter 7). However, bile acids may be deconjugated by bacteria in the small intestine and colon. Some of the unconjugated bile acids are absorbed by passive diffusion. Bile acids synthesised de novo in the liver, and absorbed unconjugated bile acids, are conjugated in the liver. In physiological fluids, bile acids form salts with Na⁺ and K⁺ ions.

Uptake of bile salts from the blood into the hepatocyte is an active process that occurs against a concentration gradient (Fig. 6.8). It derives its energy from a Na⁺/K⁺-ATPase that pumps Na⁺ out of the cell and involves a Na⁺/bile salt cotransporter system located in the sinusoidal membrane. The process is driven by the electrochemical gradient for Na⁺ set up by the pumping out of Na⁺ ions. Another mechanism for bile acid transport, which involves a transporter with a wider specificity, has also been characterised. The dif-

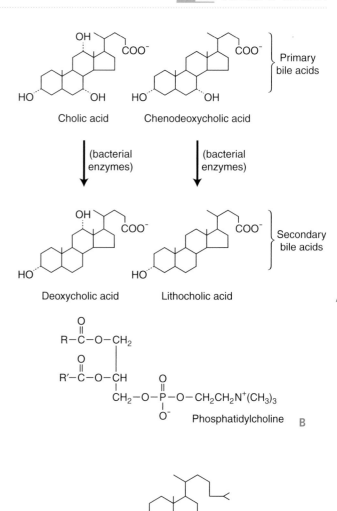

Fig. 6.7
(A) Structure of primary and secondary bile acids, and their modification by intestinal bacteria. (B) Structure of phosphatidylcholine (R = palmitic acid, R' = oleic or linoleic acid). (C) Structure of cholesterol.

ferent bile salts compete with each other indicating that they share the same transporter. Inside the hepatocyte the bile salts bind to protein, thereby keeping the intracellular concentration of free bile salts low. These proteins may be involved in transport of the bile acids through the cell.

Bile salts are secreted into the canaliculus against a considerable electrochemical gradient. The transport across the canalicular membrane is Na⁺-independent. The energy may be partly derived from the membrane potential, which is approximately 40 mV (negative inside the cell), but an ATPase-dependent pump that is specific for bile acids is

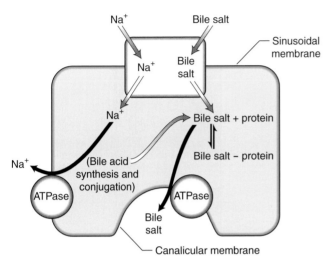

Fig. 6.8
Uptake and secretion of bile acid in the hepatocyte.

present in the canalicular membrane and this is the major mechanism for bile salt transport across this membrane (Fig. 6.8). It is distinct from the Na^+ gradient-driven bile acid uptake transporter in the sinusoidal membrane.

Bile acids are held in micelles in bile. They can be concentrated several-fold in gallbladder bile but they are still held in micellar form. Bile acids are powerful detergents, and their sequestration in micelles may reduce their detergent and cytotoxic actions.

The major phospholipid in bile is a phosphatidylcholine (lecithin) with a unique fatty acid pattern: palmitic acid forms the outer ester bond and either oleic acid or linoleic acid the inner ester bond (Fig. 6.7). The immediate source of this phospholipid is a preformed pool in the liver cell membranes. The cholesterol in bile is also mainly derived from a preformed pool but an appreciable proportion is derived via de novo synthesis in the liver. In the bile, cholesterol is not esterified to any significant extent (Fig. 6.7).

Inside the hepatocytes, the phospholipid and cholesterol probably exist as components of membranes of intracellular vesicles. The membranes of these vesicles are incorporated into the plasma membrane by fusing with it. The rate of secretion of phospholipid and cholesterol appears to be linearly related to the rate of bile salt secretion. Bile salts are secreted into the canaliculus first. The detergent action of these may be responsible for removing the other lipids from the canalicular membrane. The ratio of cholesterol to phospholipid is fairly constant (approximately 0.3 in the human). Some biliary phospholipid and cholesterol is present in bile in vesicles. These vesicles can incorporate bile salts and are gradually converted to micelles.

Micelle formation

Bile salts are essential for the formation of micelles in bile. The bile salt molecule is ampiphilic; the roughly planar ring system is hydrophobic and forms one side of the molecule. The alcohol groups, the carboxyl group, and the peptide bond of the bile acid all project from the other side, imparting a net negative charge, and therefore a hydrophilic nature to that side of the molecule (Fig. 6.9). A micelle has a hydrophilic shell region and a hydrophobic core region. Newly formed (primary) micelles are initially composed of bile salt molecules. The bile salts orientate themselves in the micelle with the hydrophobic side in the core and the hydrophilic side in the shell (Fig. 6.9). Primary micelles can sequester very little cholesterol. However, they take up phospholipid to form mixed micelles. Phosphatidylcholine is also an ampiphilic molecule; the long-chain fatty acyl chains forming the hydrophobic domain that resides in the core region of the micelle, and the phosphorylcholine group the hydrophilic domain that projects into the shell region (Fig. 6.9). The mixed micelle can hold more cholesterol than the primary micelle. In the presence of phosphatidylcholine, larger micelles tend to form than when it is absent. It is therefore known as a 'swelling' ampiphile. Cholesterol, which is extremely insoluble in water, resides in the core. As the net charge on all micelles is negative they repel each other, thereby preventing coalescence and inducing the formation of a stable suspension. The negatively charged micelle collects an outer shell of cations, mainly Na^+ ions. A micelle is disc-shaped, and its thickness approximates that of a lipid bilayer.

Two properties of bile salts determine the probability of their participation in micelle formation; the Krafft point and the critical micellar concentration. The Krafft point is the temperature below which micelles composed of the particular bile acid will not form. Most bile acids have Krafft points well below body temperature, although the secondary bile acid lithocholic acid has a high Krafft point and is incapable of forming micelles at body temperature. The critical micellar concentration is the minimum concentration of a particular acid required for micelle formation. The critical concentration is usually well below the concentration of bile acids present in bile, and micelles easily form. Micelle formation is also dependent on the phospholipid concentration, and on the ionic strength and pH of the medium; neutral or alkaline conditions are a prerequisite. The alkaline secretion from duct cells has an important role in this respect.

Micelle formation determines the volume of bile secreted. An individual micelle may be composed of 20 or so molecules of lipid but it constitutes only one

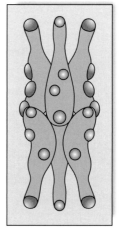

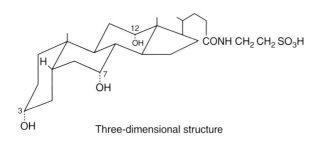

3ᵪ, 7ᵪ, 12ᵪ - Trihydroxy-5β-cholan - 24 oyl taurine
Chemical structure

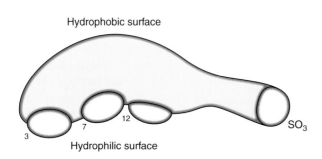

Three-dimensional structure

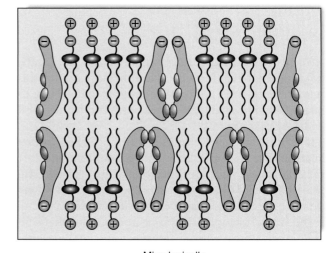

Primary micelle in water   B

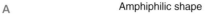

A   Amphiphilic shape

Mixed micelle   C

Fig. 6.9

(A) Electrical polarity of a conjugated bile acid. (B) Primary micelle, composed of bile salts, showing orientation of the ampiphilic lipid in the micelle. (C) Mixed micelle, containing bile acid and phospholipid, illustrating surface net negative charge and outer shell of cations (mainly Na^+ ions).

osmotic particle. Thus a simple chemical analysis of the composition of bile does not indicate its osmolarity. Bile is in osmotic equilibrium with blood plasma and any increase in its content of osmotic particles is followed by increased secretion of fluid (the choleretic effect). When biliary lipids are secreted into bile, however, micelle formation enables bile to be highly concentrated with respect to its lipid constituents without the enormous increase in volume that would accompany an equivalent secretion of water-soluble molecules.

Conjugation of metabolites and drugs

A number of other anions, in addition to bile acids, are present in bile. Their concentrations may be 10–1000 times that of their precursors in the plasma, indicating

that active transport mechanisms exist for the removal of their precursors from the blood, or for their secretion into the canaliculus. Some of these anions are of endogenous origin, such as conjugates of bile pigments or steroid hormones, and others are xenobiotics such as drugs or toxins or their metabolites. Many of these organic anions undergo biotransformation in two phases in the liver cells. Figure 6.10 shows a general scheme for these reactions. Phase 1 metabolism can be an oxidation, reduction or hydrolysis, but the most common type of phase 1 reaction is oxidative. These reactions make the molecule more polar. They are catalysed by a complex enzyme system, known as the mixed function oxygenase system, present in the endoplasmic reticulum. The most important enzyme in this system is cytochrome P-450, a haem protein that is part of the electron transfer chain, which catalyses

Gallstones Box 3

Fat malabsorption

The pale colour of the patient's stools was due to the absence of bile pigments (see below), and the greasiness to the presence of abnormally large quantities of unabsorbed fat. Elimination of abnormal amounts of fat is known as steatorrhoea. The fat causes the faeces to float, and to smell abnormally offensive because it is fermented by bacteria in the colon.

Bile acids play an important role in the digestion of lipid, and in the absorption of lipid- and fat-soluble vitamins (vitamins A, D, E, and K). Consequently in severe cholestasis, such as when the common bile duct is obstructed by gallstones, bile acids are not delivered to the small intestine and lipids are therefore not absorbed. Fat malabsorption causes flatulence and diarrhoea. The duration of the time period over which fat malabsorption is present in gallstone disease before it is treated is usually relatively short and for that reason fat-soluble vitamin deficiency is unusual, except in the case of vitamin K as body stores of vitamin K are very limited. Deficiency of this vitamin leads to deranged blood coagulation. In the long term, malabsorption of vitamin A can result in night blindness; and long-term malabsorption of vitamin D can result in osteomalacia and osteoporosis (as vitamin D is necessary for Ca^{2+} absorption). Vitamin E malabsorption has no known sequellae in the human. Restriction of dietary fat reduces steatorrhoea, but then vitamin K supplements are required.

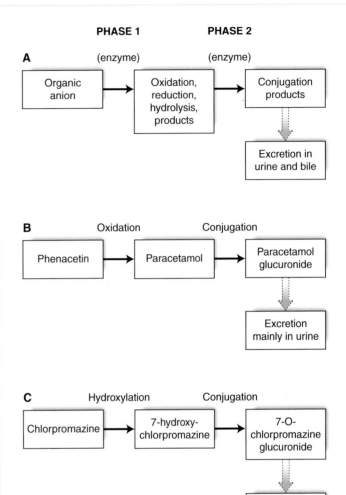

Fig. 6.10
Biotransformation of anions in the hepatocyte. (A) General scheme involving two phases. (B) A drug (phenacetin), which is metabolised in the liver, secreted into the blood, and excreted in the kidney. (C) A drug (chlorpromazine), which is metabolised in the liver and excreted in the bile.

an intermediate hydroxylation step in phase 1 oxidative reactions.

Some drug oxidation reactions involve specific enzymes. Ethanol oxidation, for example, is catalysed by alcohol dehydrogenase, and monoamine oxidase inactivates many biologically active amines, including adrenaline and serotonin. Reduction reactions are less common, but one important clinical example is the inactivation of the anticoagulation drug warfarin.

Phase 2 involves conjugation of the anion with a more strongly ionisable group that introduces a negative charge, or increases the negative charge, on the molecule, making it more hydrophilic. The most common phase 2 reaction involves the production of glucuronides. These glucuronidation reactions are all catalysed by UDP-glucuronyl transferase (Fig. 6.10). The formation of bilirubin glucuronide is described below and illustrated in Figure 6.11. Steroid hormones, thyroid hormones, bilirubin, and many drugs are converted to glucuronides in the liver. Many compounds

are conjugated to form sulphates, in the presence of glutathione. Others are conjugated to amino acids or to certain hexoses.

These transformations enable the organic anion generated to be handled by anion transporters (see below) in the canalicular membrane. The conjugates are usually more water soluble and less toxic than their precursors, although some (e.g. 7-O-chlorpromazine glucuronide) may be more toxic, and as a consequence they may damage the biliary system, or act as carcinogens (especially in the lower part of the duct system). Furthermore some conjugated drugs become less hydrophilic after being acted upon by bacteria in the colon. If they are then absorbed by passive absorp-

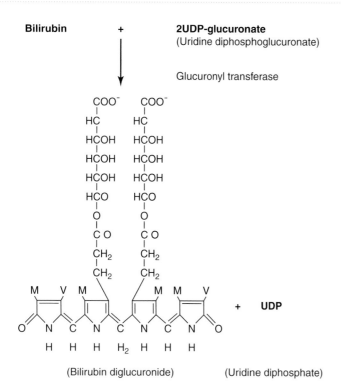

Fig. 6.11
Conjugation of bilirubin in the hepatocyte.

tion in the colon and recycled via the liver (the enterohepatic circulation), they can be difficult to eliminate from the body. Their toxicity is thereby increased. In liver diseases such as cirrhosis, in which the hepatocytes are damaged, there may be an increase in the half-life of some drugs because the capacity of the liver to metabolise and secrete them is decreased.

Determinants of preferential excretion into bile

Some organic anions are excreted preferentially via the bile and some via the urine. The processing of two important drugs to glucuronides is indicated in Figure 6.10. One of these, the analgesic drug phenacetin, is converted to paracetamol glucuronide, which is secreted by the liver into the blood to be excreted mainly by the kidney. The other, the antipsychotic drug, chlorpromazine, is converted to 7-O-chlorpromazine glucuronide, which is excreted mainly in the bile. In the human, small organic anions of molecular mass less than 500 Da are excreted exclusively by the kidney, while bigger anions are preferentially excreted into bile. Conjugation with glucuronic acid or glutathione serves to increase the molecular mass of a substance by 176 Da and 306 Da respectively, and conjugation may therefore increase the likelihood of secretion of the anion into bile. The reason for this dis-

criminatory threshold is unknown but the anion transporters in the canalicular membrane (see below) may show a molecular size specificity. Another possibility is 'molecular sieving' by tight junctions between the hepatocytes; according to this hypothesis all anions are secreted into the canaliculus but the small ones leak back into the plasma across the tight junction.

Transport of organic ions

Transport into the hepatocyte
Organic ions are transported in the blood largely by high affinity binding to albumin and consequently the concentrations in plasma of the free ions are low. However, the amount of material extracted in a single pass through the liver is often greater than that in free solution. The mechanism for this is unknown.

Uptake of cholephilic anions by the hepatocyte involves membrane carrier proteins with high affinity binding sites. Competition studies indicate that the carriers are shared by several anions. Thus bilirubin, sulphonamides, salicylates, and sulphobromophthalein share the same carrier, which is known as the organic anion transporter (oatp). Transport of anions via this mechanism is energy-requiring and can be against enormous concentration gradients. It involves a chloride antiport system.

Transport into bile
Transport of anions across the canalicular membrane into the bile can be against a 100-fold concentration gradient. The membrane potential difference, which is approximately 40 mV, intracellular negative, can only account for transport of organic anions against a 3-fold concentration gradient. At least three specific ATP-dependent active transport mechanisms are present in the canalicular membranes for the transport of organic ions. The ATP-dependent transporters and the membrane potential-dependent transporter are distinct proteins. The membrane potential-dependent transporter is a glycoprotein. One of the ATP-dependent transporters is responsible for transport of bile acids and has been described above. Another is known as the canalicular multi-organic anion transporter (cMOAT) (Fig. 6.12). It transports many organic anions, including bilirubin glucuronide and conjugates of various xenobiotics. It does not transport unconjugated bilirubin. The jaundiced mutant (Tr-) rat that exhibits hyperbilirubinaemia is deficient in this transporter. A similar defect is present in Dubin–Johnson syndrome in the human. The third transporter is actually a group of phosphoglycoproteins (Pgps), known as P-transporters, which bind ATP. They transport mainly hydrophobic, neutral

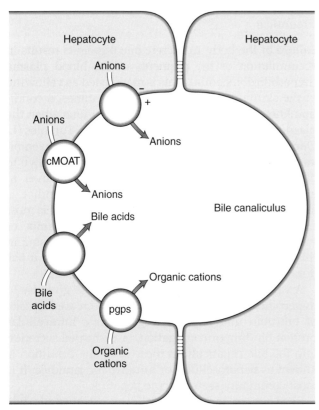

Fig. 6.12
Organic ion transporters in the canalicular membrane of the hepatocyte. cMOAT, canalicular multi-organic anion transporter, pgps, P-transporters which transport organic cations into bile.

compounds, and organic cations, into bile. One P-transporter, known as the multidrug transporter 3 (mdr-3), transports many cationic drugs across the canalicular membrane including certain peptides and anti-cancer drugs such as daunomycin. Interestingly the expression of the P-transporters is temporarily increased after partial hepatectomy.

Metabolism of bilirubin

Bilirubin, which is reddish-orange in colour, is the major bile pigment produced by breakdown of either haemoglobin or myoglobin in the reticuloendothelial system. Figure 6.13 shows the formation of bilirubin from haem, the porphyrin moiety of haemoglobin. Some of the intermediate product, biliverdin, a green pigment, is also usually present in bile, and in bile which has been stored the bilirubin reoxidises to form biliverdin, and the bile tends to go green. (These pigments are bound to albumin in the circulation.)

Free bilirubin from the blood enters the liver cells via an anion transporter that exchanges it for Cl^-. Inside the cell it is bound to specific cytoplasmic proteins,

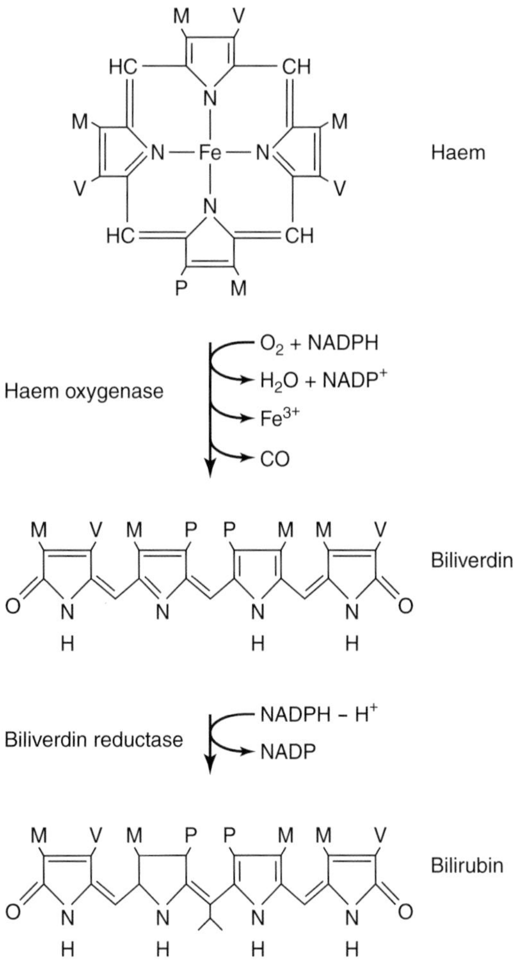

Fig. 6.13
Formation of bile pigments from haem. M, methyl, V, vinyl, P, propionyl, CO, carbon monoxide.

known as ligandins (or Y and Z proteins). It is then conjugated to glucuronic acid to form bilirubin diglucuronide, in a reaction catalysed by glucuronyl transferase (Fig. 6.11). The glucuronide is more water-soluble than free bilirubin. Some of the bilirubin glucuronide escapes into the blood and may be excreted by the kidney, but most is excreted actively via the cMOAT transporter system.

In Crigler–Najjar disease there is an inherited deficiency of glucuronyltransferase and high concentrations of unconjugated bilirubin are present in the plasma, causing jaundice. The affected individuals may develop kernicterus (deposits of pigment in the brain), which can cause nerve degeneration. Exposure to light degrades the pigment, and children born with this disease can be treated by phototherapy.

At birth, babies have little ability to conjugate bilirubin but it develops within the first few weeks of life. Thus some babies are jaundiced soon after birth, as unconjugated bilirubin is not readily excreted. This condition is known as physiological jaundice of the newborn.

Fate of bile pigments in the gastrointestinal tract

After delivery to the intestines most conjugated bilirubin is eliminated in the faeces. This is because the small intestinal mucosa is not very permeable to the conjugated metabolite. However, some may be deconjugated by the action of bacteria in the intestines and the free bulirubin formed can be absorbed to some extent, by passive diffusion into the portal blood as it is more lipid-soluble than the conjugated bilirubin. It is then returned to the liver (via the enterohepatic circulation). Intestinal bacteria can also convert bilirubin to colourless derivatives known as urobilinogens, which can be absorbed into the portal blood. These are mostly excreted in the bile but some are excreted in the urine. Urobilinogen remaining in the gut is partially reoxidised to stercobilinogen, the reddish-brown pigment responsible for the colour of the faeces. Figure 6.14 outlines the fate of excreted bile pigments.

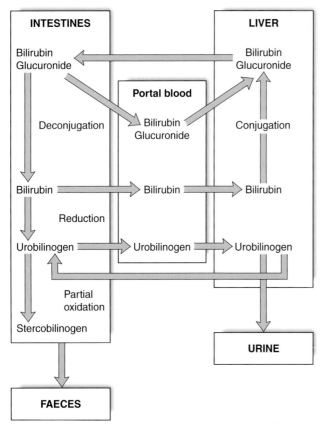

Fig. 6.14
Metabolism of bile pigments in the intestines.

Jaundice

Failure of the body to excrete bile pigments results in accumulation of the pigments in the blood plasma (hyperbilirubinaemia). This is manifested as yellowing of the skin, sclera, and mucous membranes, a condition known as jaundice. Jaundice is obvious when the plasma bilirubin concentration exceeds 34 μmoles/L. One cause of hyperbilirubinaemia is excessive haemolysis of red blood cells and haemoglobin breakdown to bilirubin. Consequently the capacity of the liver to excrete it is overwhelmed. This type of jaundice is known as prehepatic or haemolytic jaundice. It is most frequently associated with haemolytic anaemia of various types. The bilirubin present in the plasma in this type of jaundice is largely unconjugated as it has not been taken up and conjugated by the liver.

A variety of defects in the liver can also give rise to hyperbilirubinaemia. These include decreased uptake of bilirubin into hepatocytes, defective intracellular protein binding or conjugation, or disturbed secretion into the bile canaliculi. In these cases the condition is known as hepatocellular or intrahepatic jaundice. It is most commonly seen in acute hepatitis.

Blockage of the intrahepatic or extrahepatic bile ducts by, for example, gallstones, also causes jaundice as the bile is refluxed into the blood. This is commonly referred to as post-hepatic or obstructive jaundice (Case history, page 103).

Proteins in bile

Most proteins in bile are plasma proteins, although some are derived from cells of the hepatobiliary system. The plasma proteins are mostly synthesised in the liver and secreted into the blood. Some plasma proteins are normally present in bile, including unaltered active enzymes and antibodies.

Some proteins exhibit relatively low bile:plasma concentration ratios. Two non-specific pathways exist for protein transport in hepatocytes: paracellular sieving and pinocytosis (membrane vesiculation), followed by transport of the pinocytotic vesicles and exocytosis. The paracellular pathway is responsible for secretion of smaller proteins but pinocytosis does not discriminate in relation to molecular size. There are also receptor-linked pathways for the secretion of some proteins. One example is immunoglobulin A (IgA) which is transported by receptor-mediated vesicle transport in the duct cells. This protein provides immunological protection for the biliary and intestinal tracts.

Excessive secretion of these molecules across the canalicular membrane can occur when the intracellu-

Obstructive jaundice

The yellowing of the patient's sclera is due to high concentrations of conjugated bilirubin in the blood. Bile backs up in the hepatobiliary system when there is a blockage of the bile duct and it is consequently refluxed into the blood. The plasma bilirubin in this case has been conjugated by the liver cells. The presence in the blood of abnormally high concentrations of conjugated bilirubin or other constituents of bile, such as the enzyme alkaline phosphatase, indicates hepatobiliary disease. The non-clearance of bilirubin from the body may not in itself be particularly damaging. However, when jaundice is present, many other potentially toxic materials also accumulate in the blood as a consequence of their reflux from the bile or impaired secretion from the hepatocyte. This leads to impaired mental function and malaise.

The urine is dark-coloured because the bilirubin conjugates in the blood are water-soluble and are therefore excreted by the kidney. Unconjugated bilirubin binds tightly to albumin. Therefore, in healthy individuals, not much bilirubin is excreted in the urine. Conjugated bilirubin binds less tightly to albumin and when the conjugate is present in high concentrations in the blood, some of it is filtered in the glomerulus of the kidney and is only partly re-absorbed in the tubules. Thus excretion of bilirubin by the kidney (bilirubinuria) reflects the presence of bilirubin conjugates in the blood. When the bile ducts are blocked, bile pigments cannot gain entry to the gastrointestinal tract and the faeces are pale and clay-coloured (acholic).

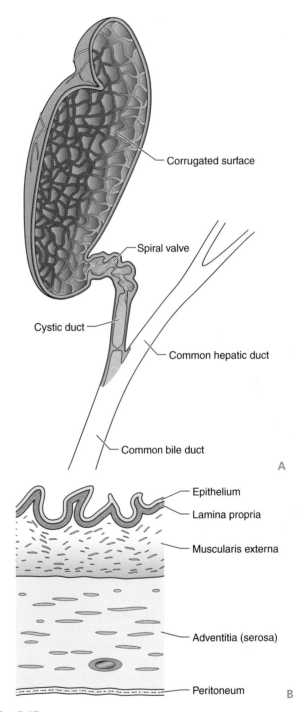

Fig. 6.15
The gallbladder. (A) Structural features. (B) Layers of the gallbladder wall.

lar microtubular guiding system directing the vesicles that house them to the sinusoidal membrane is disrupted and the secretory vesicles are misdirected to the canalicular pole of the cell. The release of some plasma membrane-derived enzymes, such as alkaline phosphatase, into bile is promoted by bile salts. This enzyme has no known function in bile but raised alkaline phosphatase in plasma is used as a biochemical marker of liver disease. It is usually elevated in any form of cholestasis, including biliary colic.

The gallbladder

Anatomy and histology

The gallbladder is a pear-shaped sac. In the human adult it is approximately 8 cm long and 4 cm wide, but it is capable of considerable distension. It is lined by a mucous membrane, which is thrown into numerous folds (rugae) when the gallbladder is contracted (Fig. 6.15). As the gallbladder fills with bile the folds flatten out. The cystic duct conveys the bile to the hepatic duct (Fig. 6.1, page 91).

The wall of the gallbladder is composed of three layers: the mucous membrane, the muscularis, and the adventitia (or serosa, see Fig. 6.15). The epithelium of the mucous membrane is composed of high columnar cells with basally located nuclei. The apical (luminal) border of the cells are provided with microvilli, consistent with their absorptive function. They resemble the absorptive cells of the small intestine. Beneath the epithelial cells is the lamina propria, which is a coat of loose connective tissue. Around the mucous membrane is a thin coat of smooth muscle, the muscularis externa. Most of the smooth muscle fibres run obliquely but some run circularly and some longitudinally. Many elastic fibres are present within the connective tissue between the muscle fibres. Outside this muscle layer is an outer coat of dense fibroconnective tissue, the adventitia (or serosa), which is covered by peritoneum.

At the neck of the gallbladder the mucous membrane is thrown into a spiral fold that has a core of smooth muscle (Fig. 6.15). This extends into the cystic duct and is known as the spiral valve. Its function may be to prevent sudden changes in the filling and emptying of the gallbladder.

Functions

The functions of the gallbladder are to store and concentrate bile, and to deliver it into the small intestine during a meal. In the human adult it has a capacity of 30–60 ml. Gallbladder bile is an isotonic solution but some of its components are highly concentrated (Table 6.1, page 95). The endothelial cells actively reabsorb Na^+ ions from the bile, by exchange for K^+ ions. The Na^+ ions are pumped into the lateral spaces between the epithelial cells. Anions, largely Cl^- and HCO_3^-, follow passively, down the electrochemical gradient. The extraction of HCO_3^- ions tends to make the gallbladder bile less alkaline. Thus gallbladder bile is less concentrated with respect to Na^+, Cl^-, and HCO_3^- than hepatic bile. The pumping of Na^+ keeps its concentration low inside the cell, and this provides the driving force for Na^+ ions to enter the cell via the apical membrane (down their concentration gradient). Transport in the apical membrane occurs partly via exchange for H^+ ions and partly by symport with Cl^- ions. As a consequence, water is transported passively, down the osmotic gradient, out of the gallbladder (Fig. 6.16). The ions and water then pass through the basement membrane into the blood capillaries.

Table 6.1 compares the composition of gallbladder bile with hepatic bile. Ca^{2+} ions are not absorbed by the gallbladder to any appreciable extent and Ca^{2+} is therefore concentrated in gallbladder bile. K^+ ions are also concentrated. The organic constituents are highly concentrated in the gallbladder, but the bile remains isosmotic with plasma. The bile pigments in hepatic bile impart a golden-brown colour to it, but gallbladder bile is almost black because the pigments are more concentrated. Bilirubin, bile acids, lecithin, and cholesterol are 5–10 times more concentrated in gallbladder bile than in hepatic bile.

Bile may be lost from the body because of a fistula between the common bile duct and the skin, as a complication of biliary surgery. This results in impaired fat absorption in the small intestine. Loss of significant amounts of K^+ ions (present in high concentrations in gallbladder bile) can also occur, and replacement with KCl has to be instigated in the clinical management of these patients.

Gallbladder contraction

The gallbladder exhibits muscle tone even in the interdigestive period. It also contracts between meals to deliver bile intermittently into the duodenum. The contractions coincide with the migrating myoelectric complex of the small intestine (see Chapter 7). These fasting contractions may reduce the likelihood of cholesterol crystals accumulating and forming gallstones.

The major stimulus for gallbladder contraction after a meal is a high blood level of CCK, the duodenal hormone that is released in response to fat in the duodenum (see Chapter 5). It acts on CCK-A receptors on the smooth muscle of the gallbladder. Gastrin, a related peptide, released by the stomach antrum in response to peptides in the food also stimulates gallbladder contraction. In addition, distension of the stomach antrum stimulates contraction via a nervous reflex. The gastric mechanisms involved in the control of bile release are presumably in preparation for when the chyme is emptied from the stomach.

Vasoactive intestinal peptide (VIP), pancreatic polypeptide (PP), and stimulation of the sympathetic nerves to the gallbladder, all cause gallbladder relax-

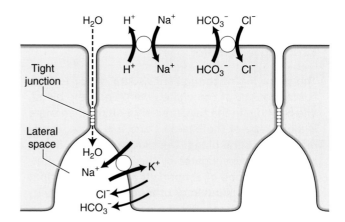

Fig. 6.16
Transport of ions in the gallbladder.

Gallstones Box 5

Composition, formation, and occurrence of gallstones

In order to understand the mechanisms of gallstone formation we need to know their composition. It has long been known that many compounds, including Ca^{2+} and bile pigments, can precipitate in bile to form stones, but 80% are formed from cholesterol.

Cholesterol stones

If the concentration of bile acids or phospholipid in the bile falls, cholesterol will not be held in micelles. The bile then becomes supersaturated with cholesterol, and this tends to precipitate out as microcrystals. These microcrystals coalesce to form gallstones. Some cholesterol stones are composed purely of cholesterol. In these cases the stones tend to be large, solitary, and pale yellow in colour. Smaller cholesterol stones are often of mixed composition but usually contain more than 70% cholesterol. These are also pale yellow but are usually multiple. They are of variable size and are laminated, with a dark central nucleus. The cholesterol crystals deposit around this nucleus, and then become hardened by the precipitation of organic salts.

Cholesterol gallstones tend to develop when there is a high ratio of cholesterol to bile acids or lecithin in the bile. This can be due to high cholesterol secretion, as a consequence of a high fat diet, or to congenital hypercholesterolaemia. They may also form if there is reduced bile acid secretion, as a consequence of bile acid malabsorption, or reduced lecithin secretion. The bile acid pool in an individual is fairly constant (see below) but in people with gallstones it tends to be smaller than average. Gallstone formation may happen at night in these individuals as bile acid secretion falls (even further) at night when blood levels are low (see below). The ratio of cholesterol to bile salts and lecithin is raised by a high fat diet, as fats are converted to cholesterol in the liver. Interestingly, however, gallstones are most common in South American women whose diet includes diosgenin-rich beans, because diosgenin increases cholesterol secretion. Inflammation of the gallbladder may also contribute by increasing reabsorption of bile salts or water in the gallbladder, thereby encouraging the cholesterol to precipitate out in the bile. Women tend to have a higher cholesterol: phospholipid ratio than men, which may account for the fact that four times more women than men suffer from gallstones. Genetic and racial factors also appear to be important. Cholesterol gallstones are also commonly found in diseases of the ileum which lead to reduced bile salt reabsorption, such as Crohn's disease (see Chapter 8).

Pigment stones

Pigment stones are usually small (a few mm in diameter), and dark brown or black in colour. When they occur, they are usually multiple. They contain between 40% and 95% pigment and less than 20% cholesterol. They constitute 20–25% of all gallstones. They can be due to an overload of unconjugated bilirubin resulting from haemolytic anaemia, burns, or crush injury. A high incidence of pigment gallstones is seen in patients with haemolytic states (such as sickle cell anaemia). The bile becomes supersaturated with unconjugated bilirubin and it precipitates out. The free bilirubin combines with calcium in the bile to form insoluble calcium bilirubinate. This forms the nidus of a stone and degradation products of bilirubin aggregate on this core to form a pigment stone. A deficit in the conjugating ability of the liver can also result in the formation of pigment gallstones. In addition, infecting organisms that contain β-glucuronidase, an enzyme which deconjugates bilirubin glucuronide, can be responsible. Until recently one form of disease where highly calcified pigment stones were present occurred in oriental countries (notably Japan). It was caused by disease of the biliary duct through infestation with parasites that contain this enzyme. Its incidence has diminished as hygiene and nutrition have improved in these countries. Unfortunately, however, as the diet has become 'westernised' the incidence of cholesterol gallstones has increased. There is also a tendency for pigment stones to form in patients with cirrhosis of the liver due to stasis in the biliary tract.

ation. Bile acids also inhibit gallbladder contraction (a feedback control).

The sphincter of Oddi

The hepatic bile duct penetrates the wall of the duodenum, at the same location as the pancreatic duct. Part of the way through the duodenal wall the hepatic duct and the pancreatic duct fuse. The lumen of the fused duct is relatively wide and this region is known as the ampulla of Vater. It opens into the lumen of the duodenum, and at the opening are the duodenal papilla. Circular smooth muscle is associated with the ampulla and with the regions of the hepatic and pancreatic ducts that are associated with it (Fig. 6.1, page 91). This constitutes the sphincter of Oddi. The closure of this sphincter prevents bile from entering the intestine. As a result the bile

Treatment with bile acids

We can now understand why gallstones can be treated by administration of bile acids. Cholesterol supersaturation in bile in patients with gallstones is often due to a diminished bile acid pool. The ingested bile acids are absorbed in the ileum and taken up by the liver and then secreted in the bile (Fig. 6.19). Thus if a bile acid is fed in substantial amounts the bile acid pool is expanded. This enables more cholesterol to be retained in micelles, rather than precipitating in the bile. The bile acids slowly dissolve the gallstones over a period of time, usually several months. Chenodeoxycholic acid (see Fig. 6.7) can be effective. Ursodeoxycholic acid (ursodiol), a derivative of chenodeoxycholic acid, which is relatively abundant in polar bear bile, is even more effective. The main side-effect of bile acid treatment is diarrhoea, secondary to incomplete absorption of the ingested bile salts. These particular bile acids are effective because they increase cholesterol sequestration in micelles and (unlike cholic acid and deoxycholic acid) they do not suppress bile acid synthesis. Ursodiol also inhibits cholesterol absorption in the intestine and decreases the synthesis of cholesterol in the liver. This causes reduced plasma cholesterol levels, and for this reason ursodiol has also been considered for the treatment of coronary heart disease.

Small gallstones disappear relatively quickly with this treatment. However, it is the large stones that are usually responsible for the symptoms of gallstone disease, so alleviation via this means takes time. Moreover most individuals with gallstones present with acute symptoms, which are often associated with a dysfunctional gallbladder. Therefore the use of bile salt therapy is limited. Life-time therapy with bile salts is required to prevent the stones recurring.

the hepatobiliary system are under physiological control; secretion of alkaline fluid from the ducts, the secretion of bile from the hepatocytes, contraction of the smooth muscle in the wall of the gallbladder to release the stored bile, and relaxation of the smooth muscle in the sphincter of Oddi which allows the bile into the duodenum.

The control of alkaline bile secretion during a meal can be divided into three phases according to the location of the ingested material:

- the cephalic phase: the response to the approach of food or the presence of food in the mouth

- the gastric phase: the response to food in the stomach
- the intestinal phase: the response to food in the duodenum.

The bile acid-dependent fraction is secreted more or less continuously, but the gallbladder usually only contracts forcefully during a meal. Thus, although secretion is continuous, bile acids usually only enter the gastrointestinal tract in appreciable amounts during a meal, when they are required.

The cephalic phase

The cephalic phase is mediated via impulses in nerve fibres in the vagus nerve. It is due to the sight and smell of food, and the activation of taste and touch receptors by the food in the mouth. In this phase there is an increase in the secretion of alkaline bile from the duct cells, which would presumably minimise the effects of increased acid secretion in the stomach during the cephalic phase. Weak contractions of the gallbladder and relaxation of the sphincter of Oddi also occur.

The gastric phase

Peptides, caffeine, or alcohol in food in the stomach, and distension of the stomach walls cause increased release of gastrin from the pyloric antrum. They also cause activation of nerve fibres in the vagus nerve. In this phase, alkaline juice secretion from the bile ducts and weak contractions of the gallbladder are stimulated via the release of gastrin and impulses in the vagus nerve.

The intestinal phase

This phase is the most important of the three phases. It is mediated largely via the peptide hormones secretin and CCK released from the walls of the duodenum into the blood. Secretin is released in response mainly to acid in the chyme. It acts on receptors on the duct cells to stimulate the release of alkaline bile. Its action is potentiated by CCK.

CCK is the most potent stimulus for gallbladder contraction. The most potent stimulus for CCK release is fat: when fat is not present in a meal, contraction of the gallbladder is in response to stimuli in the cephalic and gastric phases and is weak. CCK also causes relaxation of the sphincter of Oddi, thereby enabling the bile to flow freely into the duodenum. Bile acids exert a negative feedback control on gallbladder contraction and sphincter relaxation, by inhibiting the release of CCK from the duodenum.

Self-assessment case study: paracetamol overdose

A teenager who had just failed her examinations was discovered unconscious in her bed and rushed into hospital. An empty bottle of paracetamol (acetominaphen) tablets was found in her bedroom and it seemed likely that she had ingested a whole bottle of tablets. Her stomach was washed out as soon as she arrived in casualty. The girl's blood paracetamol levels were monitored for 12 hours and from the results it was predicted that she might suffer liver damage. She was given intravenous acetylcysteine over the following 20 hours. After about 48 hours she seemed to have recovered, but then she became aggressive, and 2 days later she started to vomit and became delirious. At the time of her relapse, she had become jaundiced, her liver was tender, and her serum transaminase levels and prothrombin levels were found to be extremely high. These and the findings of an EEG indicated that acute hepatic necrosis was present. Luckily a suitable donor liver was available and she was given a transplant. The patient's serum bilirubin levels, prothrombin time, and serum albumin were monitored to determine the progress of her recovery.

You should be able to answer the following questions:

① How is a therapeutic dose of paracetamol normally metabolised in the liver?

② Why are high levels of paracetamol toxic to the liver?

③ Why was intravenous acetylcysteine administered?

④ Why did the patient suffer a relapse after she appeared to have recovered?

⑤ Why did the patient appear jaundiced after her relapse?

⑥ Why were the patient's serum prothrombin and transaminase levels excessively high?

⑦ How can we explain the patient's aggressive behaviour?

⑧ Why was an EEG performed?

⑨ Why was a liver transplant necessary?

⑩ Why were serum bilirubin levels, prothrombin time, and serum albumin monitored after the transplantation?

⑪ Would forced diuresis or renal dialysis have been useful in this patient?

⑬ Can you suggest why alcohol ingestion should be avoided if paracetamol has been taken for a headache?

Self-assessment questions

① What are the special features of the liver's blood supply?

② What are the functions of alkaline bile secreted from the duct cells?

③ How is the alkaline secretion controlled?

④ What are the excretory functions of the hepatocytes?

⑤ How is the hepatocyte secretion controlled?

⑥ What are the functions of Kupffer cells?

⑦ What are the functions of the gallbladder?

⑧ How do cholesterol gallstones form in bile? What factors predispose an individual to develop cholesterol stones?

⑨ What causes pigment stones to form in bile in some individuals?

⑩ What is meant by 'the enterohepatic circulation'?

⑪ What purpose does deconjugation of metabolites and drugs serve?

⑫ What determines whether a compound is excreted by the liver or by the kidney?

THE SMALL INTESTINE

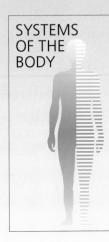

SYSTEMS OF THE BODY

Chapter objectives

After studying this chapter you should be able to:

① Describe the structure of the small intestine and the major cell types present in the mucosa.

② Understand the processes of water and electrolyte secretion and absorption in the small intestine.

④ Understand the mechanisms of diarrhoea, its consequences, and treatment.

⑤ Describe the motility of the small intestine, and its control.

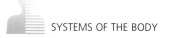

7

THE SMALL INTESTINE

Introduction

In the human most digestion and absorption occurs in the small intestine. Digestion in the stomach is dispensable and it is only preparatory. Pancreatic juice and bile from the liver enter the duodenum (Fig. 7.1). Intestinal juice is secreted along the entire length of the intestine from glands in the wall. In the normal individual, digestion is substantially complete when the chyme passes into the colon. The small intestine normally also absorbs over 95% of the water that enters the gastrointestinal tract. There is considerable reserve of function, and two-thirds of the small intestine can be removed without serious impairment of the quality of life.

Absorption is the central process of the digestive system and all other physiological processes occurring in the gastrointestinal tract subserve it. In this chapter we shall deal with the absorption of water and monovalent ions. The importance of water and electrolyte absorption in the intestines can be illustrated by the problems encountered in cholera, a condition in which there can be a massive loss of fluid from the body.

Digestion and absorption of other nutrients will be dealt with separately. We shall also consider how the contractile activity of the intestines mixes and propels the food towards the ileum.

Intestinal phase of digestion

When chyme enters the small intestine from the stomach, it causes the release into the blood of the hormones secretin and cholecystokinin (CCK) from endocrine (APUD) cells in the walls of the duodenum. Secretin stimulates secretion of alkaline pancreatic juice, alkaline bile, and alkaline intestinal juice. CCK stimulates secretion of enzyme-rich pancreatic juice. It also causes contraction of the gallbladder and relaxation of the sphincter of Oddi, which promote the entry of bile and pancreatic juices into the duodenum (Fig. 7.1). At the same time these hormones inhibit

Cholera Box 1

Cholera

An elderly man was carried by his son into a hospital, which was situated in a remote region of Bengal. The man appeared emaciated. He said he had initially been vomiting and suffering from abdominal distension. Now he was suffering from copious diarrhoea. The duty doctor noted that the man's skin lacked turgor. The man's pulse was barely detectable but his pulse rate was rapid (100 beats per minute). The younger man was also suffering from diarrhoea, but he was less severely affected. The doctor suspected that they were both victims of the latest cholera epidemic. Such epidemics are not uncommon in the region because of contamination of food and drinking water with the bacterium *Vibrio cholerae*. The elderly man was provided with electrolyte fluid via an intravenous drip. His plasma and urine K^+ and HCO_3^- concentrations were monitored. He was also given intravenous tetracycline for 2 days. The younger man was given some packets containing a mixture of salt and sugar, and a supply of clean drinking water. He was told to dissolve the salt (NaCl) and sugar (glucose) in clean water from the hospital supply and to drink large quantities of the solution over the next few days. He was given tetracycline to take by mouth. Both patients had recovered within a few days.

In this chapter we shall consider the following questions:

① What causes cholera? Why were the patients treated with tetracycline?

② Why was it necessary to monitor the patient's plasma and urine K^+ and HCO_3^- concentrations? How would the patients' acid–base status have changed? What adjustments in respiratory and renal function would be taking place in these patients in response to the changes in their acid–base status?

③ How does the *V. cholerae* bacterium cause diarrhoea? Could other treatments counteract the effect of the toxin on the crypt cells?

④ What is the rationale for treating people suffering from cholera with (a) oral fluid containing NaCl and glucose, (b) intravenous fluid? What is the likely composition of the intravenous fluid?

⑤ Why was the elderly man's pulse (a) feeble, (b) rapid? What adjustments in cardiovascular and renal function would take place in response to the hypovolaemia?

⑥ Are changes in intestinal motility involved in this condition?

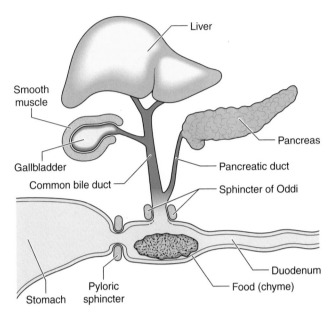

Fig. 7.1
Structures involved in the duodenal phase of digestion. Pancreatic juice and bile from the liver enter the duodenum during the intestinal phase. The entry is controlled by the pressure generated when the gallbladder contracts and by relaxation of the sphincter of Oddi. These juices, and juices from the intestinal walls, mix with the acid chyme arriving from the stomach.

Table 7.1
Control of secretion and motility during the intestinal phase

	Effect	Hormone
Secretion		
Duodenal (alkaline)	Stimulation	Secretin
Bile (alkaline)	Stimulation	Secretin
Bile (hepatocyte)	None	
Pancreatic juice (alkaline)	Stimulation	Secretin
Pancreatic juice (enzyme-rich)	Stimulation	CCK
Smooth muscle		
Stomach	Relaxation	CCK, secretin
Gallbladder	Contraction	CCK
Sphincter of Oddi	Relaxation	CCK
Intestinal	Contraction	Various

Cholera Box 2

Causes of cholera

The *V. cholerae* bacterium present in contaminated water and food produces a toxin that elicits a massive secretion of fluid and electrolytes. The effect is produced mainly in the proximal small intestine. Epidemics in the Indian subcontinent usually occur in the early summer before the monsoon breaks. The bacteria are harboured in the gallbladder in asymptomatic carriers, which may comprise up to 5% of the population in this region.

Treatment with antibiotics such as tetracycline or chloramphenicol is effective but should be regarded as ancillary to rehydration therapy (see below). Thus, tetracycline treatment decreases the average duration of the disease by 60%.

Anticholera vaccines have been developed, but these are of limited use during epidemics because it takes 2–3 weeks for them to become effective.

Bacteria are normally destroyed by gastric acid in the stomach, providing some protection for normal individuals. Increased susceptibility to the disease is seen in individuals with achlorhydra or those who have had a partial gastrectomy.

gastric emptying, which enables processing of the contents of the small intestine to occur before the next portion of chyme enters from the stomach, and prevents the intestinal chyme from becoming too acid. The latter is important because the action of pancreatic enzymes and lipid absorption require an alkaline or neutral pH.

The chyme also stimulates contraction of the smooth muscle of the intestines, which mixes the intestinal contents and propels it towards the ileum. The intestinal phase of the control of digestion is summarised in Table 7.1.

Anatomy and structure

In the adult human, the small intestine consists of approximately 6 metres of 3.5-cm diameter tubing which is coiled in the abdomen. It leads from the stomach to the colon (see Fig. 7.2). The first 25 cm or so is the duodenum. This region differs from the rest of the small intestine in having no mesentery. The adjacent region is the jejunum which comprises approximately 40% (2.5 metres) of the small intestine. The remaining distal part is the ileum. The longitudinal smooth muscle in the wall is normally partially contracted (tone). After death, when it is relaxed, the small bowel reaches a length of approximately 7.5 metres.

Duodenum

The duodenum has an essential role in mixing digestive juices, derived from the liver and pancreas, and from its own wall with the food. It forms an arc ending in a sharp bend, the duodenojejunal flexure. The head

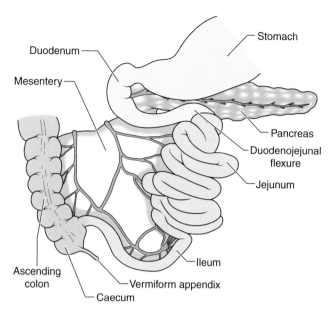

Fig. 7.2
Anatomical arrangement of the small intestine and associated structures.

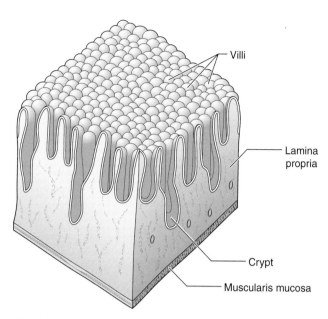

Fig. 7.3
Structure of the submucosa of the small intestine showing the relationship of the glands to the villi.

of the pancreas lies within the arc (see Fig. 7.2). At approximately two-thirds of the way down the descending part of the duodenum are two papillae. The major duodenal papilla is the location of the duct where the bile and pancreatic juice empty into the duodenum via the ampulla of Vater. The opening of the ampulla is controlled by the sphincter of Oddi (see Chapters 5 and 6). An accessory pancreatic duct, present in most individuals, opens at the tip of the lesser papilla.

The surface of the duodenum is folded. The folds are known as plicae circularis (circular folds). Most are crescent-shaped and do not disappear when the intestine is distended. The mucosa of the small intestine is covered with tiny projections, known as villi. These are tongue-shaped in the duodenum.

Two types of glands are present in the duodenal mucosa. At the base of the villi are tubular invaginations that reach almost to the muscularis mucosae, known as intestinal glands or crypts of Lieberkuhn (see Fig. 7.3). The submucosa of the duodenum contains coiled compound tubular mucous glands known as glands of Brunner, which secrete an alkaline fluid rich in mucus and are more numerous in the proximal region of the duodenum. They usually open at the base of the intestinal glands.

Jejunum and ileum

No anatomical feature separates the jejunum from the ileum. The structure of the jejunum and ileum is basi-

cally similar to that of the duodenum. However, there is a gradual decrease in diameter, in the thickness of the wall, and in the number of folds, with distance from the duodenum (Fig. 7.4). The folds are absent altogether from the terminal ileum. In addition, the villi gradually become less numerous, smaller, and more finger-like, with distance from the duodenum. Numerous lymph nodes, called Peyer's patches are present in the mucosa and submucosa of the ileum. The junction between the ileum and the large intestine is the ileocaecal junction. It consists of a ring of thickened smooth muscle, known as the ileocaecal sphincter (see Chapter 10), which reduces reflux back from the colon.

The jejunum and ileum are on a mesentery. This contains the arterial blood vessels (branches of the superior mesenteric artery) and the veno-lymphatic drainage vessels, which are supported in fatty connective tissue that is covered by mesothelium.

Blood supply

At rest approximately 10% of the cardiac output flows to the intestine. The blood vessels in the jejunum and ileum are derived from the superior mesenteric artery (Fig. 7.5). Numerous arterial branches form an extensive network in the submucosa, which supplies the wall of the intestine.

Nerves, hormones, and local paracrine factors control the intestinal circulation. Stimulation of the sympathetic nerves (which follow the arteries) causes

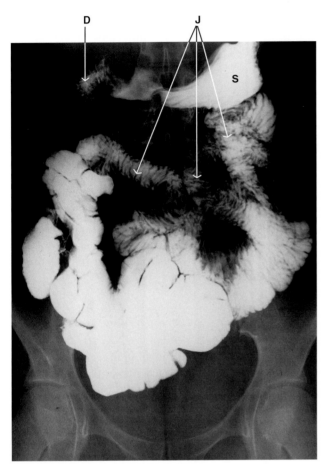

D   J

S

Fig. 7.4
An X-ray of the small bowel taken 2 hours after ingestion of barium. The mucosal outline of the jejunum (J) is clearly seen, showing the dense mucosal folds that maximise the surface area. The stomach (S) and duodenum (D) are also visible.

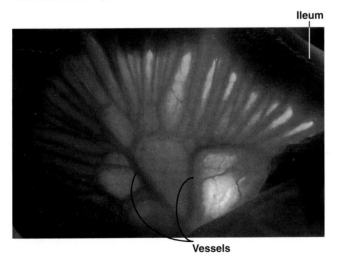

Ileum

Vessels

Fig. 7.5
A photograph of the vascular arcade in the ileum, showing the multiple arterial anastomoses in the mesentery.

vasoconstriction and reduced blood flow enabling a redistribution of blood away from the intestine. This is particularly important during low cardiac output states such as shock, or during exercise when extra blood is required for skeletal muscle. In the blood vessels of the villi, the vasoconstriction is relatively short-lived. This is due to vasodilator metabolites, such as adenosine, which accumulate during the vaso-constrictor response.

The splanchnic blood flow increases by 50–300% during a meal (functional hyperaemia). Distension of the walls of the intestine and substances present in the chyme stimulate the blood flow. Other stimuli include products of carbohydrate and lipid digestion in the proximal small intestine, and bile acids in the distal ileum. Gastrin, CCK, secretin, serotonin, and histamine all have the capacity to increase blood flow, and may be involved in this response during a meal.

The nutrients absorbed across the absorptive cells, are transported to the liver in the portal veins (Chapter 6).

Countercurrent exchange in the villi
The blood vessels of the villi (Fig. 7.6) constitute a countercurrent exchange system, whereby there is net diffusion of dissolved substances across the intersti-tium from the venule to the arteriole, or vice versa, depending on which limb has the higher concentra-tion. Thus oxygen tension is higher in the ascending arterial blood because it is extracted from the blood

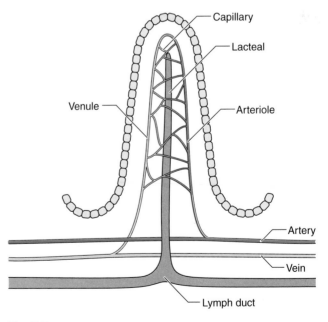

Capillary

Lacteal

Venule

Arteriole

Artery

Vein

Lymph duct

Fig. 7.6
Structural features of the villus.

in the capillaries, and it diffuses from the ascending limb to the descending limb. This results in a lower oxygen tension at the tips of the villi than at their bases. The relative hypoxia at the tip has been causally implicated in the shedding of the epithelial cells from the tips of the villi. In hypovolaemic shock, a situation where hypotension is present, the reduced perfusion pressure together with increased smooth muscle relaxation that accompanies it, leads to a reduced oxygen supply. This can cause the tips of the villi to become severely hypoxic. During hypovolaemic shock this can lead to ulceration of the intestines, which can develop within hours of the onset of hypovolaemia. Such acute ulcers are seen in patients who have suffered severe burns, especially children, and after major haemorrhage, such as where there is a leaking aortic aneurysm.

Structure of the intestinal wall

The wall of the small intestine has the same basic structure as other regions of the gastrointestinal tract (see Chapter 1). Above the serosa is the muscularis externa, which consists of two layers of smooth muscle, an outer longitudinal coat, and an inner circular coat. Preganglionic parasympathetic nerve fibres of the vagus nerve synapse with the cells of the terminal ganglia in the myenteric plexus. The postganglionic nerves stimulate muscle contraction and gland secretion (see Chapter 1). Postganglionic sympathetic nerve fibres arising largely from the prevertebral ganglia mostly innervate their target effector cells directly. The submucosal plexus contains a few parasympathetic ganglia of the vagus nerve, but postganglionic sympathetic fibres from the superior mesenteric plexus form the major proportion of the extrinsic nerves present.

Beneath the submucosa is the muscularis mucosae, which consists of two thin layers of muscle with some elastic tissue. The inner muscle layer consists of circularly disposed fibres, and the outer layer longitudinally disposed fibres. The muscularis mucosae permits localised movement of the mucous membrane. Small bundles of muscle fibres extend from it to the epithelium. Some of the fibres end on the epithelial basement membrane. Beneath the muscularis mucosa in the lamina propria is a layer of connective tissue that supports the epithelium and contains collagen, reticular fibres, and some elastic fibres. It also contains blood capillaries and lymph capillaries, which are situated close to the epithelial surface, especially in the villi (Fig. 7.6). It also contains numerous lymphatic nodules. Lymphocytes and plasma cells gain access to this layer across the epithelial membrane. These cells protect the tissue against bacteria that enter across

the epithelial membrane. The plasma cells produce IgA immunoglobulins. The innermost layer is the epithelium (described below).

The villus

The villus is regarded as the unit of absorption. Its length varies between 0.5 and 1.5 mm, depending on its location in the small intestine. The structure of the villus is depicted in Figure 7.6. Each villus contains a blood capillary network and a blind-ended lacteal (or lymph vessel). It is covered by simple columnar epithelium. Most of these cells have numerous cytoplasmic extensions at the luminal surface, known as microvilli. The microvillous surface of the intestine is known as the brush border.

Histology

The mucosa of the small intestine is simple columnar epithelium. Four cell types are present:

- absorptive cells, which produce digestive enzymes and absorb nutrients from the chyme
- goblet cells, which produce mucus that lubricates the surface and protects it from mechanical damage
- granular cells (cells of Paneth), which produce enzymes and protect the intestinal surface from bacteria
- APUD cells, which produce peptide hormones that regulate secretion and motility in the gastrointestinal tract, liver, and pancreas. The general function and structure of APUD cells are described in Chapter 1.

The four cell types arise from undifferentiated cells in the crypts of Lieberkuhn. The granular and endocrine cells remain at the bottom of the crypts but the absorptive and goblet cells slowly migrate up the sides of the villi, to the tips. Figure 7.7 shows the cell types and their typical locations in the mucosa. The cells that migrate are eventually shed from the tips. The process of migration from the crypts to the tips of the villi occurs over 3–6 days in the human. Thus most of the intestinal epithelium is renewed every few days. The columnar cells mature as they travel towards the tips of the villi, and their functions change. There is a gradual transition from base columnar cells in the crypts to villous columnar cells; their size increases progressively as they ascend the walls of the crypts and villi, and their content of free ribosomes decreases, whilst their content of rough endoplasmic reticulum increases.

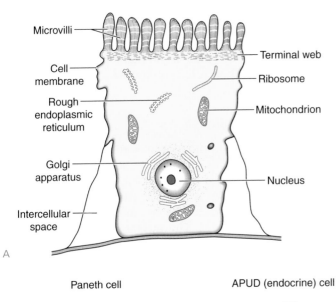

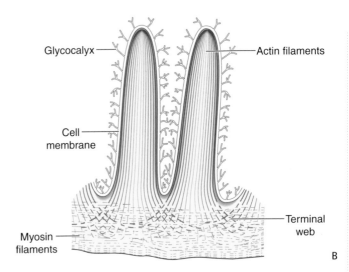

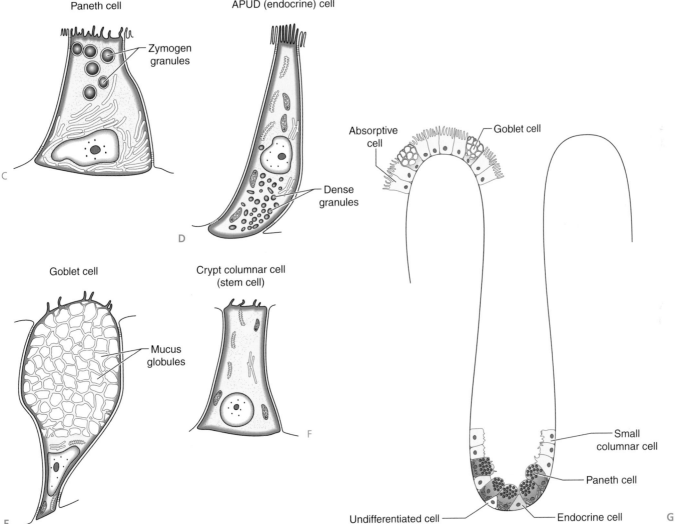

Fig. 7.7
Cell types in the intestinal epithelium. (A) Absorptive
columnar cell. (B) Structure of microvilli. (C) Paneth cell.
(D) Endocrine cell. (E) Goblet cell. (F) Undifferentiated
columnar cell. (G) Localisation of the different cell types
in the epithelium of the crypts and the villi.

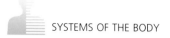
Cell types

Villous epithelium

About 90% of the cells covering the villi are the absorptive columnar cylindrical cells. Most of the rest are goblet cells, but 0.5% or less are endocrine cells. The absorptive cells have abundant cytoplasm and mitochondria but few ribosomes. They have a thick striated microvillous border and convoluted lateral cell membranes. Figure 7.7 shows the structure of an absorptive cell, and the structure of microvilli. The rough endoplasmic reticulum and Golgi saccules are well-developed in columnar cells at the base of the villi but less prominent in cells at the tips of the villi. The columnar cells produce a cell coat composed of glycoproteins, but the cells at the base of the villi are more active in this respect, as is consistent with their well-developed Golgi saccules. Some of the glycoproteins present are enzymes involved in the digestion of nutrients such as disaccharides (see Chapter 8). They act in situ but are also active after being shed into the lumen.

Crypt epithelium

The base of the crypt contains approximately equal numbers of small columnar cells and Paneth cells. The small columnar cells have sparse cytoplasm containing few mitochondria and little rough endoplasmic reticulum and a small Golgi apparatus. However, they contain numerous free ribosomes, consistent with their active protein synthesising function. They have smooth lateral membranes and are relatively undifferentiated. These are the stem cells which give rise to the other cell types.

Paneth cells are highly differentiated, possessing abundant rough endoplasmic reticulum and a prominent Golgi apparatus. They synthesise enzymes, such as lysozyme, and sequester them in zymogen granules, from which they are released into the lumen by exocytosis.

There are also oligomucous cells, which contain few mucus globules in the crypts. These are the precursors of the goblet cells. They can divide but lose this ability when they become distended with mucus after migrating up to the villus.

Endocrine cells comprise about 1% of the cells in the crypts. They have a narrow apex, and a wide basal region packed with dense argentaffin granules. Some of these cells produce hormones such as secretin, CCK, somatostatin, or endorphins. Others produce serotonin.

There are a few caveolated cells, characterised by invaginations of the cell membrane extending into the cytoplasm (caveolae). They have long microvilli, which contain long bundles of straight filaments that extend into the cytoplasm, and filaments encircling the apical region. Their role is unknown.

Intestinal secretions

An alkaline fluid containing electrolytes, mucus, and water is secreted throughout the length of the small intestine. The precise composition of the secretion, and the mechanisms that control it, vary from one region to another. It is secreted by the immature cells in the crypts of Lieberkuhn. The mechanisms involved are outlined in Figure 7.8. The key step is the active transport of Cl^- across the basolateral membrane of the cell. Cl^- is actively transported into the cell via a cotransporter protein that transports Na^+, K^+, and $2Cl^-$. The transport of Na^+ down its electrical gradient is the driving force for the operation of this transporter. The K^+ is transported back out via K^+ channels in the same membrane. This K^+ flux maintains the electrical potential difference (cytosol-negative) across the cell membranes. This potential difference contributes to the driving force for the basolateral influx of Na^+ across the basolateral membrane, and also for Cl^- transport across the luminal membrane. Cl^- is transported into the lumen via the cystic fibrosis transport regulator (CFTR, see Chapter 5), which is an electrogenic Cl^- channel in the luminal membrane. Na^+ is then transported into the lumen between the cells, down the

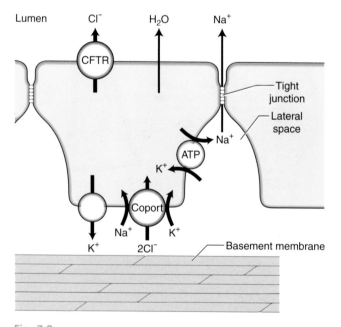

Fig. 7.8

Mechanism of secretion of electrolytes and water by the immature cells of the crypts of Lieberkühn.

electrochemical gradient produced by the extrusion of Cl^- from the cell. The opening time of the CFTR channel is prolonged by increased cAMP. Therefore secretion by the crypt cells is stimulated by substances that elevate cAMP, such as vasoactive intestinal peptide (VIP) and prostaglandins. Ca^{2+} mobilising agents such as acetylcholine potentiate the actions of these substances. There is a defect in the CFTR channel in cystic fibrosis (see Chapter 5). The first manifestation of cystic fibrosis can be postnatal constipation (meconium ileus), which is directly related to absence of the CFTR channel.

Control of secretion in the small intestine

Secretion in the small intestine can be controlled by hormones, paracrine factors, and nervous activity. Gastrin, neurotensin, serotonin histamine, prostaglandins, and a number of other hormone and paracrine factors stimulate the epithelial cells directly. The cells are innervated by secretomotor neurones, mainly from ganglia in the submucosal plexus but also from ganglia in the myenteric plexus. The submucosal neurones release ACh, VIP, substance P and serotonin, and probably other transmitters, to stimulate secretion. Parasympathetic nerves innervate neurones in the enteric nerve plexi. They enhance secretion via ACh release onto neurones in the plexi. Parasympathetic tone contributes to the basal secretion. Reflexes triggered by distension of the lumen of the small intestine, and the presence of various substances (glucose, acid, bile salts, ethanol, cholera toxin) in the intestinal chyme, stimulate secretion. These reflexes involve intrinsic and extrinsic (parasympathetic nerves).

Noradrenaline inhibits secretion in two ways: it acts directly on the epithelial cells (via α-adrenoreceptors), and it acts on neurones in the submucosal ganglia to inhibit secretory nerves that stimulate the epithelial cells. Somatostatin acts humorally on the crypt cells, as an inhibitory neurotransmitter. It is released from the enteric secretomotor nerves, and from the nerve fibres that innervate the crypt cells. It inhibits secretion by decreasing the levels of cAMP in the epithelial crypt cells. The effect of somatostatin to inhibit secretion has led to use of its analogues, such as octreotide, in the treatment of secretory diarrhoea, and to reduce fluid loss from small bowel (ileo-cutaneous) fistulae.

Absorption

Most substances are absorbed in the proximal small intestine and most of the contents of the small intes-

Cholera Box 3

Changes in electrolyte and acid–base balance

Secretions of the small intestines contain large amounts of HCO_3^-, Na^+, and Cl^- ions. K^+ is absorbed during a meal, down the concentration gradient set up by the absorption of water (see below). However, when the concentration of K^+ in the lumen is reduced below approximately 25 mM, the concentration gradient favours net secretion into the lumen. This occurs via the paracellular pathway. In diarrhoea, the luminal contents become diluted with respect to K^+ and it is transported into the lumen. Considerable losses of K^+ can occur, leading to hypokalaemia.

As HCO_3^- is secreted into the lumen, H^+ is transported into the blood, which becomes transiently acid. Excessive loss of HCO_3^- in secreted intestinal fluid causes a severe acidosis. The transient acidity in the blood is normally neutralised by the alkaline tide that accompanies the secretion of acid in the stomach (see Chapter 3). If there is excessive loss of alkaline fluid from the gastrointestinal tract, however, the acidity in the blood is proportionately increased and it cannot be buffered. This metabolic acidosis will be partially compensated in the short-term by an increased rate and depth of breathing, which results in CO_2 being blown off from the body. Longer term adjustments are brought about by reabsorption of HCO_3^- in the tubules of the kidney, and excretion of H^+.

K^+ is required for cell growth and division, enzyme action, cell excitability, muscle contraction, acid–base balance, and volume regulation. Hypokalaemia (reduced serum K^+ concentration) causes hyperpolarisation of cell membranes and reduces the excitability of neurones, cardiac muscle, and skeletal muscle. Severe hypokalaemia can cause paralysis, cardiac arrhythmias, a decreased ability to concentrate urine, and death, which is usually due to cardiac arrest.

tine have normally been absorbed by the time the chyme reaches the middle of the jejunum. However, a few substances such as vitamin B_{12} and bile salts (see Chapter 8) are actively absorbed in the ileum.

Surface area of the small intestine

The rate of transport of materials across the small intestine is proportional to its surface area. The surface area of the small intestine is vast. This organ is therefore well-adapted for absorption. Its area

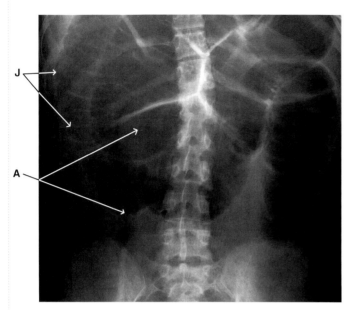

Fig. 7.11

A plain abdominal X-ray showing obstruction to the small bowel. The jejunum (J) has become grossly dilated and filled with air (A) and fluid, due to failure of membrane transport.

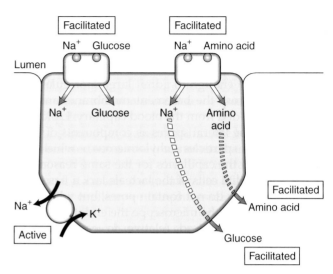

Fig. 7.12

The secondary active transport of Na^+ via the Na^+/glucose and Na^+/amino acid co-port systems in the absorptive cells of the proximal small intestine.

intestine into the blood by active mechanisms. This involves the transcellular route. It is usually transported in the absence of a chemical gradient as the chyme in the small intestine is normally isotonic with plasma, but it is obviously transported against the small electrochemical gradient present. The processes involved are illustrated in Figure 7.12. The key process is the active transport of Na^+ out of the cell, across the lateral border via a Na^+/K^+ ATPase pump, which simultaneously pumps K^+ into the cell. This maintains the low concentration of Na^+ within the cell. The Na^+ concentration gradient set up by this pump is the driving force for the transport of Na^+ from the lumen of the intestine into the cell. This diffusion across the luminal brush border of the cell is therefore down the concentration gradient. However, transport across this membrane occurs at a faster rate than it would by simple passive diffusion. This is because the Na^+ ions are transported on carrier proteins in the brush border membrane. One of these carriers is the Na^+-dependent/glucose transporter (SGLT1, see Chapter 8). It only functions if glucose, or galactose (which competes with glucose), is present in the lumen. The transporter has a binding site for glucose and a binding site for Na^+. Both binding sites must be occupied for the transport process to take place, and then both Na^+ and the hexose are transported into the cell via this co-port system (Fig. 7.12 and Chapter 8). The transport of Na^+ and glucose by this means is inhibited

by the presence of high concentrations of K^+ in the lumen. This is because K^+ occupies the Na^+ binding site to inhibit the transport process. Inside the cell, where there is a high concentration of K^+, the displacement of Na^+ from the carrier by K^+, may be responsible for Na^+ being released into the cell's cytoplasm. The transport of hexoses, including glucose, is described in more detail in Chapter 8.

Neutral amino acids also stimulate Na^+ absorption via a co-port system involving transporter molecules. This mechanism also depends on the Na^+ concentration gradient set up by the operation of the Na^+/K^+ ATPase pump in the lateral border of the cell (see Fig. 7.12 and Chapter 8).

The net rate of absorption of Na^+ is highest in the jejunum because the glucose and neutral amino acid transporters are situated mainly in this region. Sugars and amino acids produce a lesser stimulation of Na^+ absorption in the ileum where the transporters are less numerous.

The active transport of Na^+ out of the cell across the lateral border increases its concentration in the lateral spaces. Cl^- and other monovalent anions are transported down the electrical gradient created, mainly via the paracellular pathway, through the tight junctions, into the lateral spaces. This occurs in the duodenum, jejunum, and ileum, although the proportion transported via this route is greater in the duodenum, where the tight junctions are leakiest.

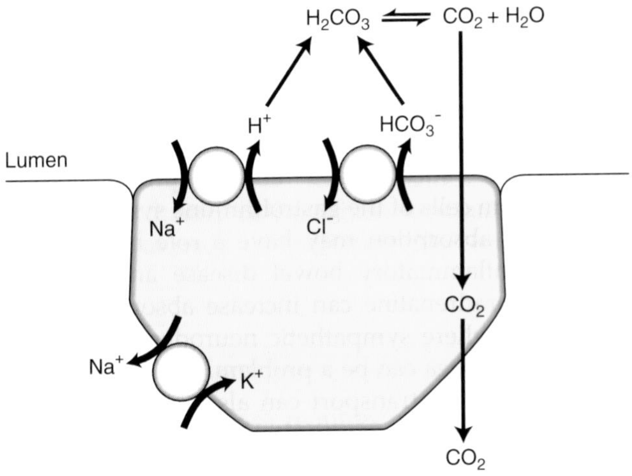

Fig. 7.13
The active transport of sodium and chloride ions via Na$^+$/H$^+$ exchange and Cl$^-$/HCO$_3^-$ exchange systems respectively, in the small intestine.

The accumulation of ions within the lateral spaces creates an osmotic gradient, and water is transported down this osmotic gradient, via the paracellular pathway, into the spaces. The spaces expand during a meal because of this increase in osmolarity. The transport of water out of the lumen results in concentration of the chyme. This increases the concentration, and therefore the concentration gradient, for ions such as K$^+$. These are then transported passively between the cells into the lateral spaces. Thus the transport of many substances ultimately depends on the active transport of Na$^+$ out of the epithelial cells.

Na$^+$ can also be actively absorbed in exchange for H$^+$, which is secreted into the lumen, i.e. via a N$^+$/H$^+$ exchange mechanism. This anion exchange operates in the small intestine and the colon. It is the major route for active Na$^+$ transport in the ileum where the glucose and amino acid transporters are less numerous than in the jejunum, and in the colon. However, the ileum and colon can absorb Na$^+$ against a higher potential difference than can the jejunum. The anion exchange mechanism is illustrated in Figure 7.13. The H$^+$ secreted into the lumen reacts with HCO$_3^-$ to form carbonic acid. The HCO$_3^-$ arises via transport out of the cells because of the operation of a Cl$^-$/HCO$_3^-$ exchange mechanism whereby Cl$^-$ is absorbed in exchange for HCO$_3^-$. Thus active transport of Na$^+$ and Cl$^-$ is coupled in this way. The carbonic acid formed in the lumen is hydrolysed to give CO$_2$ and water. CO$_2$ is lipid-soluble and it diffuses across the membranes of the cells into the blood. In this way H$^+$ and HCO$_3^-$ are effectively reabsorbed.

Cholera Box 5

Rehydration therapy

Individuals suffering from cholera are treated with (a) intravenous fluid and electrolytes, or (b) oral fluid, salt, and sugar.

Intravenous rehydration
The intravenous fluid consists of water containing electrolytes in concentrations that are isotonic with plasma. The massive fluid loss can lead to dehydration, hypovolaemia, renal failure, and death. Particular attention is paid to K$^+$ and HCO$_3^-$ replacement, as excessive losses of these ions can have rapid and dangerous consequences.

Oral rehydration therapy
The discovery of the co-port mechanisms for Na$^+$ transport in the small intestine has revolutionised the treatment of food poisoning due to *V. cholerae* or *Escherichia coli*, where excessive fluid loss and dehydration can occur. Prior to the discovery of the co-port mechanisms, approximately 50% of individuals suffering from cholera died because of collapse of the extracellular fluid volume (ECF). Treatment was by administration of large quantities of salt solution, a regime that was only partially effective. Oral rehydration therapy with a solution of glucose and common salt has dramatically reduced the death rate. The solution used should be isotonic or hypotonic, as a hypertonic load will create an osmotic gradient for the transport of more water into the lumen. Inflammation and damage to the mucosa are not normally present in cholera and the digestion and absorptive mechanisms are not affected in this disease. Therefore glucose can be replaced with table sugar (sucrose) as it is digested to glucose (and fructose). Replacement of glucose with starch can also be effective because digestion of each starch molecule results in numerous glucose digestion products, and it can therefore be ingested as a dilute solution, which does not constitute a great osmotic load.

Control of absorption

Various factors are involved in the control of water and electrolyte absorption by the cells near the tips of the villi. These include endocrine, paracrine, and nervous influences. Glucocorticoids stimulate electrolyte and water absorption in both the small and large intestines, gastrointestinal tract. This activity is tonus. Spontaneous contractions of smooth muscle occur in the absence of stretch, hormones or nervous activity, due to the uneven amplitude of the oscillating membrane potential (see Chapter 1). The inherent mechanisms of tone and rhythmicity may be augmented by a background of transmitters, such as acetylcholine released from nerves in the vicinity. This slow wave activity of the smooth muscle in the duodenum is influenced by that in the stomach. Longitudinal muscle fibres from the stomach cross the pyloric sphincter region to the duodenum (see Chapter 4). The frequency of contractions in the duodenum (approximately 12 per minute) is higher than in the stomach. Every fifth contraction of the muscle in the duodenal bulb is augmented by a contraction of the antrum due to the transmission of the slow waves via the fibres crossing the sphincter. This acts to prevent the duodenal contents flowing back into the stomach.

There is also a regular type of spontaneous contraction, known as the migrating myoelectric complex (MMC, see below), which moves distally down the intestine. Transmitters released during the progression of the MMC (see below) may be responsible for augmenting other types of spontaneous muscle activity. In addition catecholamines such as noradrenaline released from sympathetic nerves, and adrenaline released into the blood, during fasting and in times of stress, can reduce the tone of the smooth muscle.

The migrating myoelectric complex
In fasting individuals there are cycles of smooth muscle contractions with an average frequency of approximately 1.5 hours. These are the MMCs. Each cycle involves contraction of several adjacent segments of the small intestine and lasts 10 minutes or so. The contractions occur sequentially in adjacent groups of segments. They actually begin in the stomach and migrate via the proximal small intestine 'aborally' towards the colon (Fig. 7.14). In the fasting state the periodic sweeping of the contents towards the colon may clean the intestine of residual food and secretions. It may also prevent the migration of colonic bacteria into the ileum. As one sweep reaches the terminal ileum, another starts in the duodenum. MMCs also occur when a meal is being processed, but then they are more frequent and less ordered. They presumably then assist in sweeping the digested contents of the lumen towards the colon.

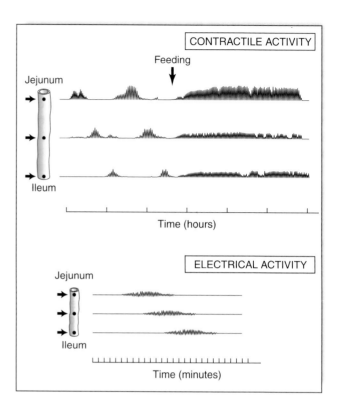

Fig. 7.14
The moving myoelectric complex.

Mixing and propulsion during a meal

Segmentation mixes the contents of the lumen when a meal is being processed, whilst peristalsis is responsible for propelling the chyme along towards the colon.

Segmentation

Segmentation involves contraction of rings of circular muscle situated at intervals along a region of the small intestine (Fig. 7.15). The contractions remain stationary. These rings of muscle then relax, and then adjacent segments contract. The overall effect is a continuous rhythmic division and subdivision of the intestinal contents, which results in a thorough mixing of the chyme in the lumen. Segmentation increases in frequency and strength when chyme enters the duodenum. It occurs more frequently in the duodenum (approximately 12 contractions per minute) than in the jejunum or ileum (approximately 8 contractions per minute). This is appropriate because the need for mixing is greatest in the duodenum where the alkaline pancreatic juice and bile mixes with acid chyme from the stomach to provide the appropriate neutral or slightly alkaline conditions necessary for digestion and micelle formation. Rhythmic (concertina-like) back and forth movements also occur, but may simply be as a result of segmentation. At any one time a

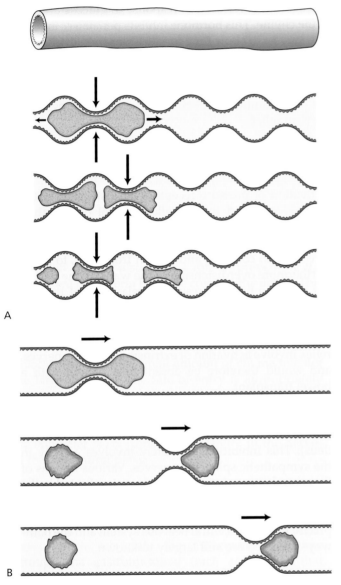

A

B

Fig. 7.15
Motility in the small intestine. (A) Segmentation, (B) peristalsis.

Peristalsis

Peristalsis involves the sequential contraction of adjacent rings of smooth muscle in the aboral direction, followed by relaxation of these rings of muscle, causing a wave of contraction that propels the chyme towards the colon (Fig. 7.14). In the human, after a meal has been eaten, peristaltic activity in the small intestine is infrequent and of low strength. Furthermore each wave of contraction travels only about 10 cm. It is for this reason that resection of segments of the intestine does not interfere with propulsion. However, there are occasional waves of intense contraction, known as peristaltic rushes, which travel the entire length of the small intestine. Both the short and the long waves are responsible for moving the chyme along the intestine towards the colon.

Contraction of the muscularis mucosae

In addition to the above types of motility due to contractions in the circular and longitudinal layers of muscle, sections of the muscularis mucosae undergo irregular contractions. These contractions assist in the mixing of the chyme. In addition the villi contract in an irregular fashion. Contractions of the villi are most frequent in the proximal small intestine. They squeeze the lacteals in the centre of the villi, thereby emptying them of lymph and enhancing intestinal lymph flow (see above).

Control of motility

Certain basic patterns of contractile activity may be programmed into the neural circuitry of the intrinsic nerve plexi. However, motility in the small intestine is under physiological control by various factors, including stretch, intrinsic nerves of the intramural plexi, extrinsic autonomic nerves, paracrine factors, and circulating hormones.

An intrinsic property of smooth muscle is reflex contraction in response to stretch of the muscle, without the involvement of nerves or hormones (see Chapter 1). This is known as the myenteric reflex. However, reflex contractile activity due to activation of pressure receptors and chemoreceptors in the walls of the intestine is probably more important when a meal is being processed by the small intestine.

Nervous control

Activation of the intrinsic nerves in the intramural plexi can control segmentation and short peristaltic

group of segments contract and this is followed by a period of rest. In the jejunum segmentation occurs as bursts of contractions that last approximately 1 minute, followed by an interval when the contractions are weak or absent. This pattern is known as the minute rhythm.

Contraction of a ring of smooth muscle forces the chyme forwards and backwards, but because segmentation is more frequent in the proximal regions, the chances of the material being pushed towards the colon are greater than it being pushed towards the stomach. Thus, although segmentation is responsible for mixing the chyme, it also aids propulsion of the chyme towards the colon.

THE SMALL INTESTINE

7

ment through the intestines and softens the rectal contents. Examples of emollients are didactyl sodium sulphosuccinate and liquid paraffin. Liquid paraffin can interfere with the absorption of fat-soluble vitamins, and for this reason it is now seldom used.

Bulk-forming agents

Bulk-forming agents, such as bran and methylcellulose, are generally the preferred treatment for constipation as they are free from side-effects, inexpensive, and probably the most acceptable and natural of the alternatives. They consist of non-digestible cellulose fibres that become hydrated in the intestines. This decreases the viscosity of the luminal contents to increase their flow through the intestines. Hydration causes them to swell, providing bulk, with consequent activation of the defaecation reflex (see Chapter 10).

Self-assessment case study: congenital chloridorrhoea

A premature infant who was born with a distended abdomen, developed diarrhoea soon after birth. The chloride content of the fluid on the infant's napkin was extremely high (95 mmol/L). The child appeared dehydrated and blood analyses showed that she was hyponatremic, hypochloremic, and hypokalaemic during the first week of life. Later she developed a metabolic alkalosis. Her faeces were acid. Fortunately she was quickly diagnosed as having congenital chloridorrhoea. In this condition the Cl^-/HCO_3^- exchanger is absent from the luminal membranes of the jejunum, ileum, and colon. The Na^+/H^+ exchanger is normal in this condition, but eventually the acidity of the luminal contents inhibits the Na^+/H^+ exchange mechanism as well. Initially, intravenous electrolyte replacement therapy was instituted, but after a few weeks, electrolyte replacement therapy (a solution of KCl and NaCl) was given orally.

After studying this chapter you should be able to attempt the following questions:

① Why are abnormally high amounts of Cl^- lost in the faeces?

② How does this defect result in diarrhoea?

③ Is the fluid likely to be due to the absence of the exchanger in the small intestine or the large intestine, or both? Explain your answer.

④ Why was it not necessary to include glucose in the oral replacement fluid?

⑤ Can you explain the development of alkalosis in the child?

⑥ Why were the child's faeces acid?

⑦ What is the basis of the oral replacement therapy with KCl and NaCl?

Self-assessment questions

① How does cholera toxin cause diarrhoea?

② How is the small intestine specialised for absorption?

③ What determines water absorption in the small intestine?

④ Can you describe three special mechanisms for the absorption of Na^+ ions in the small intestine?

⑤ Can you describe the four major mechanisms of diarrhoea?

⑥ Why is the small intestine longer after death?

⑦ What is the MMC?

⑧ What measures can be taken to alleviate constipation?

DIGESTION AND ABSORPTION

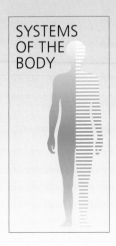

SYSTEMS
OF THE
BODY

Chapter objectives

After studying this chapter you should be able to:

① Explain the mechanisms of digestion and absorption of complex nutrients, vitamins, and minerals.

② Understand the consequences of malabsorption in intestinal diseases.

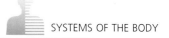
8

DIGESTION AND ABSORPTION

Introduction

Most digestion and absorption occurs in the small intestine. The transport of water, monovalent ions, and drugs was discussed in Chapter 7. In this chapter the digestion of complex nutrients, the absorption of the products of digestion, and the absorption of vitamins and minerals will be considered.

This chapter will address the consequences of disease of the small intestine for nutrition. As absorption of different nutrients can occur in different regions of the gastrointestinal tract, the regions affected by the disease process determine which nutrients will be poorly absorbed. Crohn's ileitis will be used to illustrate some of the general principles of absorption, as well as the specific problems encountered as a consequence of malabsorption of the nutrients that are normally absorbed in the terminal ileum.

Absorption

Most nutrients are absorbed at a slow rate by passive diffusion throughout the small intestine. However, many important nutrients are absorbed at a faster rate by processes that involve saturable mechanisms (see Chapter 1). The proximal small intestine, i.e. the duodenum and jejunum, is the location of most of these special mechanisms, and most substances are absorbed predominantly in the duodenum and jejunum. Figure 8.1 shows the approximate sites of absorption of many important nutrients. The important divalent cations, Ca^{2+} and Fe^{2+}, are absorbed mainly in the duodenum and jejunum. Hexoses, including glucose, galactose and fructose, are also absorbed in the duodenum and jejunum, as are amino acids, small (di- and tri-) peptides, and some water-soluble vitamins. Fatty acids, monoacylglycerols, and fat-soluble vitamins are also absorbed in the duodenum and jejunum. The main

Crohn's disease Box 1

Crohn's ileitis

A young man, 17 years of age, complained to his general practitioner that he had been suffering from abdominal pain, diarrhoea, and feelings of lassitude, as well as weight loss. The doctor examined him and found that his abdomen was distended. He ascertained that the abdominal pain was in the central and right lower quadrant. He suspected acute appendicitis and the patient was admitted to hospital. An abdominal operation was arranged. The surgeon observed that the appendix appeared normal. However, a short length of the terminal ileum was reddened, thickened, and oedematous. These features indicate terminal ileal Crohn's disease. No further surgery was performed. Following the operation, blood and faecal samples were obtained for analyses. The patient was allowed a few days to recuperate and then sent home. He was prescribed codeine for the pain, and diphenoxylate (Lomotil) for the diarrhoea, and he was started on oral steroids to reduce the inflammation. He was advised to try to keep to a nutritious diet. The acute symptoms gradually settled, but the patient suffered several relapses over the next few years, and his condition gradually progressed. He required intramuscular injections of vitamin B_{12} and iron supplements. He developed steatorrhoea (large, pale-coloured faeces). He eventually suffered an intestinal obstruction. He was maintained on intravenous parenteral nutrition for 2 weeks and during this time the symptoms diminished. However, they returned when the patient resumed normal nutrition. He was then subjected to an emer-

gency operation to remove the affected part of the ileum (which was causing the obstruction). Following the operation he made a good recovery. He resumed a normal diet and regained the weight he had lost. Later in life he developed symptomatic gallstone disease which required the removal of his gallbladder (cholecystectomy).

Upon consideration of the details of this case we can address the following questions:

① What is the basic defect in Crohn's disease and what causes it? Which parts of the gastrointestinal tract can be affected in this disease? How is it diagnosed? Which blood and faecal analyses would have assisted the diagnosis of Crohn's ileitis? Can we suggest the likely causes of the intestinal obstruction? How can the condition be treated?

② Why did this patient suffer from weight loss and tiredness? Why was this patient given intramuscular vitamin B_{12}? Why was the patient started on iron supplements?

③ Why were diarrhoea and steatorrhoea present?

④ What could be the cause of the gallstone disease in this patient?

⑤ Why was the patient maintained on parenteral nutrition for a while? What was the likely composition of the intravenous fluid used? What other measures can be taken to prevent malnutrition in this condition?

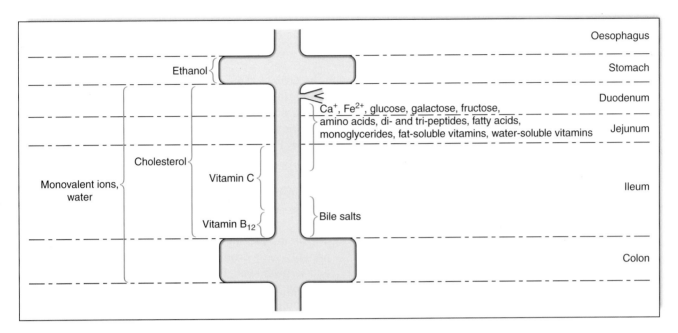

Fig. 8.1
Sites of absorption of important nutrients in the gastrointestinal tract.

exceptions are water and monovalent ions which are absorbed throughout the small and large intestines, cholesterol which is absorbed throughout the small intestine, vitamin C which is absorbed in the proximal ileum, and vitamin B_{12} and bile salts which are absorbed predominantly in the terminal ileum.

Carbohydrates

The average daily intake of carbohydrate in the human adult is probably between 250 and 800 g per day. The useful carbohydrate in the food is largely vegetable starch in potatoes, bread, pasta and rice, and to a lesser extent glycogen (animal starch) in meat and liver. These polysaccharides are composed entirely of D-glucose subunits linked together mainly by α-1,4 glycosidic linkages. In the human, over 90% of the starch in the diet is digested and absorbed. The remainder passes into the colon where it may be utilised by colonic bacteria.

Cellulose, also composed of glucose subunits, is present in the diet but is not digestible in humans and other non-ruminants because the subunits are linked by β-1,4 glycosidic bonds which cannot be hydrolysed by the enzymes in the digestive tract. Therefore it passes into the colon. Cellulose is nevertheless an important source of dietary fibre, providing bulk that stimulates intestinal motility and prevents constipation (see Chapter 10). In ruminants, cellulose is degraded by bacterial cellulases that hydrolyse the β-1,4 glycosidic linkages to produce D-glucose, which is absorbed.

There are appreciable amounts of disaccharides, including sucrose (table sugar), lactose (milk sugar), and maltose (malt sugar), in Western diets. The only free monosaccharide likely to be present in the diet is glucose, which is added to 'high energy' drinks and foods.

Dietary carbohydrate is utilised to provide energy for muscular and secretory activity and other metabolic functions. It is not 'essential' as a source of energy as calories can also be provided by fat and protein. However, a few carbohydrate substances, such as inositol, are 'essential' vitamin components of the diet, as they either cannot be synthesised in the body, or cannot be synthesised at a rate rapid enough to meet the body's requirements.

Structure of starch and glycogen

The molecular weight of vegetable starch ranges from a few thousand to 500 000. It consists of two components: amylose and amylopectin. In amylose the subunits are linked together in straight unbranched chains via α-1,4 glycosidic linkages. Amylopectin consists of branched chains, with branches occurring at approximately every 30th glucose residue. In this substance, α-1,4 linkages are present within the chains and α-1,6 linkages occur at the branch points (Fig. 8.3). Glycogen has a structure similar to amylopectin but the molecular weight is usually greater, between 270 000 and 100 000 000, and it has a more branched structure, the branches occurring every 8–10 glucose residues.

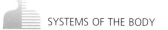
DIGESTION AND ABSORPTION

Crohn's disease Box 2

Defect, occurrence, diagnosis, and treatment

Crohn's disease is an inflammatory disorder that can affect any region of the gastrointestinal tract, from the mouth to the anus. However, the terminal ileum is the commonest site to be affected. In the mouth, aphthous ulcers of the buccal mucosa and tongue are seen. At the anus, skin tags, fissures and fistulae may be present. The disease is characterised by remissions and relapses. Macroscopically, the intestines appear red and swollen. Normal areas of tissue are usually present between the damaged areas. Because the inflammatory process involves all layers of the intestinal wall, diseased segments become grossly thickened. This can give rise to obstruction (Fig. 8.2). As the inflammation resolves, areas of secondary scarring (fibrosis) in the wall of the bowel also constitute obstructive regions. The mucous membrane appears 'cobble-stoned' due to longitudinal fissures and transverse oedematous folds. Aggregations of inflammatory cell infiltrates may be present, and the mesenteric lymph nodes may be enlarged due to re-active hyperplasia. Granulomas (aggregates of epithelial macrophages surrounded by a cuff of lymphocytes) may be present in the lymph nodes and the bowel wall.

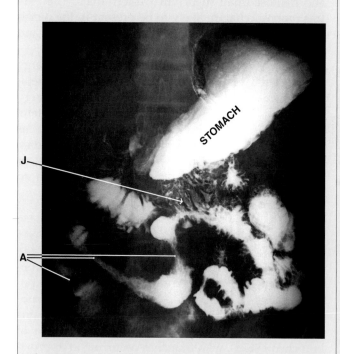

Fig. 8.2
An X-ray of the ileum, taken 15 minutes after ingestion of barium in a patient with Crohn's ileitis. Three narrowed segments of ileum are visible (strictures A). The normal mucosal folds of the proximal jejunum are also seen (J).

As Crohn's disease results in inflammation through the entire thickness of the bowel wall, and is often associated with obstruction of the faecal stream, the formation of enteric fistulae is a further feature of the disease. Fistulae may extend between different loops of the bowel (entero-enteric fistulae), or between the bowel and the skin (enterocutaneous fistulae, especially in the perianal areas). Gastrointestinal bleeding can also occur. This is usually mild but, because it is chronic, it can lead to iron-deficiency anaemia. There is also an increased incidence of malignant neoplasms in patients with Crohn's disease, especially in the small and large bowel. This may be related to the chronic damage of the bowel mucosa.

Crohn's disease is most commonly first diagnosed in young adults. The highest frequency is seen in Caucasians, and in the Western world. In the United Kingdom it affects approximately 50 individuals per 100 000 of the population, but its prevalence is higher because it is a chronic disease. The cause is unknown, but it is probably multifactorial. As it is an inflammatory disease infectious organisms, including the measles virus and *Mycobacterium pseudotuberculosis*, have been variously implicated.

Autoimmunity has also been suspected because there is an association with known autoimmune conditions such as arthritis and eczema. Inherited factors are also implicated because of the high concordance in monozygotic twins, and in families. Crohn's disease in children can lead to growth retardation and delayed sexual development, probably because of poor nutrition.

The diagnosis of Crohn's disease is difficult because all the salient features are seen in other disorders. A combination of histology, endoscopy, and radiology is usually employed. Evidence from blood analyses, including leukocytosis, elevated sedimentation rate, and thrombocytosis, is indicative of an active inflammatory process. Radiological evidence of the sites of involvement, and the chronic remitting course of the patient's illness also assist the diagnosis. However, a definitive diagnosis requires histological assessment of the bowel and identification of granulomata.

The management of patients with this disease includes i) treatment of the symptoms (diarrhoea, pain), ii) treatment with anti-inflammatory and immunosuppressive agents, iii) management of the patient's nutritional status, including enteral and parenteral nutrition (see below) and iv) surgical treatment of complications such as luminal obstruction.

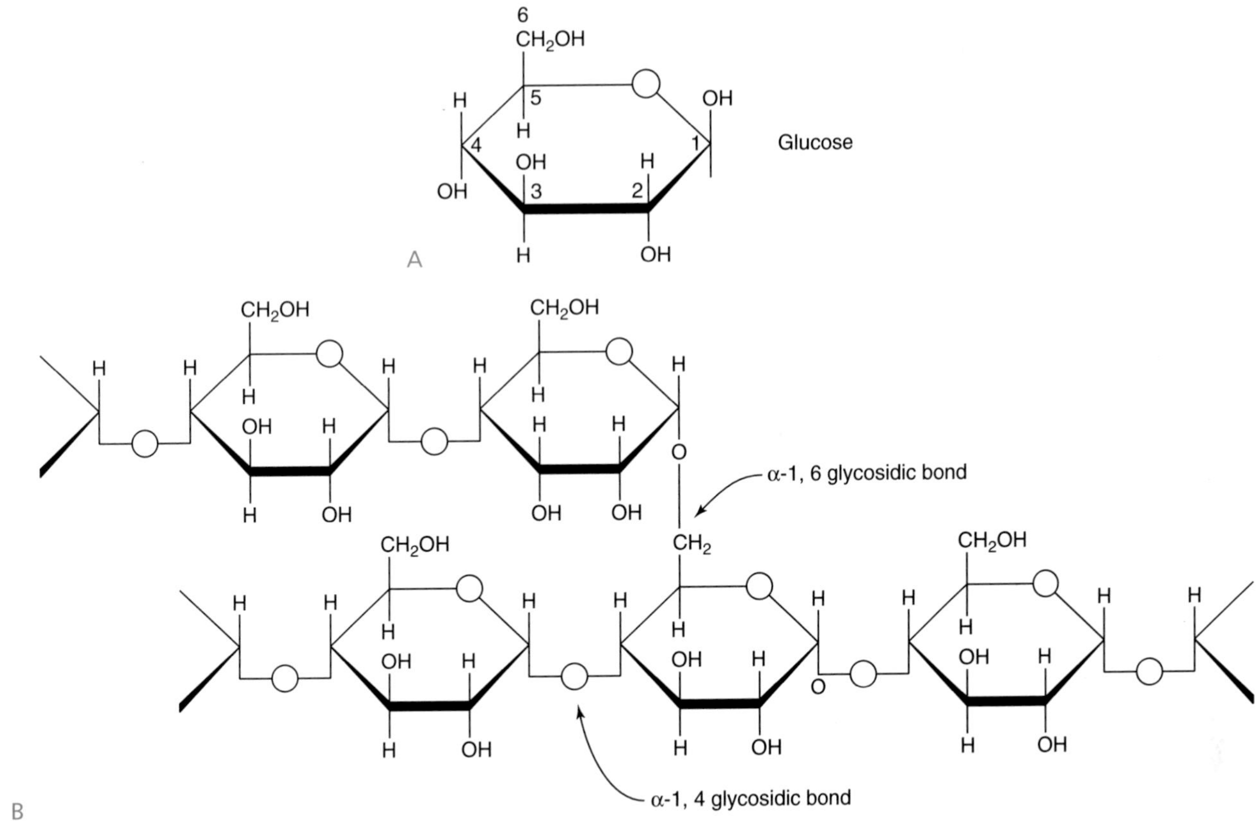

Fig. 8.3
(A) Structure of glucose showing the conventional numbering system for the carbon atoms. (B) Portion of an amylopectin molecule showing α-1,4 and α-1,6 glycosidic linkages.

Digestion of carbohydrate

In the gastrointestinal tract there are several enzymes that degrade starch and glycogen. These include the α-amylases secreted by the salivary glands and the pancreas, and isomaltase and glucoamylase which are integral components of the intestinal absorptive cell membranes. Maltose, sucrose, and lactose can also be degraded to their component monosaccharides by enzymes situated in the brush border of the upper small intestine (see below).

α-Amylases

α-Amylases split the α-1,4 glycosidic linkages in amylose to yield maltose and glucose, but they do not act on maltose, a disaccharide composed of two glucose subunits linked by an α-1,4 linkage. In theory, α-amylase will ultimately degrade a solution of amylose to maltose, and glucose which can be released from the ends of the chains (Fig. 8.4). Intermediate oligosaccharides (dextrins) are formed in the process. α-Amylases also attack amylopectin and glycogen at their α-1,4 linkages. Intermediate unbranched oligosaccharides and branched oligosaccharides (α-

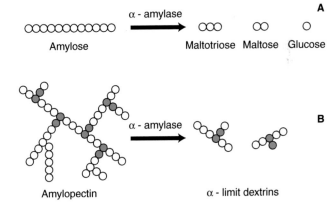

Fig. 8.4
Degradation of (A) amylose and (B) amylopectin, by α-amylases. The filled circles indicate glucose subunits with α-1,6, glycosidic linkages.

limit dextrins) are formed. Thus a mixture of products is produced (Fig. 8.4).

Salivary amylase starts the digestion of starch. It continues to act for up to half an hour in the interior of the food bolus after it has arrived in the stomach. It is even-

137

tually inactivated at the low pH produced by the gastric acid when it penetrates the food bolus. It can digest up to 50% of the starch present in food. Pancreatic juice, which contains a second α-amylase, is released into the duodenum when a meal is present in the digestive tract. Pancreatic amylase continues the digestion of starch and glycogen in the small intestine. It is produced in larger amounts than salivary amylase. The α-amylases from the two sources appear to be identical in their catalytic properties, despite having different amino acid sequences. They both require Cl⁻ for optimum activity and act at neutral or slightly alkaline pH values.

Role of brush border enzymes

The intestinal isomaltase (α-1,6 glycosidase) splits α-1,6 linkages in the branched poly- and oligosaccharides produced by amylase action in the small intestine. The combined action of α-amylase and α-1,6 glycosidase can degrade amylopectin and glycogen to a mixture of maltose and glucose, but there are other enzymes present in the brush border which function to speed up and complete the process of starch digestion. These are:

- glucoamylase, which degrades small unbranched oligosaccharides
- maltase and isomaltase, which degrade maltose and isomaltose respectively.

All of these enzymes have access to the mixture of polysaccharides, oligosaccharides, and disaccharides in the chyme in the small intestine during a meal.

The enzymes available to digest disaccharides are:

- maltase, which degrades maltose to glucose (see above)
- sucrase, which degrades sucrose to glucose and fructose
- lactase, which degrades lactose to galactose and glucose (Fig. 8.5).

Sucrase and isomaltase are synthesised as a single polypeptide chain inside the cell, and this is inserted

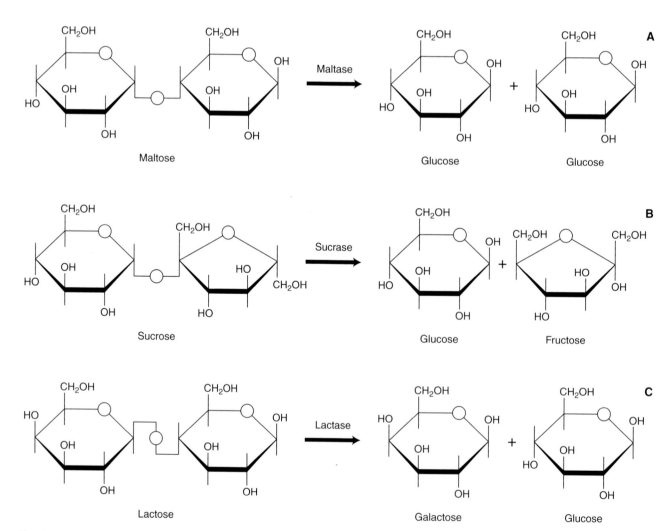

Fig. 8.5
Degradation of disaccharides by brush border disaccharidases. (A) Maltose, (B) sucrose, (C) lactose.

intact into the brush border plasma membrane. Pancreatic protease cleaves the polypeptide chain at a site between the active centres of the two enzyme moieties, but they remain non-covalently associated in the membrane. When sucrase is incorporated into artificial membranes it binds sucrose at one face and releases glucose and fructose on the other side of the membrane. This has led to speculation that it is both a hydrolytic enzyme and a transport molecule. The other brush border enzymes do not appear to behave in this way. These disaccharidases are all present in the brush border of the enterocyte, and it seems that the digestion of disaccharides and small oligosaccharides actually occurs in the membrane itself. This has been inferred from the fact that after administration of a solution of a disaccharide to an animal very little free glucose can be detected in the lumen, yet the disaccharide molecules are too large to diffuse through the pores in the membrane, and disaccharide molecules cannot be detected in the blood. It seems likely that the brush border enzymes occupy positions in the membrane which are adjacent to the hexose carriers. The release of monosaccharides occurs on the surface of the membrane and these are then transferred to the adjacent carrier molecule for transport into the cell (Fig. 8.6).

Monosaccharide absorption

The most abundant monosaccharides in dietary carbohydrate are the hexoses, D-glucose, D-galactose, and D-fructose, the products of digestion of starch, sucrose and lactose. Both L-hexoses and D-hexoses are absorbed slowly by passive diffusion in the gastrointestinal tract. However, the plasma membrane of cells is relatively impermeable to polar molecules such as monosaccharides and the transport of these sugars into the enterocyte by passive diffusion is therefore slow. Glucose, galactose, and fructose are absorbed by saturable mechanisms, mainly in the duodenum and jejunum. This is accomplished by membrane-associated transporters located in the brush border and basolateral membranes of the mature enterocytes. These bind the sugars and transfer them across the cell membranes and deliver them to the interstitial fluid in the lateral spaces, from where they are taken up into the adjacent capillaries to enter the portal blood.

Pentoses are smaller than hexoses but they are absorbed at a slower rate than glucose, galactose and fructose, indicating that they are probably absorbed by passive diffusion.

Hexose transporters

There are two types of hexose transporter in mammalian cells: Na$^+$/glucose cotransporters which are involved in the secondary active transport of glucose, and Na$^+$-independent facilitative hexose transporters. Two forms of the Na$^+$-dependent transporter have been identified. These are SGLT1 and SGLT2, but only SGLT1 is present in the small intestine. There are at least five functional isoforms of facilitative transporter (GLUT1, GLUT2, GLUT3, GLUT4, and GLUT5). All mammalian cells express at least one of these transporters. The most studied is GLUT4, an insulin-sensitive glucose transporter present in muscle and adipose tissue (see Chapter 9). GLUT1, GLUT2, and GLUT5 are all present in the enterocyte. Figure 8.7 shows the structures of the SGLT1 and GLUT1 transporters, and their conformations in the membrane. The two molecules exhibit many similar features. The specificity of the transporters is shown in Table 8.1.

The uptake of glucose across the enterocyte plasma membrane involves the binding of glucose to the Na$^+$/glucose cotransporter SGLT1, as described in Chapter 7. SGLT1 is present only in mature enterocytes in the upper regions of the villi. Galactose also binds to this carrier, but fructose does not. Glucose and galactose transport into the epithelial cell is via secondary active transport. The energy required is derived from the coupling of sugar transport to

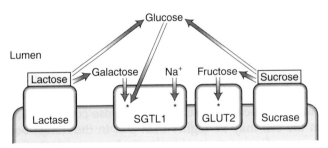

Fig. 8.6
Disaccharidases and hexose transporters in the brush border membrane. The enzymes reside in the brush border in close proximity to the hexose transporters. Disaccharides and oligosaccharides are degraded in the membrane by the enzymes, and the products are either transferred to other enzymes for further degradation or, in the case of monosaccharides, to the appropriate transporter.

Table 8.1
Specificity of transporters for hexoses in the enterocyte

Transporter	Glucose	Galactose	Fructose
SGLT1	+	+	−
GLUT1	+	+	−
GLUT2	+	+	+
GLUT5	−	−	+

Protein

In the Western hemisphere, the amount of protein in the average diet exceeds that required for nutritional balance. The dietary requirement for protein in the human adult is between 30 and 50 g per day. Protein is required to supply the eight 'essential amino acids', which the body cannot synthesise or cannot synthesise rapidly enough, and to replace nitrogen lost in the urine. In addition to that which is ingested, 10–30 g of protein (enzymes, mucins etc.) are secreted into the digestive tract each day. An additional 25 g or so are derived from epithelial cells that have been shed into the lumen. Most of this protein is digested and absorbed; approximately 10–20 g, derived from cell debris and colonic microorganisms, is eliminated in the faeces each day.

Digestion

Proteins are high molecular weight substances composed of up to 20 different amino acids, joined together in peptide linkages (Fig. 8.9). In the adult, most protein is degraded in the digestive tract to small peptides and amino acids. This is accomplished by a variety of proteolytic enzymes. These can be divided into two categories: endopeptidases and exopeptidases. Endopeptidases cleave peptide bonds in the centre of the peptide chains, the initial products being mostly large peptides, which are subsequently degraded to oligopeptides. Exopeptidases cleave bonds at the ends of the peptide chain, splitting off amino acids one by one, in a stepwise manner: carboxypeptidases act at the C-terminal, and aminopeptidases at the N-terminal. Enzymes that specifically attack dipeptides and tripeptides are also present. The combined actions of these enzymes digest proteins to small peptides and amino acids.

Digestion in the stomach

Pepsin is an endopeptidase secreted by the stomach as an inactive precursor, pepsinogen, which is activated by gastric juice (see Chapter 3). It favours peptide linkages where aromatic amino acids are present. It is responsible for the digestion of only approximately 15% of dietary protein. Protein digestion is not impaired in the absence of pepsin because other proteases are available.

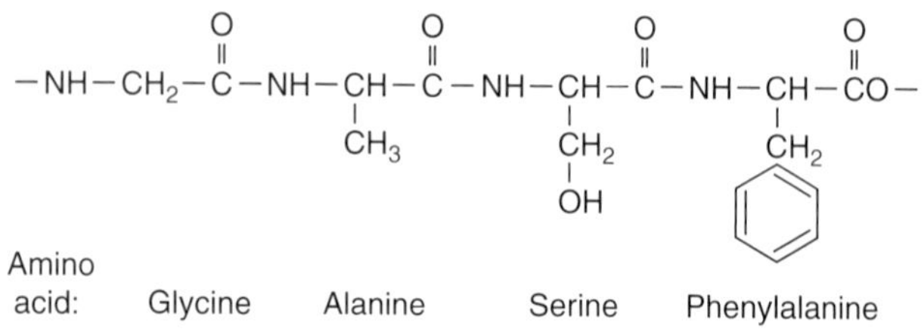

Digestion in the small intestine

Pancreatic juice contains three endopeptidases, trypsin, chymotrypsin, and elastase (Fig. 8.10). Trypsin prefers peptide linkages where the carboxylic acid group is provided by a basic amino acid, and chymotrypsin linkages where the carboxylic acid group is provided by an aromatic amino acid. Elastase degrades elastin. Pancreatic juice also contains two carboxypeptidases (A and B). Carboxypeptidase A has the highest specificity for bonds where the C terminal amino acid is basic, such as lysine or arginine. The pancreatic enzymes are secreted as inactive precursors which are converted to the active enzymes in the duodenum (see Chapter 5). They all have slightly alkaline pH optima. At least 50% of the protein ingested is normally degraded in the duodenum.

A number of peptidases reside in the brush border of the enterocyte. They are most abundant in the cells in the jejunum. The active sites of these enzymes face the intestinal lumen and they act in situ, upon contact with the protein in the chyme. Enterocyte peptidases also act in the lumen where they are present as components of

Fig. 8.9
Part of a peptide chain showing three peptide linkages.

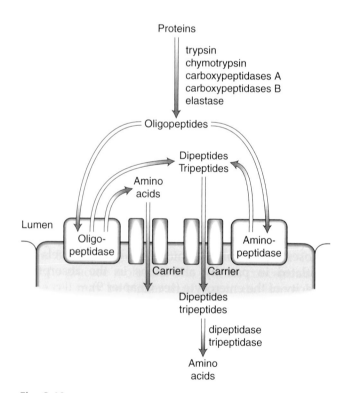

Fig. 8.10
Digestion of proteins and peptides, and absorption of di- and tripeptides and amino acids in the enterocyte.

disintegrating cells that have been shed from the tips of the villi. One of the brush border enzymes is leucine aminopeptidase. Others are oligopeptidases, which degrade small peptides such as tetrapeptides. There is also a dipeptidyl aminopeptidase, which removes dipeptides from the N-terminal of proteins.

The products of proteolytic digestion are tetrapeptides, tripeptides, dipeptides, and some amino acids. Tripeptides, dipeptides, and amino acids are transported into the epithelial cells. The dipeptides and tripeptides are degraded to amino acids by cytosolic tripeptidases and dipeptidases in the endothelial cells (see below). These relationships are represented in Figure 8.10.

Absorption of protein products

Mechanisms exist in the digestive tract for the absorption of both small peptides and amino acids. In addition, traces of intact protein are absorbed in some human adults.

Amino acids

The transport of amino acids across the membranes of the enterocytes into the blood can occur via passive diffusion, facilitated diffusion, or active transport. Relatively hydrophobic amino acids such as tryptophan are transported to an appreciable extent by passive diffusion. Only the L-isomers of amino acids are absorbed by facilitated diffusion and active transport. They are absorbed in the jejunum and the upper ileum. Carrier systems for amino acids exist in the brush border and the basolateral border (Table 8.2). At least seven specific transport systems are present in the brush border membrane, and at least three are present in the basolateral membrane. The transport of most amino acids occurs against a concentration gradient, and therefore depends on active mechanisms. Each carrier is shared

by a group of amino acids. Those which share the same transport mechanism compete with each other for a binding site on the carrier protein. The membrane locations of the transporters that have been characterised are indicated in Table 8.2.

Five of the known amino acid transport systems in the brush border are Na^+-dependent co-porters, which operate in a manner resembling that of the SGLT1 glucose transporter (see above and Chapter 7). The pumping of Na^+ ions across the basolateral membrane produces concentration and electrical gradients that favour Na^+ transport into the cell. This provides the driving force for the operation of the co-transporters in the brush border. These are therefore secondary active transport mechanisms. The five transporters have the following specificities:

1. small neutral amino acids
2. neutral amino acids, basic amino acids, and cystine
3. acidic amino acids
4. imino-amino acids
5. β amino acids (mainly taurine).

The other two brush border transporters do not require the presence of Na^+ ions in the lumen. One of these transports neutral amino acids, basic amino acids and cystine, and the other transports basic amino acids.

Three transporters in the basolateral border are collectively responsible for the facilitated diffusion of neutral and basic amino acids into the lateral spaces (Fig. 8.11). These transporters are present in many different types of cell. Acidic amino acids such as glutamate and aspartate are utilised by the enterocyte as energy substrates, and do not appear to be transported out of the cell by specific carrier mechanisms. The basolateral membrane also expresses carriers that transport amino acids from the fluid in the lateral spaces into the enterocyte, where they are used for protein synthesis. These systems

Table 8.2
Carriers involved in amino acid absorption in the enterocyte

Location	Carrier	Na^+-dependence	Amino acid specificity
Brush border	B	Yes	Neutral
Brush border	$B^{0,+}$	Yes	Neutral, basic, and cystine
Brush border	Imino	Yes	Imino (proline, hydroxyproline)
Brush border	X_{AG}	Yes	Acidic
Brush border	β	Yes	β, mainly taurine
Brush border	$b^{0,+}$	No	Neutral, basic, cystine
Brush border	y^+	No	Basic
Basolateral border	asc	No	Small neutral
Basolateral border	y^+	No	Basic
Basolateral border	L	No	Large, hydrophobic neutral

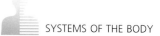

8

DIGESTION AND ABSORPTION

be formed in the skin from 7-dehydrocholesterol, under the influence of sunlight. Vitamin D_3 is converted to 1,25-dihydroxy vitamin D_3 via reactions occurring in the liver and kidneys. This vitamin behaves as a hormone in the body, and it circulates via the blood to control Ca^{2+} metabolism and homeostasis in various tissues. It is a steroid molecule that binds to nuclear receptors in the enterocytes of the small intestine to stimulate the synthesis of the brush border and cytosolic binding proteins. It also stimulates the synthesis of the basolateral Ca^{2+}-ATPase pump. Absorption of Ca^{2+} ions is also stimulated by parathyroid hormone, another hormone intricately involved with Ca^{2+} homeostasis in the body. The mechanism of action of parathyroid hormone in the small intestine is not clearly understood, although one effect is to stimulate the formation of 1,25-dihydroxy vitamin D_3. By these mechanisms the body maintains a balance between Ca^{2+} absorption and utilisation. Excess absorption results in increased Ca^{2+} excretion in the urine, which can lead to precipitation of insoluble salts such as calcium oxalate, which in turn can lead to formation of urinary tract stones.

Bile salts indirectly facilitate the absorption of Ca^{2+} ions by promoting the formation of micelles in the lumen of the small intestine (see below and Chapter 6). This is partly because vitamin D is fat-soluble and its absorption depends on micelle formation, and partly because bile salts help to hold fatty acids in the micelles, thereby preventing them from forming insoluble Ca^{2+} soaps, which cannot be absorbed. Thus bile salt deficiency can result in negative Ca^{2+} balance (see Chapter 6). Another consequence of calcium soap formation is that Ca^{2+} is not available to precipitate oxalic acid, a constituent of certain foods such as rhubarb. As a consequence, in bile salt deficiency where calcium soaps are formed, oxalic acid can be absorbed up to 5 times more rapidly than normal. Calcium oxalate kidney stones can also develop in such individuals because of the high levels of oxalate in the blood.

Calcium absorption is facultatively regulated to meet the needs of the body. The ability to absorb Ca^{2+} ions via enhanced active transport is increased by calcium deprivation. Young and growing people absorb Ca^{2+} more rapidly than do mature and elderly people. Lactating women require Ca^{2+} for milk production, and they absorb Ca^{2+} avidly.

Rickets and osteoporosis

Calcium deficiency leads to rickets in children and osteoporosis in adults. These diseases can be caused by a deficiency of vitamin D or a diet low in calcium. It has been shown in animals with rickets caused by vitamin D deficiency, that their brush border membranes are deficient in IMCal transporter molecules.

However, if vitamin D_3 is administered, the binding protein appears in the brush border within 90 minutes of the vitamin being ingested.

Iron

The average dietary intake of iron in the adult is approximately 20 mg per day. The proportion which is absorbed is regulated to meet the body's needs. Iron deficiency results in iron-deficiency anaemia, a condition in which haemoglobin synthesis is defective. It causes tiredness because the body's requirement for oxygen is not being met. In the normal adult very little iron is required because most of the iron released from erythrocytes at the end of their lifetime is recycled. The adult male or non-menstruating female loses approximately 0.6 mg per day. Menstruating women lose on average approximately 1.2 mg per day (averaged over the monthly cycle). The amount absorbed in the small intestine is equal to the amount lost; i.e. probably only 3–4% of the amount ingested, but its rate of absorption is increased when more iron is required, for example after a haemorrhage.

Iron is ingested in several forms. The major component in normal meat-eating individuals is haem, the product of proteolytic degradation of haemoglobin and myoglobin in the intestines. Haem contains iron in the divalent ferrous iron (Fe^{2+}) form. Fe^{2+} and ferric iron (Fe^{3+}) salts are usually present in the food. Thirty to 50% of the iron present in haem is released in the stomach lumen. Iron tends to form insoluble complexes that are only slowly absorbed, such as hydroxides, phosphates and bicarbonate, with the anions present in digestive secretions. It also forms insoluble complexes with tannins, phytins, and fibre present in the food. These complexes are more soluble at low pH and their absorption is stimulated by the presence of gastric acid. Furthermore various components of food such as ascorbate (vitamin C) form soluble complexes with iron, thereby preventing it from forming insoluble complexes. Ascorbate also reduces Fe^{3+} to Fe^{2+}. Fe^{2+} has a lower tendency to form insoluble complexes and so is better absorbed than Fe^{3+}. Fe^{2+} also binds to gastroferritin, a protein secreted by the oxyntic cells of the stomach (see Chapter 3), which keeps it in an absorbable form. Removal of the stomach can lead to the development of iron-deficiency anaemia as a consequence of the absence of gastric acid and gastroferritin (see Chapter 3).

Haem and Fe^{2+} ions, but not Fe^{3+} ions, are absorbed in the small intestine. Figure 8.14 illustrates these processes. The haem molecule consists of a porphyrin moiety containing bound Fe^{2+}. It is absorbed intact into the enterocyte via facilitated diffusion. Once inside the cell the Fe^{2+} ions are liberated from the molecule in a

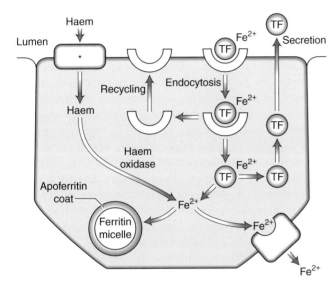

Fig. 8.14
Fe^{3+} transport in the absorptive cell. TF, transferrin.

reaction catalysed by xanthine oxidase (haem oxidase). The free Fe^{2+} ions produced are then processed in the same way as inorganic Fe^{2+} ions absorbed from the lumen.

A small amount of Fe^{2+} is transported in ionic form into the blood, but most of it is absorbed by combination with transferrin, a protein secreted into the lumen by the epithelial cells of the duodenum and jejunum. Each molecule of transferrin binds two Fe^{2+} ions. The complex binds to a transferrin receptor in the brush border membrane of the epithelial cells in the duodenum and jejunum. The receptor-transferring–iron complex is internalised via endocytosis. The receptor then releases the complex inside the cell, and Fe^{2+} ions are then released from the complex. The transferrin and the receptor are resecreted into the intestinal lumen. Most of the liberated Fe^{2+} ions enter a store within the cell (see below) but some of them bind to a receptor on the lateral border of the cell and are actively transported into the blood. In the blood the receptor binds to another transferrin molecule, which transports it to the tissues. The transferrin in the blood is similar but not identical to that released (from the epithelilal cell) into the intestinal lumen.

Iron is stored within the enterocyte as a salt, in combination with apoferritin, a β-globulin made up of 24 subunits. The synthesis of apoferritin is stimulated by iron. The complex of Fe^{2+} salts with apoferritin is known as ferritin. Ferritin forms a micelle that consists of ferric hydroxyphosphate surrounded by apoferritin subunits. Each micelle can contain as many as 4000 atoms of iron. When iron ingestion is increased, more iron is bound in the mucosal cells, partly because iron stimulates the synthesis of apoferritin, and so absorp-

tion into the blood is increased only slightly. The iron complexes in the enterocyte comprise a storage pool which is not usually absorbed. The iron in this pool is lost when the cells which contain it are shed from the villi. The cells disintegrate in the intestinal lumen and the liberated iron is eliminated in the faeces. Ferritin is the principal storage form of iron in tissues. It contains around 27% of the body's iron.

Mucosal cells, which are loaded with iron, have a reduced ability to take up iron. This prevents the absorption of excessive amounts, which can be toxic. Haemachromatosis is a condition that develops when there is prolonged excessive absorption of iron. It may be caused by excessive dietary intake, and is characterised by excessive deposits of ferritin and haemosiderin (another iron binding protein) in tissues. It can result in pigmentation of the skin, pancreatic damage leading to 'bronze' diabetes, cirrhosis of the liver, and (as a consequence) a high incidence of hepatic carcinoma. Ideopathic haemochromatosis is a congenital disorder characterised by a high rate of iron absorption in the presence of elevated, rather than depleted, body stores. In this condition the mucosal regulatory mechanism is impaired.

Haemorrhage

The amount of iron absorbed in the small intestine increases following a haemorrhage, but not until 3 days after the haemorrhage has taken place. This delay is due to the time taken for the absorptive cells to migrate from the crypts to the tips of the villi where they become mature. The message to increase the rate of iron absorption is given to the dividing cells in the crypts but they cannot absorb iron until they reach the tips of the villi.

The rate of iron absorption is also increased in iron-deficient individuals. One reason for this is that they have an increased number of transferrin receptors in their brush border membranes, but other mechanisms for increasing iron absorption may also be available.

Chronic iron deficiency results in iron-deficiency anaemia, a condition in which the red blood cells are characteristically small (microcytes) and contain a low concentration of haemoglobin (hypochromia). It may be of dietary origin, or due to chronic blood loss. 'Silent' chronic bleeding from the gastrointestinal tract is a feature of all gastrointestinal cancers, and for this reason any adult with unexplained iron deficiency should be investigated for tumours of the large bowel, stomach, and oesophagus.

Water-soluble vitamins

The water-soluble vitamins required by the body are vitamin C (ascorbate), which prevents scurvy and is present largely in fresh fruit, components of the vitamin B 'complex', including thiamine, riboflavin, biotin, pantothenic acid, niacin, pyridoxine, inositol, choline, and importantly folic acid and cobalamin (vitamin B_{12}). In the main, members of the B complex are found together in nature. Furthermore the overt manifestations of deficiency of members of this group, such as muscle weakness, fatigue and growth retardation, dermatitis and neuropathy, overlap. Water-soluble vitamins are required as cofactors in many metabolic reactions.

Most water-soluble vitamins are absorbed to an appreciable extent by simple passive diffusion, but for many, specific mechanisms are also available, although these are not all clearly understood.

Pyridoxine (vitamin B_6) appears to be transported solely via passive diffusion and then metabolised within the epithelial cell, but other known water-soluble vitamins can be absorbed by specialised saturable mechanisms. Biotin, inositol, choline, and riboflavin are absorbed by facilitated diffusion in the proximal small intestine, whilst pantothenic acid, thiamin, inositol, and nicotinic acid are absorbed by active Na^+-dependent mechanisms in the proximal small intestine. Folic acid (pteroylmonoglutamic acid) and pteroylpolyglutamates are absorbed by carrier-mediated facilitated diffusion in the jejunum. The polyglutamates are cleaved within the enterocytes to pteroylmonoglutamate. 5-Methyltetrahydrofolate, another dietary source of the vitamin, is absorbed by passive diffusion.

Ascorbate is absorbed mainly in the proximal ileum using a secondary active transport mechanism involving co-port with Na^+ ions, in the brush border. The operation of the Na^+/K^+ ATPase in the basolateral border provides the gradient for Na^+ transport into the cell.

Vitamin B_{12}

Vitamin B_{12} exists as four metabolically important forms in food – cyanocobalamin, hydroxycobalamin, deoxyadenosylcobalamin, and methylcobalamin – which are mostly bound to protein. This vitamin is required for red cell maturation. For this reason pernicious anaemia develops in vitamin B_{12} deficiency. The dietary requirement for vitamin B_{12} is close to the maximum absorptive capacity, but large quantities of the vitamin are stored in the liver and these stores would normally be sufficient for at least 3 years if the vitamin ceased to be absorbed (as after gastrectomy, see Chapter 3). Some is lost in the bile secreted by the liver, although most of this is reabsorbed.

The cobalamins are released from their protein complexes, in the stomach, by the action of pepsin. They are then rapidly bound to cobalamin-binding glycoproteins known as R proteins which are secreted in saliva and gastric juice. These complexes are degraded by pancreatic proteases. In pancreatic insufficiency when proteolytic enzymes are deficient, the complexes with R proteins are not degraded and the vitamin is not absorbed. Vitamin B_{12} then combines with another glycoprotein, intrinsic factor, which is secreted by the stomach (see Chapter 3). This complex is resistant to proteolytic degradation. The formation of the vitamin B_{12}–intrinsic factor complex is necessary for the vitamin to be absorbed via active transport in the terminal ileum. The complex is a dimer of intrinsic factor that binds two vitamin B_{12} molecules. The brush border membrane of the ileal epithelial cells contains receptors for the vitamin B_{12}–intrinsic factor dimer complex. It seems likely that the complex is split after binding to the receptor and vitamin B_{12} then enters the cell by an active transport mechanism. One possible scheme for its absorption is shown in Figure 8.15. The vitamin does not appear in the blood until 4 hours after it has been ingested. This delay may be due to its sequestration in mitochondria where it is metabolised. The mechanism of transport across the basolateral border is not known but most of the vitamin B_{12} appearing in the portal blood is bound to a globulin, transcobalamin II. This protein is synthesised by the cells in the ileum, as well as by the liver. The vitamin B_{12}–transcobalamin II complex is taken up

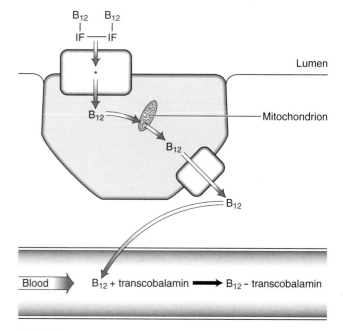

Fig. 8.15
Possible scheme for vitamin B_{12} absorption.

by receptor-mediated endocytosis in the liver and other tissues.

Vitamin B_{12} is also absorbed passively to some extent throughout the small intestine. Probably only 1–2% of the ingested vitamin is absorbed in this way, but if massive doses are eaten, enough can be absorbed to prevent pernicious anaemia. There is a shorter lag time involved in absorption by the passive mechanism than via the receptor-mediated mechanism.

Pernicious anaemia

Deficiency of intrinsic factor is the most common cause of pernicious anaemia. Historically, intrinsic factor extracted from hog stomach was administered in this condition, and the vitamin was then absorbed normally. Many patients developed antibodies to intrinsic factor in their blood and it was once believed that these may be antibodies to the foreign intrinsic factor. This led to the belief that the vitamin B_{12}–intrinsic factor complex was absorbed intact. However, it is now known that pernicious anaemia can be an autoimmune disease and so patients can have high antibody titres in their blood even when exogenous intrinsic factor has not been ingested (see below). Nowadays the vitamin is injected intramuscularly. This is usually only necessary once every 3 months, as it is stored in the liver.

Pernicious anaemia is usually due to atrophy of the gastric mucosa leading to the almost complete inability of the stomach to secrete intrinsic factor, HCl, and pepsinogen. It is only the lack of intrinsic factor that is serious if the gastric mucosa is atrophied, because pepsinogen and acid (which activates pepsin) are not essential (see above).

The complexity of vitamin B_{12} absorption is illustrated by the existence of three types of pernicious anaemia seen in childhood; an autoimmune condition, similar to that described above, a congenital deficiency of intrinsic factor with normal secretion of pepsinogen and acid, and congenital vitamin B_{12} malabsorption syndrome. In the latter, gastric function and release of intrinsic factor are normal but the absorption of vitamin B_{12} in the ileum is impaired, due to a defect in the receptors which bind the vitamin B_{12}–intrinsic factor complex.

Lipids

Dietary lipids

The range of fat ingested by an individual varies enormously. In Western countries it is probably between 25 and 160 g per day. Most ingested fat is neutral lipid (triacylglycerol) present in butter, margarine, cooking oil, meat etc. In addition some phospholipid and some

---

Crohn's disease Box 3

Anaemia

Anaemia is common in individuals with Crohn's disease, and contributes to the patient's lassitude and feelings of tiredness. There are a number of reasons for the development of anaemia in Crohn's disease:

① The nutrients absorbed specifically in the terminal ileum are vitamin B_{12} and bile acids (see below). Pernicious anaemia (caused by vitamin B_{12} deficiency) takes some years to develop in Crohn's disease as the liver stores of vitamin B_{12} are usually adequate for several years. However, if a large part of the ileum is diseased or resected, vitamin B_{12} deficiency will eventually develop, unless measures are taken to prevent it. The vitamin is administered if necessary, by intramuscular injections to bypass the gastrointestinal tract. The red blood cells fail to mature in vitamin B_{12} deficiency, and pernicious anaemia eventually results (see Chapter 3). It is characterised by a low red cell count, and high mean red cell volume (as immature red cells are larger than normal mature cells, i.e. they are 'macrocytic').

② Iron-deficiency anaemia is often present in Crohn's disease due to small but prolonged blood loss. It is characterised by a low blood haemoglobin concentration and small red cells (microcytes). Iron-deficiency anaemia is likely to be more severe if the proximal small intestine, where iron is absorbed, is affected, or if the patient restricts the consumption of meat.

③ Folate deficiency, which leads to macrocytic anaemia, can also occur if the jejunum is affected.

④ The abdominal pain and gastrointestinal colic experienced in Crohn's disease can inhibit food intake. The resultant dietary deficiencies will compound the problems due to malabsorption in this condition and can also contribute to the development of anaemia (especially iron-deficiency anaemia).

---

cholesterol ester, components of plant and animal cell membranes, are also present in the food, together with small amounts of other lipids.

Fat-soluble vitamins and essential fatty acids

Certain lipid molecules are 'essential' in the diet, as they are required in the body, but cannot be synthesised. These include the fat-soluble vitamins A, D, E and K, and the essential fatty acids. Deficiency of vitamin A results in hyperkeratosis of the skin, and xerophthalmia, a disturbance of epithelial tissues. In the human an early symptom of this condition is night blindness due to abnormal responses of the retinal rods. Vitamin D is required for Ca^{2+} absorption (see below) and for normal calcium and phosphate metabolism. Deficiency of vitamin D and the resultant Ca^{2+} deficiency leads to abnormalities in bones and teeth, parasthesiae (due to impaired nerve conduction), skeletal pain, and tetany (due to impaired muscle function). Vitamin E is an important antioxidant and deficiency in rodents causes sterility and muscle weakness, but its role in the human is not entirely clear. Vitamin K deficiency causes bleeding diathesis, due to defective blood coagulation as a result of failure to synthesise prothrombin which is required for blood clotting. Part of the vitamin K requirement of an organism may be supplied by bacteria which colonise the intestines. The essential polyunsaturated fatty acids linoleic acid (C18:2) and γ-linoleic acid (present in evening primrose oil), linolenic acid (C18:3), and arachidonic acid (C20:4) are required for the proper functioning of the nervous system. Under normal circumstances, less than 6 g of fat are eliminated in the faeces per day and most of this arises from bacterial cells and cell debris. If larger amounts of fat are eliminated the condition is known as steatorrhoea (see below) and indicates a deficiency in fat absorption.

Lipid solubility

Some lipids, for example short-chain fatty acids (with a carbon chain of less than 10), and some polyunsaturated complex lipids containing short-chain fatty acids or polyunsaturated fatty acids, are soluble in water. These are absorbed by passive diffusion. They dissolve in the membrane and are transported down their concentration gradients into the cell, and then into the portal blood. The transport of water-soluble lipids into the blood is a rapid process.

The digestion and absorption of most lipids are achieved by a variety of highly complex processes that enable the body to overcome the fact that most lipid is insoluble in water, but has to be transferred from the gut lumen to the lymph and eventually the blood via aqueous media; the chyme in the lumen, the cell's interior, the interstitial fluid, the lymph, and eventually the blood. A further problem is that the enzymes which catalyse the breakdown of the complex lipids, i.e. lipases, phospholipases, and cholesterol esterases, are all water-soluble and insoluble in lipid, but have to gain access to the lipid molecules before they can hydrolyse them. The mechanisms enabling these problems to be

overcome will be described after the reactions involved in the digestion of lipids have been outlined.

Digestion

The digestion of triacylglycerol is catalysed by lipases (glycerolester hydrolases). The major lipase in the digestive tract is secreted by the pancreas. Minor lipases are present in saliva (lingual lipase) and gastric juice, but these are probably only important when the pancreatic enzyme is absent or inactive. The pancreatic enzyme cleaves the ester bonds on positions 1 and 3 in the triacylglycerol molecules, in a stepwise manner, with the formation of 1,2 diacylglycerol and 2,3 diacylglycerol intermediates. The ultimate products are 2-monoacylglycerol, which is absorbed without further degradation, and fatty acids. The overall reaction is given in Figure 8.16.

Cholesterol esterase is secreted in pancreatic juice. In intestinal chyme, it forms dimers that are resistant to proteolytic digestion, and cleaves the ester bond in cholesterol ester with the formation of free cholesterol and fatty acid (Fig. 8.16). It also acts more slowly to hydrolyse triacylglycerol, lysophospholipids, monoacylglycerols, and esters of fat-soluble vitamins.

Phospholipase A_2 is secreted in pancreatic juice as an inactive precursor. It is activated in the small intestine (see Chapter 5). It cleaves the ester bond at the 2 position in many phospholipids, including phosphatidylcholine (lecithin), phosphatidylserine, and phosphatidylethanolamine, to give fatty acid and lysophospholipid. The hydrolysis of phosphatidylcholine is shown in Figure 8.16.

Emulsification

The process of emulsification is essential for the efficient digestion of lipids. It enables the enzymes involved to gain access to their lipid substrates. If oil is added to water it forms a layer on top of the water because it is insoluble, and is less dense than water. If some lipase is added it dissolves in the water layer and will only attack the lipid at the lipid–water interface. Therefore the rate of lipid hydrolysis is proportional to the surface area of the lipid–water interface. In the small intestine the surface area of the lipid–water interface is increased by the process of emulsification, whereby the large droplets of lipid are broken down into tiny droplets that can be held in a stable suspension. The lipid–water interface is consequently increased enormously, enabling lipid digestion to proceed at a rapid rate.

The process of emulsification requires conjugated bile acids, which coat the lipid droplets and prevent

1. Triacylglycerol

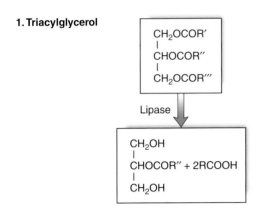

2. Cholesterol ester

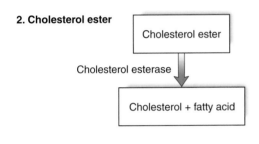

3. Phospholipid

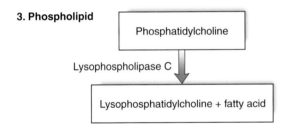

Fig. 8.16
Digestion of complex lipids in the small intestine.

them coalescing together. These substances are secreted in bile. Within 20 minutes of the beginning of a meal the gallbladder contracts and empties concentrated bile into the duodenum. The structure and release of the bile acids is discussed in Chapter 6. The emulsified droplets are 0.5–1.0 mm in diameter. A neutral or slightly alkaline environment is required for emulsification. This is normally provided by the intestinal chyme in which the alkaline secretions mix with the acid from the stomach and neutralise it.

Lipase is essentially inactive in the presence of bile acids, but colipase, a small protein (MW 10 000) present in pancreatic juice, forms a complex with lipase and bile acid, and this enables the colipase–lipase complex to spread over the surface of the minute droplets and hydrolyse the triacylglycerol present. Triacylglycerol is hydrolysed on the surface of the emulsion droplets and the products of digestion, monoacylglycerol and fatty

acids, are liberated from the droplets into the aqueous medium. The hydrolysis of triacylglycerol under these circumstances is more rapid than the absorption of its products. A small proportion of the fatty acids released from the droplets is water-soluble (see above), and this can be absorbed directly into the blood. However, most free fatty acids and monoacylglycerols are insoluble in water. They would soon saturate the chyme and separate out into large droplets again, if it were not for a process known as micelle formation.

Micelle formation

A micelle is a lipid particle 4–6 nm in diameter which consists of an aggregate of approximately 20 lipid molecules. Bile acids are required for micelle formation. Bile itself contains micelles composed of bile salts, cholesterol and phosphatidylcholine (see Chapter 6) but in the small intestine the micelles have a more heterogeneous composition. The process of micelle formation is discussed in Chapter 6. In the small intestine, the initial constituents of the micelles in the duodenum are bile salts and 2-monoacylglycerols. These micelles then sequester other fat-soluble substances, such as long-chain fatty acids, cholesterol, fat-soluble vitamins, and phospholipids. An individual micelle may contain several or all of these molecules, although fatty acids are quantitatively the most important. Cholesterol, long-chain fatty acids and fat-soluble vitamins, which are highly insoluble in water, are maintained in the core region of the micelle. Monoacylglycerol and lysophospholipids orientate themselves so that their acyl chains are in the core region, and their more polar regions project towards the aqueous phase (i.e. in the shell region). Bile salts are present in the shell region. The polar groups on the bile salt impart a negative charge to the surface of the micelles. This causes mutual repulsion between different micelles, keeping them in stable suspension in the chyme. The negatively charged shell collects cations such as Na^+, which form an outer shell around the micelle. When the bile acid concentration is at, or above, its critical micellar concentration, the bile acid and insoluble lipids such as monoacylglycerol aggregate as micelles. With increasing bile acid concentration more monoacylglycerol molecules are carried as micelles. In the normal human the critical micellar concentration is usually well below the concentration actually present, and micelles easily form. There are certain disease states, however, such as obstructive jaundice (see Chapter 6), where the concentration is too low. The critical micellar concentration (see Chapter 6) is higher for unconjugated bile acids than for conjugated bile acids. Consequently if a considerable fraction of the bile acids is deconjugated in the intestinal lumen by bacterial action, micelle formation may be impaired.

Most fatty acids and monoacylglycerol are absorbed in the duodenum and upper jejunum, while the bile acids are absorbed more distally in the ileum. Cholesterol can be absorbed throughout the length of the small intestine, although a considerable proportion of it escapes into the colon. Thus the composition of the micelles changes as they move down the small intestine; their content of fatty acids and monoacylglycerol diminishes whilst their proportional content of bile acids increases.

The constituent lipid molecules of micelles move back and forth between the micelles and the aqueous solution with great rapidity. The aqueous chyme is kept saturated with lipid molecules by the movement of fatty acids and monoacylglycerol from the micelles into the solution. Thus the micelles serve as a reservoir of these products so that the aqueous phase in contact with the enterocyte brush border is always saturated with lipid molecules and a dynamic equilibrium between the micelle and the solution is established. The dissolved fatty acids can be absorbed. However, the micelles first have to diffuse across the 'unstirred layer' to the enterocyte cell membrane.

The unstirred layer

The unstirred layer is a layer of fluid in contact with the epithelial surface, which does not readily mix with the bulk of the chyme. It is 200–500 mm thick. Micelles and nutrients have to diffuse through this layer to the surface membrane of the enterocyte. Thus there is a concentration gradient of nutrients across the unstirred layer with the lowest concentration at the epithelial surface. A pH gradient also exists across the unstirred layer, with the fluid in contact with the brush border being slightly more acid than the bulk of the chyme. This promotes the absorption of fatty acids as they tend to be less ionised, and therefore more easily absorbed across the lipid membrane.

Fate of lipid in the epithelial cell

Lipids can dissolve in the lipid of the brush border membrane and easily diffuse across it. The transported lipids are metabolised within the cell and used in the resynthesis of complex lipids (Fig. 8.17). Triacylglycerol is synthesised via both the α-glycerolphosphate pathway, which also operates in liver and other tissues, and via the monoacylglycerol pathway, which involves direct esterification of monoacylglycerol by fatty acyl-S-CoA, a pathway restricted to the mucosal

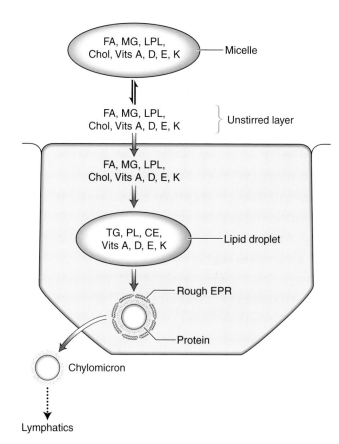

Fig. 8.17
Transport of lipids in the enterocyte. MG, monoacylglycerol, LPL, lysophopholipid, TG, triacylglycerol, PL, phospholipid, FA, fatty acids, Chol, cholesterol, Vits, vitamins, CE, cholesterol ester.

cell (Fig. 8.17). Phospholipid is synthesised by esterification of lysopholipid with fatty acyl-S-CoA and cholesterol ester by esterification of free cholesterol with fatty acyl-S-CoA (Fig. 8.18). The complex lipids are formed in the smooth endoplasmic reticulum of the enterocyte. The complex lipid molecules aggregate together to form droplets within the cell. The phospholipids form at the surface of the droplets, with their polar heads oriented towards the exterior of the droplets. The droplets become surrounded with rough endoplasmic reticulum and the ribosomes synthesise a β-lipoprotein, which, together with the phospholipid, forms a coat around the droplets (Fig. 8.17). The droplet with its protein and phospholipid coat is known as a chylomicron. Chylomicrons vary in size from a few nm to 750 nm in diameter. The different lipids, including the fat-soluble vitamins, are sequestered together in the same chylomicrons. In individuals with the inherited disorder β-lipoproteinaemia, synthesis of β-lipoprotein is defective or absent and then only large chylomicrons, if any, are formed, and fat absorption is impaired.

Crohn's disease Box 4

Steatorrhoea

In Crohn's disease of the ileum, fat absorption is usually impaired. This is largely a consequence of defective bile acid absorption (which occurs mainly in the ileum, see below), which results in a low total bile acid pool.

Bile acids are important for both the emulsification of lipid nutrients and micelle formation. Moreover bacterial overgrowth is seen in the small bowel in Crohn's disease if the flow of intestinal contents is obstructed, and this can result in deconjugation of bile acids by the bacteria. Unconjugated bile acids exhibit a higher critical micellar concentration, and therefore micelle formation may be impaired, compounding the fat malabsorption seen in the disease. Moreover the intestinal and mesenteric lymphatics may be extensively involved in Crohn's disease, and this can also contribute to impaired fat absorption. The unabsorbed fat is eliminated in the faeces (a condition known as 'steatorrhoea'). Malabsorption of complex lipids leads to a reduced calorie intake, but this may not be important if carbohydrate absorption is unaffected.

In Crohn's disease, severe malabsorption of the fat-soluble vitamins A, D, and K occasionally results in hyperkeratosis of the skin (due to vitamin A deficiency), Ca^{2+} malabsorption (due to vitamin D deficiency), which in turn can result in demineralisation of bone and tetany (see above), and blood clotting defects (due to vitamin K deficiency).

The chylomicrons are extruded from the lateral surface of the cell and taken up into the lymph in the lacteals. After a meal the intestinal lymph becomes milky due to the presence of chylomicrons. The uptake of chylomicrons into the lymph is stimulated by the adrenocorticoid hormones, and fat absorption is depressed in adrenalectomised animals.

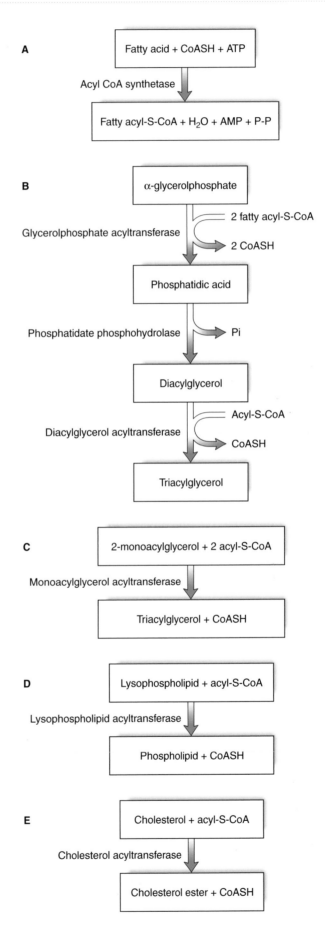

Fig. 8.18
Synthesis of complex lipids in the small intestine. (A) formation of acetyl-S-CoA, (B) synthesis of triacylglycerol via the α-glycerol phosphate pathway, (C) synthesis of triacylglycerol via the monoacylglycerol pathway, (D) synthesis of phospholipid from lysophospholipid, (E) synthesis of cholesterol ester from cholesterol.

Bile acids

Modification of bile acids in the small intestine

Bile acids are modified by intestinal bacteria. Primary bile acids are converted to secondary bile acids by dehydroxylation (see Chapter 5). Therefore excessive bacterial action can lead to a greater proportion of secondary bile acids in the bile acid pool. In addition, a portion of the bile acids can be deconjugated by bacterial enzymes with the release of the amino acid moieties. Conjugated bile acids have lower pKa values than the unconjugated acids, and are therefore more ionised and more water-soluble at the slightly alkaline pH of the intestinal chyme. As they are ionised they exist as salts with Na^+ and other cations.

Absorption

Bile acids are absorbed from the ileum into the portal blood and transported to the liver (see Chapter 6). The absorption in the small intestine is by both active and passive mechanisms. The active transport occurs only in the terminal ileum, and only ionised conjugated bile acids are absorbed by this active process. It is very efficient and normally only approximately 5% of conjugated bile acids reach the colon. The active transport is via a co-port carrier molecule in the brush border membrane, which also transports Na^+, in a manner similar to that in the hepatocyte (see Chapter 6). The driving force for the transport across the brush border is the electrochemical gradient created by the pumping of Na^+ out of the cell. The process whereby bile acids are transported out of the enterocyte has not yet been characterised.

Un-ionised conjugated bile acids are more fat-soluble than the ionised (conjugated) molecules. Glycine is a weak acid and a fraction of the glyco-conjugates is un-ionised and therefore fat-soluble. A small amount of it is absorbed passively through the lipid membrane. Taurine conjugates are almost completely ionised at the pH of the small intestine and are therefore not absorbed in this way. Excessive deconjugation of conjugated bile acids by intestinal bacteria leads to decreased absorption and a greater loss to the colon with a resulting decrease in the size of the bile acid pool. However, unconjugated bile acids are more fat-soluble than conjugated bile acids and a proportion is absorbed by passive transport in the intestines.

Bile pigments

Bile pigments are lipid substances with limited solubility in aqueous solution. Unconjugated bilirubin is more lipid-soluble than conjugated bilirubin, and it

---

Crohn's disease Box 5

Bile acid malabsorption

Bile acids are normally actively absorbed in the terminal ileum, and recycled via the enterohepatic circulation (see Chapter 6). They are essential for lipid absorption. In Crohn's ileitis a reduced bile acid pool is present because bile acid absorption in the ileum is impaired. This is largely due to the reduced surface area available for absorption and loss of bile acid transporters. However, if bacterial overgrowth is present, enzymes in the bacteria can deconjugate the bile acids, and unconjugated bile acids are not as rapidly absorbed as the conjugated derivatives. If excessive bile acids are lost in the faeces, the liver cannot replace them by de novo synthesis rapidly enough to replace them. This results in fat malabsorption (see above).

A reduced bile acid pool can result in cholesterol not being held in micellar suspension and it precipitates out to form gallstones (cholelithiasis, see Chapter 6). Disruption of the enterohepatic circulation of bile acids is probably the reason there is an increased incidence of gallstone disease in individuals with Crohn's disease.

The diarrhoea present in Crohn's disease is partly 'osmotic' (see Chapter 7), due to quantities of unabsorbed nutrients and bile acids creating an osmotic gradient for water transport into the lumen. However the diarrhoea is also due to the stimulation of propulsive motility by bile salts entering the colon. In addition unabsorbed fats entering the colon can be hydroxylated by bacteria, and the hydroxylated fats can stimulate colonic motility.

---

can be absorbed by diffusion across the lipid membrane of the enterocyte. Bacterial action in the intestines deconjugates some of the conjugated bile pigments with the result that some bile pigment is reabsorbed into the portal blood. The metabolism of bile pigments by bacteria and their absorption via the enterohepatic circulation is described in Chapter 6.

Fat malabsorption

Fat digestion and absorption is a very complicated process necessitating the proper functioning of many organs, including the liver, the pancreas, and the small intestine. For this reason many different defects of digestion and absorption can result in malabsorption of fats and steatorrhoea. Some of these defects and the diseases responsible are listed in Table 8.3. Malab-

Table 8.3
Some defects in fat digestion and absorption

Disease site	Defect	Consequence
Liver or biliary tract (e.g. gallstone disease, cirrhosis)	Deficiency of conjugated bile acids and HCO_3^-	Impaired emulsification Impaired micelle formation
Pancreas (e.g. chronic pancreatitis)	Deficiency of lipase and HCO_3^-	Impaired digestion
Intestines (e.g. Crohn's disease, coeliac disease)	Reduction in surface area	Impaired absorption
β-Lipoproteinaemia	Impaired protein synthesis	Impaired chylomicron formation
Lymphatics (obstruction)	Impaired transport to lymph	Impaired transport to blood
Adrenals	Deficiency of adrenocorticoid hormones	Impaired transport to lymph

sorption diseases include Crohn's disease, coeliac disease and a somewhat similar condition known as tropical sprue, Whipple's disease which is due to a bacterial infection, various conditions caused by parasitic infestation and abetalipoproeinaemia (see above). Malabsorption of fat can be overcome by ingestion of water-soluble short-chain fatty acids, which are easily absorbed into the portal bloodstream from the small bowel.

Malabsorption can result from:

1. enzyme deficiency (often inherited)
2. bile salt deficiency (liver disease)
3. drug therapy
4. infection
5. mucosal disease of the small bowel (coeliac disease).

Enzyme or bile salt deficiency will result in failure to break down long-chain fatty acids, allowing them to pass into the large bowel without being absorbed. Drugs such as cholecystyramine have the same effect by binding bile salts thereby preventing them from forming micelles. Disease of the mucosa reduces the absorption of digested fatty acids due to reduction in the surface area for absorption and impairment of transport mechanisms. This can occur in inherited disorders such as coeliac disease, or acquired disease such as Crohn's disease. Occasionally radiotherapy may damage the mucosa and lead to malabsorption.

The manifestations of malabsorption syndrome may be local to the gastrointestinal tract, and include steatorrhoea, diarrhoea, and abdominal distension, or systemic effects. Systemic effects include:

1. weight loss
2. anaemia due to deficiency of iron, vitamin B_{12}, or folate
3. bleeding disorders due to vitamin K deficiency
4. peripheral neuropathy, dermatitis, and hyperkeratosis, due to deficiency of vitamin A or vitamins of the B complex

Crohn's disease Box 6

Treatment of malnutrition

In Crohn's ileitis, malnutrition is due to many different factors. Malabsorption of fat and fat-soluble vitamins as a consequence of defective bile acid absorption is often a major problem. Iron-deficiency anaemia can result from chronic bleeding. If the proximal small intestine is involved, lactase deficiency, resulting from loss of mature enterocytes, can occur leading to milk intolerance (see above). There can also be a severe loss of protein, including albumen, across the region of ulcerated mucosa in the intestine. This can result in hypoalbumenaemia and ascites (a fluid transudation into the peritoneum). Deficiencies of vitamins of the B complex can lead to a red tongue, cracked lips, dermatitis, and peripheral neuropathy.

Thus blood tests for anaemia should be carried out, and plasma albumen and vitamin concentrations should be determined.

Vitamin supplements can be given when there is evidence of deficiencies. Medium-chain triacylglycerols, which contain fatty acids that can be absorbed directly into the blood in the absence of bile acids, can be substituted for long-chain triacylglycerols in the diet, and this reduces the steatorrhoea. Total parenteral nutrition (intravenous feeding) can be used in extreme cases to rest the bowel and allow healing. It involves the intravenous administration of amino acids, glucose, and lipid in amounts sufficient to meet the protein and energy needs of the individual, and electrolytes, vitamins and minerals in amounts sufficient to meet the estimated daily requirements. In patients with Crohn's disease total parenteral nutrition can lead to positive nitrogen balance, weight gain, and temporary remission of symptoms.

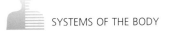
8

DIGESTION AND ABSORPTION

5. effects on the musculoskeletal system which lead to osteopaenia and tetany, due to deficiency of vitamin D and Ca^{2+}

6. endocrine disorders resulting from general malnutrition

7. oedema caused by deficient protein absorption.

Self-assessment case study: coeliac disease

A 25-year-old woman visited her doctor and complained of diarrhoea and flatulence. She also said she had recently lost a considerable amount of weight, and felt weak and exhausted most of the time. She also suffered from back pain. Upon questioning she said her faeces were bulky, greasy, and foul-smelling. She recalled that she had had persistent diarrhoea throughout childhood but the symptoms had disappeared during adolescence. She was referred to a gastroenterologist. The consultant arranged for blood and faecal analyses. The faecal tests confirmed the presence of steatorrhoea. The blood tests indicated that she had iron-deficiency anaemia, and folate deficiency, as well as Ca^{2+} deficiency. Her blood electrolyte concentrations and prothrombin clotting time were within the normal range. The consultant suspected coeliac disease and arranged for an endoscopy (telescopic visualisation of the duodenum) to be performed. A biopsy of the mucosa was taken at the examination which showed flattening of the villi and excess plasma cells in the submucosa (Fig. 8.19). In view of these findings the consultant told the patient to exclude wheat, rye, barley, and oat flours from her diet, but to try to ensure that it was nutritionally balanced. She was prescribed iron, folate, and vitamin D supplements. This diet was not easy to follow as so many food products contain the flours, but after a few weeks the patient was vastly improved. She had gained weight and was no longer feeling constantly tired.

Coeliac disease is due to an abnormal reaction to gluten, a constituent of wheat flour that damages the enterocytes, causing atrophy of the villi and malabsorption. The damage is due to an abnormal immune response to gliadin, a component of gluten. The cells cannot be replaced quickly enough by stem cell division in the crypts, and many of the cells present are immature and therefore do not absorb nutrients effectively. The duodenum and proximal jejunum are usually more severely affected than the ileum. The production of duodenal hormones such as CCK and secretin, may also be deficient.

After reading this chapter you should be able to answer the following questions:

① Why was steatorrhoea present in this patient?

② What are the likely causes of diarrhoea in coeliac disease?

③ What is the cause of malabsorption of nutrients in this condition?

④ Why was iron-deficiency anaemia present?

⑤ If the duodenum and proximal jejunum were the only regions of the small intestine involved, which nutrients are likely to be malabsorbed?

⑥ What problems result from deficiencies of these nutrients?

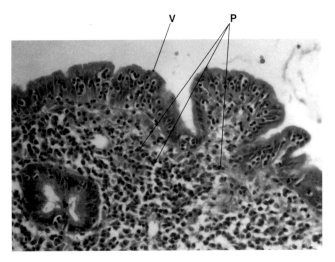

Fig. 8.19
Section through the jejunal mucosa, showing the flattened villi (V), and plasma cell infiltrate (P) typical of coeliac disease.

⑦ How would a defect in CCK and secretin release affect the functioning of the digestive system?

⑧ Why was the patient's clotting time measured?

⑨ Is milk intolerance likely to be a complication in this condition?

⑩ Why were the patient's blood electrolyte concentrations measured?

Self-assessment questions

① Which enzymes are available for starch digestion in the digestive tract?

② How is glucose absorbed in the enterocyte?

③ Which products of protein digestion are absorbed in the small intestine?

④ What is the mechanism of vitamin B_{12} absorption in the ileum?

⑤ What are the roles of vitamin D in the process of Ca^{2+} absorption?

⑥ In which forms can iron be absorbed in the small intestine?

⑦ What is the role of xanthine oxidase in iron absorption?

THE ABSORPTIVE AND POSTABSORPTIVE STATES

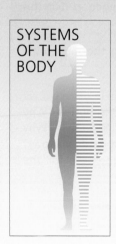

SYSTEMS
OF THE
BODY

Chapter objectives

After studying this chapter you should be able to:

① Understand how nutrients are utilised during the absorptive state to provide energy, and how energy is provided when nutrients are not being absorbed.

② Consider how the absorptive and postabsorptive patterns of metabolism are controlled by hormones, and how this control is impaired in diabetes mellitus.

Introduction

The nutrient state of the blood depends on whether or not a meal is being processed in the gastrointestinal tract. When nutrients such as glucose and lipid are being absorbed, and their levels in the blood are high, the pattern of energy metabolism is known as the absorptive state. In this state a fraction of the blood glucose is used by various tissues to meet their immediate energy needs. The excess glucose and the absorbed lipid are stored as glycogen in liver and muscle, and lipid in adipose tissue. These stores can be used to provide energy between meals or during fasting, a pattern of energy metabolism known as the postabsorptive state. The change from one pattern of metabolism to the other is brought about by changes in the blood levels of insulin and other hormones. The importance of maintaining the appropriate patterns of metabolism can be illustrated by considering the metabolic defects present in insulin-dependent diabetes mellitus (IDDM, or type I diabetes), in which the secretion of insulin is severely impaired. In this chapter we shall mainly consider the metabolic abnormalities present in diabetes, and their consequences.

The absorptive state

In the absorptive state, the nutrients entering the blood from the gastrointestinal tract are hexose sugars (glucose, fructose, galactose) and amino acids. The liver is the first port of call for these absorbed nutrients. It initially takes up a large fraction of the nutrients, thereby altering the composition of the blood before it is circulated to the rest of the body. The nutrients remaining in the blood are taken up by adipose tissue, muscle, and other tissues. Most lipids are absorbed from the small intestines into the lymph as components of chylomicrons. They enter the venous blood at the thoracic duct, and are then metabolised and stored in adipose tissue.

Fate of absorbed carbohydrate

Absorbed carbohydrate consists of glucose, galactose, and fructose. However, the liver converts fructose and galactose to glucose, which it then releases into the blood. It is expedient therefore to consider absorbed carbohydrate as glucose. Figure 9.1 illustrates the various fates of glucose during the absorptive state.

Diabetes-IDDM Box 1

Insulin-dependent diabetes mellitus

A 12-year-old girl was taken to see her doctor. Her parents were worried because she seemed listless and was losing weight. They said she also seemed to be drinking a lot and was frequently having to pass urine. The doctor noticed that her breathing was rapid and shallow, and that her breath smelled of acetone. The patient provided a sample of urine. Clinistix tests on the urine sample indicated the presence of glucose and ketones. An appointment was made for her to attend a diabetes clinic. She was told to fast from the previous evening before she attended for the appointment. A blood sample was taken and the blood glucose concentration was found to be 11.1 mmol/L. This is above the normal range (3.5–7.0 mmol/L), indicating the presence of severe hyperglycaemia (high blood glucose). Severe hypo-insulinaemia (low plasma insulin), metabolic acidosis and ketoacidosis (high levels of ketone bodies in the blood) were also noted. The results confirmed that the patient was severely diabetic. She was later taught how to inject herself with insulin, which had to be done three times a day, before meals. Although the information was not volunteered, the girl had recently had to have a number of teeth filled.

After considering the details of this case we can address the following questions:

① Is this patient likely to be suffering from IDDM or non-insulin-dependent diabetes mellitus (NIDDM, type 2 diabetes)? What are the basic defects in each condition? Would the levels of plasma insulin be low in both conditions? Why had this young patient required so many teeth filled?

② What is the explanation for the listlessness of this patient?

③ How is blood glucose normally controlled in the absorptive state, and how is this changed in diabetes mellitus?

④ What are the mechanisms causing the high urine output (polyuria) in this patient?

⑤ Why did the patient's breath smell of acetone? Why was her urine analysed for ketone bodies? Why was this patient's acid–base status changed? Why was her breathing abnormal (rapid and shallow)? How would the body normally compensate for the acidosis?

⑥ Are hormones other than insulin also affected in diabetes?

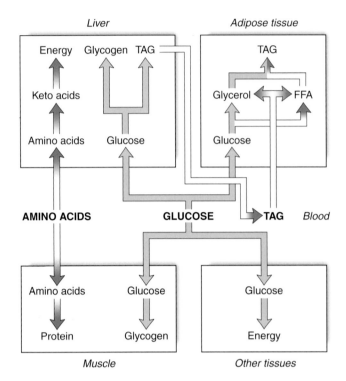

Fig. 9.1
Energy metabolism in the absorptive state. TAG, triacylglycerol, FFA, free fatty acids.

where it is converted to fatty acids and α-glycerolphosphate, which are used in the synthesis of triacylglycerol. The α-glycerolphosphate pathway for triacylglycerol synthesis is outlined in Chapter 8.

Thus, during the absorptive phase, glucose is used for energy production by most tissues of the body, and the excess is stored in muscle and liver as glycogen, and in adipose tissue as fat. These relationships are outlined in Figure 9.1.

Fate of blood triacylglycerol

Absorbed triacylglycerol is carried in the lymph as droplets partially coated with protein, known as chylomicrons (see Chapter 8). The triacylglycerol synthesised from glucose in the liver is also released to circulate in the blood, but as components of very low density lipoproteins (see above). The blood enters the adipose tissue where the lipids present in both very low density lipoproteins and chylomicrons are hydrolysed to fatty acids and glycerol by a lipoprotein lipase present in the endothelial surfaces of the capillaries. Most of the fatty acids produced are taken up into the adipose cells by passive diffusion, although a small fraction circulates to the liver and other tissues. The glycerol produced is either taken up by the adipose tissue cells (adipocytes) or transported to other tissues. In adipocytes, the fatty acids and glycerol are reconstituted to triacylglycerol via the α-glycerol phosphate pathway (see Chapter 8), and stored in the cells. Thus, during the absorptive state, triacylglycerol in adipose tissue arises from three sources: absorbed glucose, very low density lipoproteins released from the liver, and dietary triacylglycerol present in chylomicrons. These relationships are summarised in Figure 9.1.

Adipose tissue is abundant in the body and is widely distributed in subcutaneous, perirenal, mesenteric, and other regions. An adipocyte contains a small amount of cytoplasm, which surrounds a large lipid droplet. There is very little water present in adipose cells. Lipid has a very low density. It provides a very efficient storage form of energy: 1 gram of triacylglycerol containing more than twice as many calories as 1 gram of glycogen or protein. Moreover, a 70 kg man has approximately 15 kg triacylglycerol, which provides 135 000 kcal of energy but only approximately 0.2 kg of glycogen, providing only 800 kcal of energy.

Fate of absorbed amino acids

In the absorptive state, a fraction of the absorbed amino acids is taken up by the liver and converted to keto acids, which are oxidised via the citric acid cycle and other pathways. Keto acids are the liver's main

A large fraction of the absorbed glucose enters the various cells of the body where it is used for the production of energy. During the absorptive state glucose is the main fuel for most of the tissues of the body, which utilise it by glycolysis (Fig. 9.8, page 165), the citric acid cycle, and other pathways.

The rest of the absorbed glucose is used to provide stores of energy for later use during the postabsorptive (fasting) state (see below). The tissues that store most of the body's energy are liver, adipose tissue, and muscle. Glucose is taken up by all of these tissues in the absorptive state.

Some of the glucose taken up by the liver is converted to glycogen, which is then stored in the liver and some is converted to triacylglycerol. The glucose provides both the glycerol and the fatty acid moieties of triacylglycerol. Some of the triacylglycerol synthesised in the liver is stored there, but most is released into the blood as a component of very low density lipoproteins, which are metabolised and stored in adipose tissue (see below). Very little glucose and fat is utilised for energy in the liver itself. (The liver's main source of energy in the absorptive state is amino acids, see below.)

Another fraction of the blood glucose enters skeletal muscle where it is converted to glycogen for storage in the muscle. A further fraction enters adipose tissue,

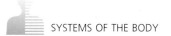

source of energy in the absorptive state. Excess keto acids can be converted to triacylglycerol in the liver. The conversion of amino acids to keto acids involves deamination, with the formation of ammonia, which is converted to urea in the liver. The urea is released from the liver into the blood, and subsequently excreted by the kidneys.

Amino acids not taken up by the liver enter other tissues, such as muscle, where they are utilised for protein synthesis. Muscle is quantitatively the most important tissue in this respect. Protein is not a particularly labile source of energy, but it is broken down and used for energy during prolonged fasting. Figure 9.1 summarises the events occurring in the absorptive state.

Insulin

Insulin has a central role in the control of metabolism. If it is injected, the absorptive state is duplicated, and if its levels are very low, as in untreated IDDM, the pattern of metabolism that predominates is an exaggerated version of that seen in the postabsorptive state. Insulin is a polypeptide (MW 6000), consisting of two peptide chains connected together by two disulphide bridges (Fig. 9.2). The prohormone precursor of insulin is a single peptide chain (MW 9000) known as proinsulin, which is converted to insulin by proteolytic cleavage. This results in the removal of a peptide, known as C-peptide. In the prohormone, C-peptide connects the two peptide chains of insulin (Fig. 9.2). Both insulin and the C-peptide are stored in granules in the β-cells of the pancreas.

The release of insulin into the blood is stimulated by eating and inhibited by fasting, and insulin is largely responsible for promoting the pattern of metabolism seen in the absorptive state. High levels of glucose and amino acids in the blood (as when a meal is being processed) are the primary stimuli for insulin secre-

tion. The hormone acts on most tissues of the body, but muscle, adipose tissue, and liver are quantitatively the most important. However, some tissues, such as brain and erythrocytes, which are obligatory utilisers of glucose for fuel, are not sensitive to insulin.

Control of insulin secretion

Insulin is a protein hormone secreted by the islets of Langerhans in the pancreas. It is released by exocytosis in response to raised intracellular Ca^{2+} levels (see Chapter 5). The second messengers involved include cAMP, but intracellular inositol trisphosphate and diacylglycerol, which activates protein kinase C, are also increased. The release of insulin from the pancreas is controlled to a large extent by the levels of glucose and amino acids in the blood perfusing the pancreas. Other factors such as hormones and neurotransmitters potentiate or inhibit the effects of the blood nutrients on insulin secretion.

Control by glucose

The secretion of insulin in response to an increase in blood glucose is under feedback control. After a meal the blood glucose increases as it is absorbed from the gastrointestinal tract. This results in stimulation of insulin secretion from the β-cells of the islets of Langerhans. These cells respond to both the actual glucose concentration, and the rate of change of glucose concentration in the blood. The effect is due to the uptake and intracellular metabolism of glucose in the β-cells. Glucose is transported into these cells via the GLUT2 transporter. The enzyme glucokinase, which catalyses glucose 6 phosphate formation from glucose, the rate-limiting step in glycolysis (see Fig. 9.8, page 165), is a key mediator in the β-cells. However 3-carbon compounds such as glyceraldehyde, which are intermediates formed downstream from glucose 6 phosphate in the glycolytic pathway, are as potent as glucose in stimulating insulin release. The mechanism depends on the generation of ATP via glucose metabolism. Closure by ATP of an ATP-sensitive K^+ channel, which results in depolarisation of the cell, causes a voltage-dependent Ca^{2+} influx. Elevated intracellular Ca^{2+} then causes insulin exocytosis.

Suphonylureas such as tolbutamide, which are used to treat non-insulin-dependent diabetes (NIDDM, see below) stimulate insulin secretion by binding to a component of the K^+ channel in the membrane, and directly closing it. On the other hand, diaxozide which is used to treat hyperinsulinaemia, opens the K^+ channel and reduces insulin secretion.

Insulin lowers blood glucose by promoting its uptake into cells (see below). Thus as the concentra-

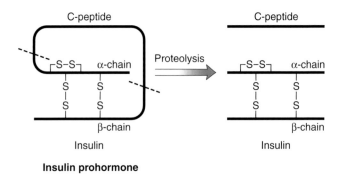

Fig. 9.2
Proteolytic processing of the insulin prohormone to insulin and C-peptide.

Diabetes-IDDM Box 2

Defect and cause

The patient was probably suffering from IDDM (type 1 diabetes). This condition mostly affects young people, the commonest age of onset being between 10 and 14 years, whereas NIDDM usually affects people in middle or later life. Hyperglycaemia is a characteristic of both conditions. In IDDM it is due to severely reduced secretion of insulin as a result of necrosis of the pancreatic β-cells. In NIDDM, extensive destruction of β-cells does not occur, and the plasma insulin level can be normal or elevated early in the course of NIDDM as a result of stimulation of the β-cells by the raised blood glucose. In the patient described above, insulin levels were low. In NIDDM there is severe resistance of the tissues to the actions of insulin. However, except in the advanced stages, the extent of the metabolic disturbance is usually less severe in NIDDM than in IDDM. Thus, for example, ketoacidosis (see below) is not usually a feature of NIDDM.

IDDM affects both sexes equally, but there is a slightly earlier peak in age of onset in girls than boys. It is more prevalent in Caucasians than non-Caucasians, and more prevalent in people living in the Northern hemisphere than in the Southern hemisphere. There is a higher incidence of first diagnoses in winter than summer. The frequency of the disease has been increasing during the last 50 years or so. However, only approximately 15% of diabetic patients suffer from IDDM (less than 0.3% of the population). Most of the rest suffer from NIDDM, but rarer forms of diabetes exist.

IDDM may be due to an autoimmune process. Circulating antibodies to cytoplasmic proteins of the β-cell are present in most patients, although these particular antibodies may be a secondary phenomenon, as they disappear early in the disease. Evidence for a more direct involvement of antigens that react with intracellular enzyme protein, such as glutamic acid decarboxylase, is emerging. There is also strong evidence for defects in cell-mediated immunity in IDDM.

The aetiology of IDDM is largely unknown, although in some cases it may be due to a viral infection. Viruses which have been implicated are Coxsackie B virus, mumps, and rubella.

Evidence has been reported implicating environmental toxins in some cases. In this respect it has been known for many years that alloxan and streptozotocin can cause β-cell necrosis and diabetes in rodents. One possible culprit is nitrosamines found in some smoked foods, which have been shown to be toxic to pancreatic β-cells in animals. Bovine serum albumin present in cow's milk has also been implicated, as antibodies to this protein are more common in the blood of diabetic than non-diabetic patients. In addition, antibodies present cross-react with a peptide known as p69, which is often present on the surface of β-cells during infectious episodes.

There is also evidence that a genetic predisposition to the disease exists in some families. Thus in identical twins, there is a 30–50% concordance for IDDM. However, the genetic influence decreases as the age of diagnosis increases, indicating the importance of other factors.

Secondary complications are neuropathy (sensory and motor), retinopathy, nephropathy, and cardiovascular defects such as ischaemic heart disease, cerebrovascular disease, and peripheral vascular disease.

---

tion of insulin in the blood rises, the concentration of glucose falls, and the stimulus for insulin secretion is removed. As a consequence, the concentration of insulin falls. The feedback control of insulin secretion by plasma glucose is summarised in Figure 9.3.

The concentration of plasma insulin normally parallels the rise and fall in the levels of plasma glucose. This is illustrated in Figure 9.4, which shows the results of a glucose drink in a fasting individual. Concentrations of glucose above 5 mmol/L are effective in increasing insulin release. The response to an oral glucose load (glucose tolerance test) is used to diagnose diabetic states, where the fasting glucose concentration is not sufficiently raised to give a clear diagnosis on its own. It may also be used to diagnose hypoglycaemic states (see Diabetes-IDDM Box 3, page

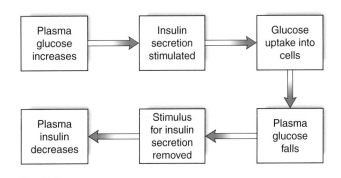

Fig. 9.3
Feedback control of insulin release.

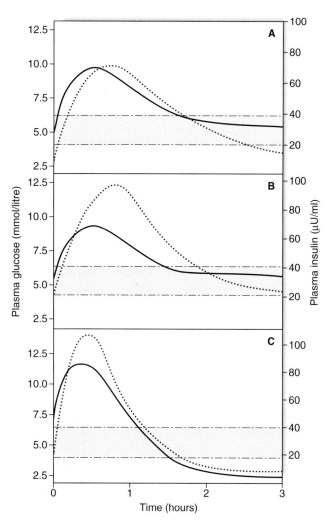

Fig. 9.4

Glucose (solid line) and insulin (dotted line) responses to a carbohydrate meal in (A) a normal individual, (B) an obese individual, (C) an individual with reactive hypoglycaemia. The shaded areas show the normal range for plasma glucose concentration.

163). After a high carbohydrate meal, the levels of plasma glucose may rise rapidly. This causes a rapid secretion of insulin from the β-cells, with an earlier and higher peak than after a more balanced meal. This results in a rapid fall in plasma glucose to levels that may be lower than normal (hypoglycaemia). This effect is exaggerated in some individuals, whose β-cells produce an excessive insulin response to the rise in plasma glucose. They are said to have 'reactive hypoglycaemia'. Various symptoms result from hypoglycaemia, including tremor, hunger, weakness, unco-ordinated movements, blurred vision, and impaired mental ability. Such people need to control their blood glucose levels by limiting their intake of carbohydrates and eating small meals at frequent intervals. Patients

who have undergone gastrectomy can have similar symptoms due to rapid entry of food into the small intestine. This situation is discussed in Chapter 3.

Control by amino acids

Insulin secretion is also controlled by the levels of amino acids in the blood. Thus after a high protein meal, which results in a high level of amino acids, insulin secretion is increased. The most potent amino acids in this respect are arginine, leucine, and alanine. The mechanism whereby these amino acids exert this effect first involves their transport into the β-cells. The cationic amino acids depolarise the membrane and open voltage-gated Ca^{2+} channels. The resulting Ca^{2+} influx then stimulates insulin secretion.

Control by hormones

Glucagon stimulates insulin release and somatostatin inhibits it. Glucagon is produced by the α-cells and somatostatin by the D cells in the pancreas (see Chapter 5). The actions of these hormones on insulin release from the pancreatic β-cells may be local paracrine effects, or they may act locally via the blood in the islet capillaries.

Oral administration of glucose causes a greater increase in blood insulin levels than the same glucose load injected into the blood. The mere presence of food in the gastrointestinal tract elicits an increase in insulin secretion (known as the 'incretin effect'). This indicates that insulin secretion is controlled by factors originating in the gastrointestinal tract (the enteroinsular axis). The duodenal hormones gastric inhibitory peptide (GIP) and the C-terminal fragment of glucagon-like peptide 1 may be responsible. However, cholecystokinin (CCK), gastrin, and secretin have also been implicated. These hormones are all secreted during a meal (see Chapters 4 and 5), but the stimulus for their release is not an increase in the level of blood glucose.

Control by nerves

The islets of Langerhans are innervated by both parasympathetic and sympathetic nerves. Stimulation of the vagus (parasympathetic) nerve fibres which innervate the β-cells potentiates insulin release via acetylcholine acting on muscarinic receptors. The effect is dependent on the presence of glucose. It is phospholipase C-mediated and involves Ca^{2+} uptake into the β-cells. Stimulation of the sympathetic nerves inhibits insulin release via noradrenaline acting on α_2-adrenergic receptors.

Actions of insulin in the absorptive state

The actions of insulin during the absorptive state are indicated in Figure 9.6. It acts on membrane receptors

Diabetes-IDDM Box 3

Diagnosis and treatment

Tests that may be performed to assess the diabetic status of an individual include plasma and urine glucose, plasma insulin, and plasma and urine ketone bodies. Glucose in blood and urine can be measured by an automated colorimetric procedure, which involves the conversion of glucose to a coloured derivative in the presence of the enzyme glucose oxidase. Insulin is measured by radioimmunoassay, using an antibody to insulin. Ketone bodies are estimated by a colorimetric test for acetone after its reaction with salicylaldehyde, which converts it to a coloured derivative. In untreated IDDM, blood and urine glucose concentrations are high, plasma insulin concentration is very low, or undetectable. In severe cases, plasma and urine ketone concentrations are high.

Glucose tolerance test

The diabetic status of an individual can be diagnosed by an oral glucose tolerance test. The patient fasts overnight and then drinks a solution containing 75 g of glucose in 250–300 ml of water. A 'fasting' sample of blood is obtained immediately prior to the glucose load and then further blood samples are obtained at 30-minute intervals thereafter, for 2 hours. Figure 9.5 shows the results of such a test in a normal individual, in a patient with IDDM, and a patient with NIDDM. In a normal individual the fasting plasma glucose level is usually within the range 3.5–7.0 mmol/L. After an oral glucose load it increased to reach a peak between 30 and 60 minutes later, and had returned to normal by 2 hours. In the diabetic patient, the fasting level of glucose was abnormally high. After the glucose load the plasma glucose increased even further to a very high level, and thereafter fell very slowly back to the (elevated) resting level. However, an oral glucose tolerance test is not usually required to diagnose IDDM because raised blood glucose and the presence of ketonuria and ketonaemia are sufficiently indicative of the condition.

IDDM is treated by injections of insulin. If inadequate insulin is administered, the patient may become comatose as a result of ketoacidosis, electrolyte imbalance, and dehydration (see Diabetes-IDDM Box 5, page 171). However, an overdose of insulin can also lead to coma as a result of the hypoglycaemia produced. Therefore the amount of insulin administered must be carefully adjusted to bring the blood glucose level back to normal. Figure 9.4 shows the changes in plasma glucose following an oral glucose load in a person with reactive hypoglycaemia, a condition in which there is hypersecretion of insulin. The response resembles that seen in an individual who has been injected with too much insulin.

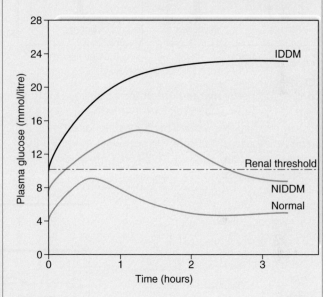

Fig. 9.5

Glucose tolerance curves in a normal subject, a subject with IDDM (type 1 diabetes mellitus), and a subject with NIDDM (type 2 diabetes mellitus). The renal threshold for glucose reabsorption in the kidney tubules, and glucose excretion in the urine is indicated.

in many cells to promote the uptake of glucose, amino acids, K^+, Mg^{2+}, and PO_4^{3-}. In addition it stimulates or inhibits rate-limiting steps in many pathways involved in energy metabolism. It directly stimulates the entry of glucose into muscle and adipose tissue, but not liver. This is a primary action of insulin. However, an increase in intracellular glucose speeds up the reactions in which it is utilised, via the mass action effect due to the increased supply of the reactant. These are secondary effects of insulin. Thus glucose oxidation, and lipid and glycogen synthesis are all stimulated in insulin-sensitive tissues when blood insulin levels increase because more glucose enters the cell.

In addition to the secondary effects of insulin on metabolism, it also exerts primary effects by directly stimulating rate-limiting reactions in a variety of pathways. Insulin stimulates key reactions involved in the utilisation of glucose for energy production via the

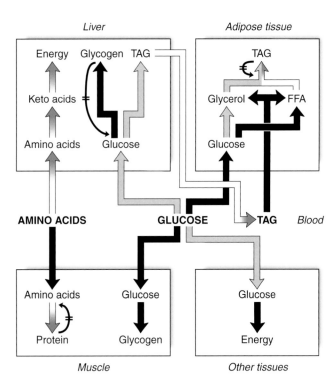

Fig. 9.6

Control of energy metabolism in the absorptive state by insulin. The bold arrows indicate the pathways and uptake mechanisms stimulated by insulin, and the arrows crossed out indicate the pathways inhibited by insulin. TAG, triacylglycerol, FFA, free fatty acids.

citric acid cycle, and in its utilisation for the synthesis of glycogen and triacylglycerol. At the same time it inhibits glycogenolysis, gluconeogenesis, and lipolysis.

Insulin also directly stimulates the uptake of amino acids into muscle and other tissues. This results in increased synthesis of protein by a mass action effect. In addition it directly inhibits the breakdown of protein. Some of the pathways influenced by insulin are shown in Figure 9.6.

The overall effect of insulin in the absorptive state is to provide glucose for utilisation as energy, to promote the storage of excess carbohydrate and fat in forms (which can be used later to provide calories in the postabsorptive state) and to increase protein synthesis (Figure 9.6).

The insulin receptor

Insulin binds to a receptor in the cell membrane of insulin-responsive tissues, to exert its physiological effects. The receptor is a transmembrane glycoprotein with both extracellular and cytoplasmic faces. Figure 9.7 shows the effects of activation of the receptor by insulin. It is a tetramer composed of two α- and two β-subunits. The α-subunit is situated on the extracellular face of the membrane. Insulin binds to a site on the α-subunit. The β-subunit spans the membrane, but

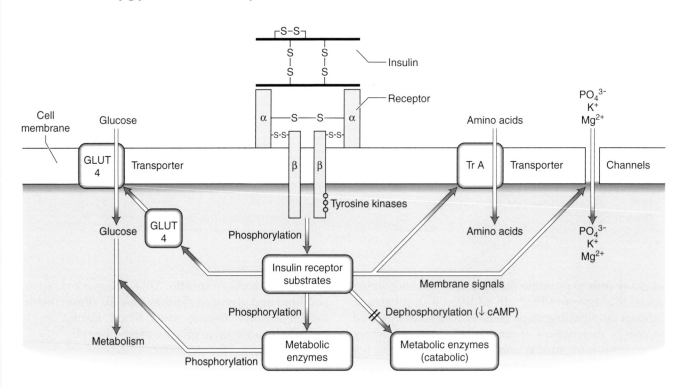

Fig. 9.7

The effects of activation of its receptor by insulin. GLUT 4, hormone-sensitive GLUT 4 glucose transporter, Tr A, amino acid transporter A.

most of it comprises a tail on the intracellular face. Each α-subunit is bound to a β-subunit by a disulphide bridge, and the two αβ-dimers are joined extracellularly through the α-subunit by another disulphide bridge. The receptor is a tyrosine kinase enzyme. When it is not bound to insulin, it is enzymatically inactive, but when it combines with insulin, a conformational change occurs that results in the exposure of three intracellular phosphorylation sites on the β-subunit tail. These sites can be autophosphorylated, using ATP as the substrate, and this results in activation of the enzyme. The phosphorylated receptor kinase can then activate tyrosine residues on intracellular proteins, simply known as insulin receptor substrates. When these proteins become phosphorylated, they in turn phosphorylate a number of intracellular kinases and phosphatases. These activated enzymes then stimulate glucose and amino acid uptake, and a number of rate-limiting reactions in various metabolic pathways. These actions determine the net direction of those pathways. However, activation of the receptor also suppresses the levels of intracellular cAMP, which results in suppression of various catabolic processes and gluconeogenesis (see below). The nature of all the post-receptor events stimulated by insulin has not been fully elucidated. After activation of the receptor, it is endocytosed, and either degraded, or recycled.

Glucose entry into cells

Basal glucose uptake into muscle, and adipose tissue is via the GLUT1 transporter. However, facilitated glucose transport involves GLUT4, an insulin-sensitive member of the GLUT transporter family (see Chapter 8). This transporter is bound to endosomes in the cytosol, and it cycles between the cytosol and the cell membrane (Fig. 9.7). When insulin levels in the blood are low, most of the transporters reside bound to the endosomes in the cytosol. Activation by insulin of its receptor stimulates the translocation of the transporters from the cytosol into the membrane, resulting in an increase in the number of transporters in the membrane. This event may involve the formation of phosphatidylinositol phosphates by the action of phosphatidylinositol-3-kinase, one of the enzymes activated by the receptor tyrosine kinase. In addition, insulin increases the synthesis of the GLUT4 transporter, and possibly also its activity. At low insulin concentrations, glucose transport is the rate-limiting step in the utilisation of glucose. After a meal, when high concentrations of insulin are present, glucose transport into cells can be stimulated up to 20-fold. Reactions in the intracellular metabolic pathways then become rate-limiting for the utilisation of glucose.

Glycolysis

Insulin increases the utilisation of glucose via glycolysis by increasing the synthesis of a number of enzymes. This pathway serves as an example of one in which there is extensive involvement of insulin (Fig. 9.8). In this pathway, insulin increases the synthesis of liver glucokinase, phosphofructokinase, pyruvate kinase, and pyruvate dehydrogenase, enzymes which catalyse key steps in the pathway. In addition it inhibits the synthesis of glucose-6-

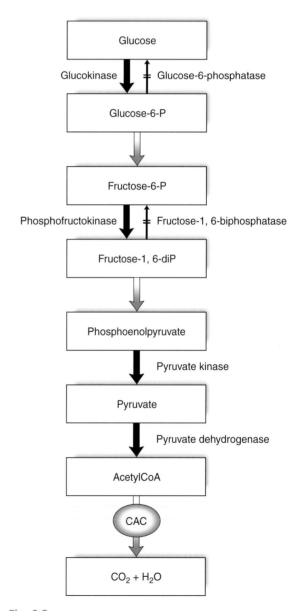

Fig. 9.8
Control of glycolysis by insulin. The bold arrows indicate the enzymes whose synthesis is stimulated by insulin, and the crossed arrows indicate those whose synthesis is inhibited by insulin.

phosphatase and fructose-1,6-bisphosphatase which catalyse reactions which oppose the utilisation of glucose via glycolysis.

Glycogen synthesis

Increased entry of glucose into cells stimulates glycogen synthesis by a mass action effect, but insulin also stimulates glycogen synthesis directly, by stimulating the activity of glycogen synthase, the rate-determining enzyme of the pathway. In addition insulin promotes the synthesis in liver (but not muscle) of glucokinase, which catalyses the formation of glucose-6 phosphate (see above). This action enables more glucose to enter the glycogenic pathway in liver, in addition to stimulating the glycolytic pathway, in other tissues (see above). Insulin also inhibits hepatic glucose-6 phosphatase, thereby inhibiting the release of free glucose into the blood.

Triacylglycerol synthesis

Figure 9.6 indicates the effect of insulin on the synthesis of triacylglycerol from glucose in adipose tissue. It stimulates fatty acid synthesis from glucose by activating several of the enzymes involved in the pathway, including pyruvate dehydrogenase, which catalyses the conversion of pyruvate to acetylCoA in the mitochondrion. AcetylCoA is then directed to fatty acid synthesis, because insulin activates acetylCoA carboxylase, which diverts the acetylCoA to the synthesis of fatty acid in the cytosol.

Inhibition of glycogenolysis, lipolysis, and gluconeogenesis

Insulin suppresses the mobilisation of body energy stores. It inhibits glycogen and triacylglycerol breakdown and gluconeogenesis by decreasing the level of intracellular cAMP. cAMP is a second messenger, which activates an intracellular cascade, which leads to phosphorylation of enzymes involved in key steps in the catabolic pathways. Figures 9.9 and 9.10 outline the intracellular cascades involved in glycogenolysis and lipolysis. cAMP phosphorylates a protein kinase, which then phosphorylates critical enzymes involved in these pathways. Thus lowering the levels of cAMP by insulin causes a reduction in the activity of the protein kinase, and this leads to decreased activity of these key enzymes and suppression of the metabolic pathway. Insulin decreases cAMP via activation of a membrane-associated phosphodiesterase, which hydrolyses it to 5'AMP.

Amino acid transport and protein synthesis

Insulin facilitates the uptake of amino acids into cells via the amino acid transporter A, a sodium-dependent carrier that transports neutral amino acids and imino

A. Glycogenolysis

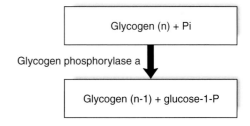

B. Activation of glycogen phosphorylase

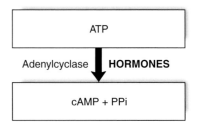

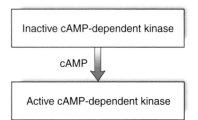

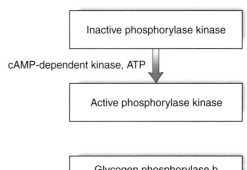

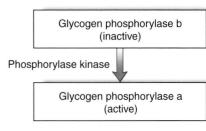

Fig. 9.9

Control of glycogenolysis by hormones. The number of glucose residues in glycogen is denoted by 'n'. In the absorptive state the formation of cAMP (bold arrow) is inhibited by insulin. In the postabsorptive state it is stimulated by adrenaline, glucagon, growth hormone, and cortisol.

A. Lipolysis

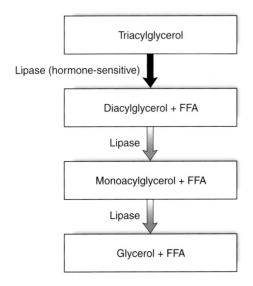

B. Activation of hormone-sensitive lipase

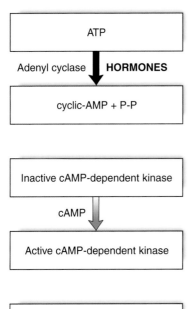

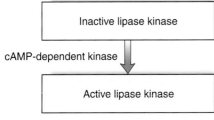

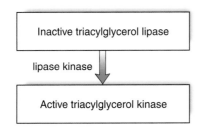

acids (see Chapter 8). Insulin controls the synthesis of mRNA for many specific proteins, increasing some and suppressing others. It stimulates the synthesis of mRNA for certain enzymes involved in glycolysis (for example hepatic glucokinase and pyruvate kinase, see above), and repressing the synthesis of mRNA for others involved in gluconeogenesis (for example phosphoenolpyruvate carboxykinase and glucose-6 phosphatase). It also stimulates DNA synthesis, cell division, and cell differentiation. The mechanisms involved in these actions of insulin are not well understood.

Insulin sensitivity

The magnitude of the effects produced by insulin depends not only on its concentration in the plasma, but also on the sensitivity of the tissues to it. The responsiveness of tissues to insulin varies even in normal individuals. Thus for example habitual exercise increases tissue sensitivity insulin. It is pertinent to note here, however, that glucose is taken up into muscle during acute exercise by an insulin-independent mechanism, which has not yet been elucidated.

Insulin sensitivity is decreased in obese individuals, leading to abnormally slow uptake of glucose into tissues after a meal (Fig. 9.4, p. 162). Relatively high amounts of insulin are secreted in response to the resulting elevated plasma glucose. The elevated insulin tends to maintain the fasting concentration of plasma glucose within the normal range. The mechanisms underlying changes in insulin sensitivity in obesity are not clear.

Non-insulin-dependent diabetes

In the United Kingdom, NIDDM is known to affect approximately 2.5% of the population, and surveys of adults indicate that in at least another 2.0% the condition is present, but undiagnosed. It affects more men than women (ratio 3:2) and is much more prevalent in ethnic minority groups, especially those originating from the Indian subcontinent (typically 7.0%), than in Caucasians.

Fig. 9.10

Control of lipolysis by hormones. In the absorptive state the formation of cAMP (bold arrow) is inhibited by insulin. In the postabsorptive state it is stimulated by adrenaline, glucagon, growth hormone, and cortisol.

Diabetes-IDDM Box 4

Metabolic state

In untreated IDDM, insulin levels may be very low, and the uptake of glucose into muscle, adipose tissue and other tissues is therefore impaired. Consequently plasma glucose is high, and the utilisation of glucose for energy by insulin-sensitive tissues, and for glycogen and fat synthesis, is reduced.

As insulin also inhibits glycogenolysis and lipolysis these catabolic processes occur at an increased rate in IDDM. Increased glycogenolysis in liver results in glucose production. Increased glycogenolysis in muscles results in lactate release into the blood, and this is used by the liver for glucose production by gluconeogenesis. Increased lipolysis results in fatty acids and glycerol being released into the blood. The glycerol is taken up and used to produce glucose via gluconeogenesis. Thus these processes all result in further increases in blood glucose, and exacerbate the hyperglycaemia. The fatty acids formed in the adipose tissue are released into the blood and taken up by various tissues and oxidised to acetylCoA. If the levels of fatty acids are excessive, acetylCoA production in the liver exceeds the capacity of the citric acid cycle to oxidise it and the excess is converted to ketone bodies (Fig. 9.11), which are released into the blood, resulting in high levels of plasma ketone bodies and ketosis. Metabolic acidosis can result from the high levels of acid ketone bodies and fatty acids in the blood plasma.

Amino acid uptake into tissues is also reduced in IDDM, due to very low insulin levels, and protein breakdown is increased. This results in an excessive conversion of amino acids to glucose via gluconeogenesis in the liver. Thus the overall effect of these metabolic dis-

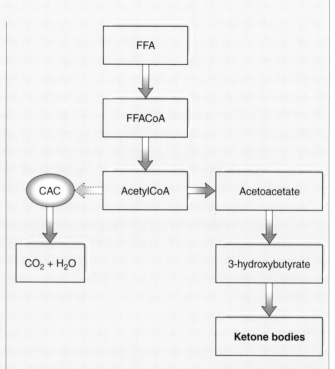

Fig. 9.11
Ketone body formation in the postabsorptive state. The dashed arrow indicates where the build up of acetylCoA diverts it away from the citric acid cycle in the mitochondrion towards ketone body formation in the cytosol.

turbances is elevated levels of glucose, ketone bodies, and fatty acids in the plasma. This pattern of metabolism is an exaggeration of that seen in the postabsorptive state.

In NIDDM the levels of insulin in the blood may be normal or elevated, but tissue sensitivity to insulin is subnormal (insulin resistance). Obesity is a predisposing factor for NIDDM. The resistance to insulin involves not only glucose uptake into muscle and adipose tissue, but also resistance to the metabolic actions of insulin, such as its effect on glycogen synthesis in muscle and liver and its effect to inhibit lipolysis in adipose tissue. In consequence circulating glucose and plasma free fatty acids are increased. The cause of the resistance to insulin is unknown, except in a few cases where there is a structural abnormality of the receptor or an intracellular protein that is involved in the response. NIDDM can usually be controlled by following a calorie-restricted diet and by exercise, which increase tissue sensitivity to insulin. If these measures are insufficient, oral drugs, such as tolbutamide, are used.

In NIDDM, the β-cell mass may eventually be diminished by up to 40%, whereas in IDDM these cells are completely destroyed. Insulin secretion is eventually impaired, although it may be initially increased in response to the hyperglycaemia.

In both NIDDM and IDDM there is a predisposition to vascular disease and hypertension, high cholesterol and high very low density lipoproteins (VLDL), neuropathy, retinopathy, and nephropathy. It may be pertinent that some of these problems, for example hypertension, are associated with obesity, even in non-diabetic individuals.

Postabsorptive state

Some tissues, such as brain and erythrocytes, can only survive if glucose is delivered to them for fuel. They cannot utilise other nutrients rapidly to any significant extent. Lack of glucose causes brain damage, coma, and death within minutes. During the postabsorptive state when glucose is not being absorbed from the gastrointestinal tract, the plasma levels of glucose are maintained within a physiological range. This is brought about in two ways. First, glucose is generated by glycogen breakdown via glycogenolysis and gluconeogenesis. Second, many tissues can utilise substrates other than glucose, such as fatty acids, for energy provision. This spares the available glucose for the tissues which are obligatory utilisers of it. However, in starvation, when the blood glucose falls slowly, the nervous system is able to adapt after a few days to use ketones as a source of energy.

Glucose-supplying reactions

The reactions that supply glucose to the blood during the postabsorptive state are outlined in Figure 9.12. During the postabsorptive state glycogen stored in the liver is broken down to glucose, which is liberated into the blood. Muscle glycogen is also broken down in

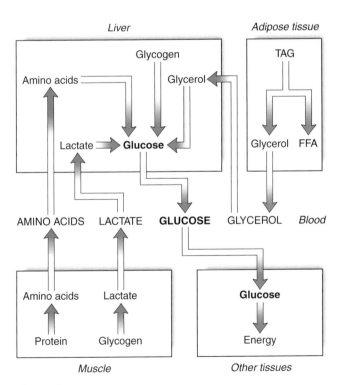

Fig. 9.12
Glucose-supplying reactions in the postabsorptive state. TAG, triacylglycerol, FFA, free fatty acids.

the absorptive state, but muscle lacks glucose-6-phosphatase (the enzyme which converts glucose 6 phosphate to free glucose), and so in muscle glucose 6 phosphate is broken down to lactate and pyruvate, which are released into the blood. These metabolites are taken up by the liver and then converted to glucose (via gluconeogenesis, see below), which is liberated into the blood. The stores of glycogen in liver and muscle can amount to 600–800 g in the postabsorptive state. This source of glucose is sufficient to meet the energy needs of the body for only 4 hours or so.

In any prolonged period of fasting the stored glycogen is used up and gluconeogenesis becomes the more important process for generating glucose and maintaining plasma levels. Lactate provides one substrate for gluconeogenesis, but in prolonged fasting, amino acids derived from protein broken down in muscle and taken up by the liver are quantitatively the most important substrate for the generation of glucose via gluconeogenesis. Glycerol derived from triacylglycerol in adipose tissue and taken up by the liver is also converted to glucose via gluconeogenesis.

Glucose-sparing reactions

Most of the energy requirement of the body during the postabsorptive state is derived via glucose-sparing reactions which utilise the energy stored as triacylglycerol during the absorptive state. Fat is broken down to glycerol and free fatty acids in adipose tissue. The glycerol is used for gluconeogenesis in liver (see above), but the fatty acids are taken up by many other tissues and oxidised to CO_2 and water via the fatty acid oxidation pathway and the citric acid cycle.

In the postabsorptive state the liver takes up a portion of the fatty acids from the blood. In the liver, free fatty acids can be converted to acetylCoA, which is degraded to CO_2 and water by fatty acid oxidation and the citric acid cycle, with the production of energy. However, when large quantities of fatty acids are being produced, as in the postabsorptive state (or diabetes), the rate of acetylCoA formation can exceed the capacity of the liver to utilise it via the citric acid cycle. The acetylCoA is then converted to ketone bodies (Fig. 9.11). Some of the ketone bodies are used for energy purposes in the liver, and the rest are liberated into the blood and taken up by other tissues and utilised via the citric acid cycle after conversion to acetylCoA. The ketone bodies are acetone, acetoacetate, and β-hydroxybutyrate. The production of acetone during the fasting state accounts for the distinctive breath odour of fasting people (and type 1 diabetic patients, see later). Thus the liver uses ketone bodies for energy production, and ceases to use amino acids during the postabsorptive state, thereby sparing

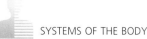

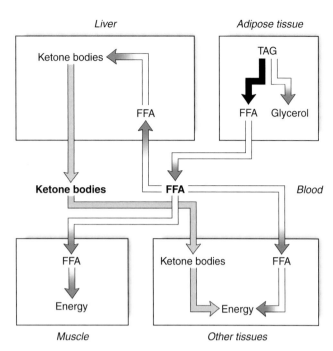

Fig. 9.15
Effect of hormones on glucose-sparing reactions in the postabsorptive state. The bold arrow indicates the stimulation of lipolysis by adrenaline, glucagons, and growth hormone in the postabsorptive state. The effect of cortisol on lipolysis is permissive.

Table 9.1
Hormones secreted in the postabsorptive state

Hormone	Origin
Glucagon	α-cells of the pancreas
Adrenaline	Adrenal medulla
Cortisol	Adrenal cortex
Growth hormone	Anterior pituitary
Adrenocorticotropin (ACTH)	Anterior pituitary
Thyroid stimulating hormone (TSH)	Anterior pituitary

The hormones listed are collectively responsible for the pattern of energy metabolism that pertains in the postabsorptive state. They are all secreted either directly, or indirectly, in response to low blood glucose.

release of growth hormone. An increase in plasma glucose inhibits growth hormone release. Other pituitary hormones are also released in response to low blood glucose via an effect on the hypothalamus to cause secretion of releasing factors that act on the pituitary cells to stimulate the secretion of the hormones. Thus low blood glucose causes the release of corticotrophin releasing factor (CRF) from the hypothalamus, which in turn stimulates the release of ACTH from the pituitary. ACTH is therefore increased in the blood during the postabsorptive state. ACTH in turn causes the release of hormones such as cortisol from the adrenal cortex. Table 9.1 lists some of the hormones involved in the postabsorptive state, which are released in response to low blood glucose.

effects of this group of hormones oppose the actions of insulin and facilitate the postabsorptive state.

Release of hormones in the postabsorptive state

Adrenaline is released from the adrenal medulla by the activity in the preganglionic sympathetic nerves that innervate it. Sympathetic nerves are stimulated by low blood glucose. For this reason low blood glucose precipitates the symptoms associated with the activation of the sympathetic nervous system, such as an increase in anxiety levels and palpitations. These symptoms are observed by many individuals in the late afternoon when blood sugar tends to be low.

Glucagon is produced by the α-cells of the islets of Langerhans. Its release is regulated by the levels of plasma glucose. Low plasma glucose stimulates glucagon release and high blood glucose inhibits it. Thus blood glucagon levels are high during the postabsorptive period. The release of growth hormone from the pituitary is also stimulated by low blood glucose. This is possibly due to activation of glucoreceptors in the hypothalamus, which results in the release of growth hormone releasing factor (GHRF) which, in turn, acts on the pituitary to stimulate the

Actions of hormones in the postabsorptive state

Effects on glucose-supplying reactions
The effects of hormones on glucose-supplying metabolic pathways in the postabsorptive state are shown in Figure 9.14. Growth hormone and cortisol inhibit the uptake of glucose by reducing the number of GLUT4 transporters in the cell membrane. For this reason patients with growth hormone producing tumours can develop diabetes. Moreover, in diabetic animals, removal of the pituitary, which secretes growth hormone, reduces the severity of diabetes.

Adrenaline and glucagon stimulate glycogen breakdown to glucose in liver, with the liberation of glucose into the blood. In addition, adrenaline, but not glucagon, stimulates glycogen breakdown in muscle to lactate and pyruvate. These products are released into the blood, taken up by the liver, and converted to glucose via gluconeogenesis, and the glucose is then released into the blood. The action of these hormones on glycogen breakdown is via stimulation of the rate-limiting step, which is catalysed by phosphorylase, by increasing the levels of cAMP, which activates a kinase, which in turn activates phosphorylase kinase, leading to activation of phosphorylase itself (see Fig. 9.9, page 166). In addition, cortisol stimulates glucose-6-phosphatase, resulting in increased release of glucose into the blood. Furthermore glucagon and cortisol stimulate gluconeogenesis from amino acids in liver. Cortisol also stimulates the breakdown of protein to amino acids in liver.

Effects on glucose-sparing reactions

Figure 9.15 shows the effects of hormones on glucose-sparing metabolic pathways in the postabsorptive state. Adrenaline, glucagons, and growth hormone stimulate lipolysis in adipose tissue, thereby increasing the free fatty acid concentration in the plasma. Cortisol has a permissive effect on lipolysis, i.e. it has no effect by itself but it potentiates the effects of adrenaline, glucagon, and growth hormone. The sympathetic nerves to adipose tissue are also stimulated by low blood glucose. These nerves release mainly noradrenaline which, like adrenaline, increases lipolysis in adipose tissue. The effects of adrenaline and noradrenaline are exerted on the rate-limiting step in the lipolyis pathway, i.e. the hydrolysis of triacylglycerol to diacylglycerol and free fatty acid, which is catalysed by the 'hormone-sensitive' lipase. The effect of these hormones involves an increase in the intracellular levels of cAMP, which triggers an intracellular cascade of reactions (Fig. 9.10, page 167) similar to that seen for the activation of phosphorylase (see above). The subsequent hydrolysis of diacylglycerol to monoacylglycerol and free fatty acid, and of monoacylglycerol to glycerol and free fatty acid, by other lipases, is extremely rapid. Table 9.2 summarises the effects of hormones to control glucose-supplying and glucose-sparing reactions in the postabsorptive state.

Comparison with postabsorptive state

The pattern of metabolism in untreated IDDM is an exaggeration of that seen in the postabsorptive state. Insulin levels are low and therefore glucose uptake into tissues is reduced, and glycogenolysis, lipolysis and gluconeogenesis, which are no longer inhibited by insulin, increase. These events result in increases in plasma glucose, plasma fatty acids, and ketone bodies. Furthermore, in diabetes, in spite of the presence of hyperglycaemia, there are increases in many of the hormones associated with the postabsorptive state, including plasma catecholamines, glucagon, cortisol, and ACTH, and sometimes growth hormone. Increases in secretion of these hormones accompanies various types of stress, and they are prob-ably partly due to activation of the sympathetic nervous system. Thus for example, stimulation of the preganglionic sympathetic nerves to the adrenal medulla causes the release of adrenaline into the blood, and stimulation of the sympathetic nerves to the α-cells of the pancreas causes release of glucagon. However, in IDDM, the predominating mechanism causing the release of these hormones (which are normally suppressed by hyperglycaemia) are largely unknown.

There is also reduced amino acid uptake into tissues and increased protein breakdown in diabetes, due to both insulin deficiency and elevated concentrations of stress hormones.

In non-diabetic subjects, in the postabsorptive state, the plasma glucose and ketone bodies do not normally exceed the threshold for reabsorption in the kidney, so these metabolites do not appear in the urine.

Table 9.2
Control of the postabsorptive state

Effect	Adrenaline	Glucagon	Growth hormone	Cortisol
Plasma glucose	↑	↑	↑	↑
Glucose uptake			↓	↓
Glycogenolysis	↑	↑		
Gluconeogenesis		↑		↑
Plasma FFA (Lipolysis)	↑	↑	↑	↑

Effects of some of the hormones, released in the postabsorptive state on aspects of energy metabolism, which result in either increases in blood glucose, or the provision of energy substrates (FFA, free fatty acids) that spare glucose for the tissues dependent on it for their energy requirements.

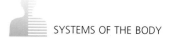
THE ABSORPTIVE AND POSTABSORPTIVE STATES

Self-assessment case study: starvation

A round-the-world yachtsman was blown off course and his boat sank. He managed to get into the yacht's dinghy and to retrieve a large container of drinking water from the boat. After 7 weeks without food he was rescued by a passing liner. His water supply had lasted, but he was weak and emaciated.

You should be able to answer the following questions using your knowledge of the metabolic pattern in the postabsorptive state:

① What metabolic processes would have been occurring to enable this man to maintain his plasma glucose levels?

② Why is it important that plasma glucose does not fall too far?

③ Would you expect the man's plasma insulin levels to be low?

④ Would you expect the man's acid–base status to be disturbed? Explain your answer.

⑤ Would you expect this man to be excreting glucose and ketone bodies in his urine? Is it likely that acetone would be detectable on his breath?

⑥ Would you expect the man's plasma glucagon levels to be high or low? Explain your answer.

⑦ Would it be advisable for the rescued man to drink a concentrated solution of glucose?

⑧ What treatment would you recommend for the starving yachtsman?

Self-assessment questions

① What is the major fuel used by most tissues of the body in the absorptive state?

② What are the direct actions of insulin in (a) the liver, (b) the muscle, and (c) adipose tissue?

③ What are the secondary effects of insulin?

④ How is glucose transported into muscle and adipose tissue?

⑤ What is meant by the 'feedback' control of plasma glucose by insulin?

⑥ What is the mechanism whereby insulin increases glucose transport into adipose tissue and muscle?

⑦ What are the glucose-supplying processes that occur in the postabsorptive state?

⑧ What are the glucose-sparing processes that occur in the postabsorptive state?

⑨ What are the major distinguishing features of (a) IDDM, (b) NIDDM?

⑩ How do adrenaline and glucagon promote glucose-sparing reactions in the postabsorptive state?

THE COLON

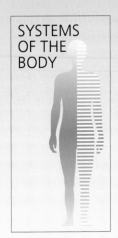

SYSTEMS
OF THE
BODY

Chapter objectives

After studying this chapter you should be able to:

① Understand the functioning of the large intestine.

② Understand the consequences of disease of the large intestine.

10

Introduction

The colon is the last 150 cm or so of the gastrointestinal tract. It is a tube of approximately 6 cm in diameter that extends from the ileum to the anus. Its main function is to store faecal material and regulate its release into the external environment. The colon also absorbs water and electrolytes from the chyme, with the result that the faecal material becomes more solid as it passes through the colon. In addition, the colon produces a thick mucinous secretion, which lubricates the passage of the faecal material through it. It also provides an environment for bacteria, some of which synthesise an important part of the vitamin requirement of the body.

Disease of the colon can result in diarrhoea, or constipation, or both. In this chapter, Hirschsprung's disease will be used to illustrate the importance of the motor function of the colon. It is a condition in which there is an absence of intramural ganglion cells from the wall of the colon, usually in a distal region.

Anatomy

The arrangement of the large intestine and its associated structures is shown in Figure 10.1. It can be

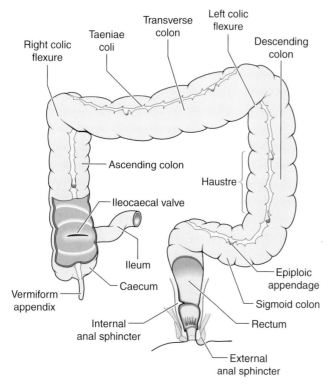

Fig. 10.1
Anatomical features of the large intestine.

Hirschsprung's disease

Case history

A newborn infant was observed to have a distended abdomen. He had passed very little meconium in the 2 days since he had been born. The doctor examined the infant's rectum by inserting a finger. The examination revealed that the rectum was empty. However, when the doctor withdrew her finger, there was a gush of meconium, and decompression of the abdomen. The obstruction reoccurred within a day or so. By this time the child had started to vomit excessively. The symptoms were relieved by an enema. A biopsy of the rectum was performed and Hirschsprung's disease was diagnosed. An abdominal operation was arranged. The surgeon removed the distal large bowel and sutured the remaining colon to the lower rectum. The child made a good recovery, and his symptoms disappeared.

After examining the details of this case, we might ask the following questions.

① Why was the infant's abdomen distended, and why had he passed no meconium since he was born?

② What is the defect in this condition, and what causes it? What did the biopsy reveal?

③ Why was it necessary to resect a segment of the infant's intestine?

④ How does this abnormality affect motility in the colon?

⑤ How does the abnormality affect defaecation?

These questions will be addressed in this chapter.

divided into various regions: the caecum, the ascending colon, the transverse colon, the descending colon, the sigmoid colon, and the rectum. The rectum is the portion beyond the sigmoid colon. The lumen of the colon becomes narrower towards the rectum. The lumen of the rectum, which is wider, provides a reservoir for faecal material, prior to defaecation.

The caecum forms a blind-ended pouch below the junctions of the small intestine and the large intestine. The appendix is a small finger-like projection from the end of the caecum, which has no known function in the human. It has a thick wall and a very narrow lumen that often collects debris.

In the large intestine the outer longitudinal smooth muscle layer is arranged in three prominent bands, known as taeniae coli. These bands are shorter than the other longitudinal muscle coats of the colon. There is also a segmental thickening of the circular smooth

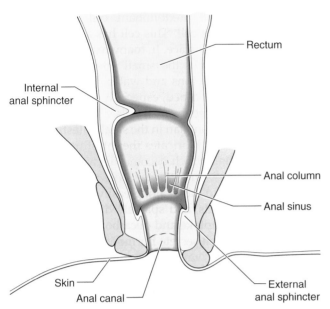

Fig. 10.2
Structure of the anal canal.

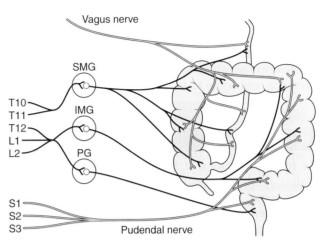

Fig. 10.3
Autonomic innervation of the colon. Grey-filled lines indicate parasympathetic nerves, and solid black lines indicate sympathetic nerves. T10, T11, T12, thoracic segments, L1, L2, lumbar segments, S1, S2, S3, sacral segments, of the spinal cord. SMG, superior mesenteric ganglion, IMG, inferior mesenteric ganglion, PG, pelvic ganglion.

muscle. Together these features impart a sacculated appearance to the organ. It has no villi (only projections). Its luminal surface is therefore smoother than that of the small intestine. The consequence of this is that the surface area of the colon is only one-thirtieth that of the small intestine.

The anal canal is the terminal portion of the rectum. It begins at a region where the rectum suddenly becomes narrower. The surface of the upper portion of the anal canal exhibits a number of vertical folds, known as anal (or rectal) columns (Fig. 10.2). These folds are relatively more pronounced in children than in adults. The depressions between the anal columns are known as anal sinuses. The sinuses end abruptly at the lower ends of the columns (the dentate line) where there are small crescent-shaped folds of mucosa oriented around the wall. These folds are termed anal valves. The anal canal is surrounded by sphincter muscles that control the release of faecal material. The internal sphincter is a thickening of the circular layer of the muscularis externa. The external sphincter, which consists of several parts, is composed of striated muscle. The arrangement of the sphincters is shown in Figure 10.2.

Innervation

The ascending colon, and most of the transverse colon is innervated by the parasympathetic vagus nerve. Beyond that the pelvic nerves innervate the colon. These are the sacral outflow of the parasympathetic nervous system. Figure 10.3 illustrates the extrinsic innervation of the large intestine. The cholinergic parasympathetic nerves synapse with neurones in the intramural plexi. They also synapse directly on the smooth muscle of the colon and the internal anal sphincter. Excitatory cholinergic neurones are also present in the ganglia of the submucosal and myenteric intramural plexi.

The colon is also innervated by adrenergic sympathetic nerves from the lower thoracic and upper lumbar segments of the spinal cord. These nerves synapse with inhibitory nerves in the intramural plexi. They also synapse directly with the smooth muscle of the colon and internal anal sphincter. The external anal sphincter is innervated by somatic motor fibres in the pudendal nerves. It is controlled both reflexly and voluntarily.

Contraction of the levator ani, an external skeletal muscle, constricts the lower end of the rectum. The contraction of another external skeletal muscle, the puborectal muscle, which is attached to the external side of the wall of the anal canal, pulls the upper canal forward. This produces a sharp angle between the rectum and the anal canal, and prevents faeces from entering the anal canal until defaecation is initiated. The levator ani and the puborectal muscle are innervated by somatic motor fibres in the pudendal nerve.

Terminals of afferent sensory nerve fibres are present in the mucosa, submucosa, and muscle layers of the colon. The colon is fairly insensitive to painful stimuli but it is very sensitive to changes in pressure. Stretching of the colon as a consequence of overdistension results in abdominal pain, but removal of lesions, such

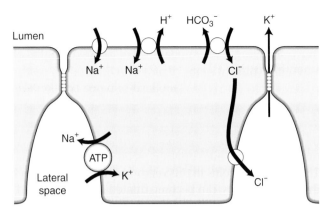

Fig. 10.6
Absorption and secretion of ions in the epithelial cell of the colon.

synapses with neurones in the intramural plexi. Stimulation of the sympathetic nerves suppresses secretion in the colon via adrenaline and somatostatin release. For this reason somatostatin analogues can be administered to treat secretory diarrhoea (see Chapter 8).

Absorption and digestion

Ions and water

The absorption of ions and water occurs mainly in the proximal region of the colon. The net absorption of Na^+ and Cl^- occurs via exchange mechanisms (Fig. 10.6). These mechanisms are similar to those in the ileum. However, in the colon the transport of Na^+ across the luminal membrane occurs via an electrogenic Na^+ channel. This produces an electrical potential of about 30 mV (lumen-negative) across the mucosa.

The electrical potential caused by Na^+ absorption promotes the secretion of K^+ into the lumen (see above), but K^+ is also absorbed in the distal colon, where the transport is via exchange with H^+ ions. The latter is an active process, involving an anionic exchange mechanism similar to that for H^+/K^+ exchange in the stomach.

The absorption of water and ions is under both neural control via the enteric nerve plexi and hormonal control. Aldosterone increases net water absorption in the colon by both stimulating the synthesis of the electrogenic Na^+ channel in the luminal membrane of the epithelial cell and by increasing the number of Na^+,K^+-ATPase molecules in the basolateral membrane. Glucocorticoids also stimulate the transport of Na^+ ions by increasing the number of ATPase pumps, and angiotensin stimulates the absorption of water and Na^+ in the colon. Vasopressin (antidiuretic hormone, ADH) decreases water absorption.

Products of bacterial action

The human body is composed of approximately 10^{14} cells, but only 10% of these are human cells. The rest are microbial cells that colonise the body surfaces and the gastrointestinal tract. The gastric acid of the stomach destroys most microflora, and the stomach and small intestines are only sparsely colonised by them. Most of the flora that colonise the gastrointestinal tract reside in the large intestine. A large number of bacteria are lost in the faeces, and human faeces contain approximately 10^{11} bacteria per gram. More than 99% of the bacteria in faeces are rod-shaped, non-sporing, anaerobes. Apart from anaerobic bacteria, lactobacilli and coliforms also colonise the large intestine.

The bacteria in the large intestine synthesise certain vitamins that are required by the body. These are vitamins of the B complex, including thiamin, riboflavin, and vitamin B_{12}, and vitamin K. The synthesis of vitamin K is especially important because the average diet does not contain enough of this vitamin for normal blood clotting. In fact animals bred in germ-free conditions develop clotting defects. The vitamins are probably absorbed by passive diffusion in the large intestine. Vitamin K is fat-soluble, and therefore may be absorbed fairly readily. A small proportion of the synthesised vitamins may be refluxed into the small intestine, and absorbed in that region.

Intestinal bacteria also have digestive actions. Thus they convert primary bile acids to secondary bile acids, and deconjugate conjugated bile acids. The lipid solubility of these substances is greater than that of the primary bile acids, and a proportion of them are absorbed in the colon. The reactions involved have been described in Chapter 6. Colonic bacteria also convert bilirubins to urobilinogens (see Chapter 6).

Absorption of drugs

Some drugs can be administered via the rectum. This route can be used to produce a local effect. Thus anti-inflammatory drugs can be used in this way to treat ulcerative colitis. This route can also be used for drugs that produce systemic effects. It can be appropriate in patients who are suffering from vomiting, and cannot take medicine by mouth, such as may be the case following an operation. However, the rectal route may be unreliable in controlling the quantities of a drug absorbed into the circulation.

Motility

The motor function of the large intestine serves both to mix the contents of the lumen, and to propel them towards the anus. The chyme entering the large intestine is semi-liquid, but water is absorbed from it, and the residual matter gradually becomes solid, as it passes along the colon. A major function of the distal large bowel (particularly the rectum) is to store faecal material. The passage of the luminal contents through the stomach and small intestine usually takes less than 12 hours, but the residue from a meal can remain in the large intestine for over a week, or more. However, normally 80% has been extruded by the end of the fourth day. The expulsion of material from the colon is highly variable, being under both autonomic and somatic control.

Mixing

Mixing or kneading of the contents of the large intestine is due to contractions of the circular muscle. These contractions result in the formation and reformation of sacs, known as haustrae. This type of segmental motility is known as haustration. The rectum is more active in segmental contractions than the colon (Fig. 10.9, page 183).

Propulsion

Movement of material along the large intestine is effected by segmental propulsion, peristalsis, and peristaltic mass movements. Segmental propulsion involves sequential haustration. Several segments may contract simultaneously, propelling the contents along. Although this can result in the material being propelled in both directions, it is usually pushed in the caudad direction. Material is displaced through several haustrae, approximately every 30 minutes.

Mass movements involve the simultaneous contraction of large segments of the ascending and transverse colon, which can propel the contents one-third to three-quarters of the length of the colon in a few seconds. Peristalsis involves waves of contraction that travel towards the anus, pushing the contents slowly along. At rest these waves travel at approximately 5 cm per hour, but the speed increases to approximately 10 cm per hour after a meal. There are also additional peristaltic movements in the descending colon which deliver the faecal material into the rectum.

Effect of food

Ingested material can affect motility in the large intestine in two ways. Firstly, food that contains large amounts of indigestible material causes stimulation of mechanoreceptors in the walls of the colon, resulting in its rapid transit through the large intestine. This is how 'fibre' in the diet prevents constipation. Secondly, some substances (for example, laxatives) stimulate chemoreceptors in the walls to stimulate motility.

Distension

The volume of faeces entering the colon can be increased if fibre is ingested. Fibre consists of poly-meric substances such as cellulose, hemicelluloses, pectins, gums, mucilages, and lignins. Most of these are polysaccharides, although lignin is a phenyl-propane polymer. These substances are found in bran, fruit, and vegetables. Western diets are low in fibre compared to diets in many other parts of the world such as rural Africa, and the relative lack of fibre in the diet probably accounts for the higher prevalence of many diseases of the large intestine in Western populations. These diseases include constipation, diverticular disease, haemorrhoids, polyps, cancer of the colon, and irritable colon. Adding fibre to the diet prevents or remedies constipation, eases haemorrhoids, and relieves the symptoms of diverticular disease. It is interesting also in this respect that Seventh Day Adventists living in the United States, who are predominantly vegetarian, have a very low incidence of cancer of the colon.

Adding fibre to the diet prevents constipation partly because it increases the bulk of the material entering the colon. This increases the stimulation of the smooth muscle, and decreases the transit time for the passage of material through the colon. Moreover, polysaccharides take up water and swell to form gels. This makes the faeces softer and more easily moved through the colon and anus. Haemorrhoids are caused in constipated individuals who strain to defaecate whilst the anal sphincters are relaxed. Thus dietary fibre relieves this condition, by reducing the need for straining during defaecation. The reasons for the other beneficial effects of fibre are not clear. However, it is possible that constipation leads to the accumulation of carcinogens and other toxins, which may cause cancer and inflammatory disease respectively. Thus adding fibre to the diet should help to prevent these conditions developing, by preventing constipation and diluting any carcinogens present.

Intestinal gas can also stimulate motility in the colon, mainly by causing distension. The gases that can be present include carbon dioxide, hydrogen, oxygen, methane, and nitrogen. These gases do not smell. The odour associated with expelled gas is due to traces of other substances, such as ammonia, hydrogen sulphide, indole, skatole, short-chain fatty acids, and volatile amines. A normal individual releases approximately 500 ml of gas per day. The gases are partly swallowed air, but they can also be derived from substances in the food, or are produced in the lumen by neutralisation of gastric acid, or by bacterial fermentation processes. They can also arise via diffusion from the blood.

Laxatives

Some ingested substances stimulate motility in the colon via activation of chemoreceptors. An example of such a compound is senna bisacodyl. The increase in motility is mediated via the myenteric plexus. This plexus can be damaged by prolonged high doses of laxatives.

Emotions

The effect of emotions on colonic motility has been studied in patients who have been provided with a colostomy. It has been shown that anger and resentment increase motility, whilst depression decreases it. The mechanisms involved are not clear, but they presumably involve autonomic nerve fibres.

Control of motility in the colon

The smooth muscle cells of both the longitudinal layer and the circular layer exhibit spontaneously oscillating membrane potentials. In the longitudinal layer the amplitude of the oscillations sometimes reaches the threshold level for action potential generation, resulting in spontaneous contractions of the muscle. In the circular layer, however, contractions do not usually occur unless the muscle is stimulated by nerves, which release transmitters such as acetylcholine in the vicinity of the pacemaker cells. Acetylcholine increases the time course of the slow wave oscillations, and these longer waves elicit contractions (Fig. 10.7).

Haustration and segmentation occur most of the time, although they are not perceived, but the frequency of these movements diminishes during sleep. They are spontaneous contractions modified by various factors such as stretch, which increases the strength of the contractions (see Chapter 1). Other factors that control colonic motility include extrinsic autonomic nerves, intrinsic nerves in the intramural nerve plexi, and hormones.

Nervous control

Motility in the colon is controlled by intrinsic nerves of the intramural plexi and by extrinsic autonomic nerves. Figure 10.8 illustrates these pathways. Intrinsic nerves, which release acetylcholine or substance P stimulate motility, and intrinsic nerves, which release purines, VIP, and nitric oxide (NO) inhibit it. The importance of the intrinsic nerve plexi to the normal functioning of the colon is illustrated by the problems which occur in Hirschsprung's disease (see Case history 10, page 178) and Chaga's disease (trypanosomiasis). Both conditions are characterised by an absence of intramural ganglion cells in a narrowed region of the colon. Hirschsprung's disease is a congenital abnormality, whilst the defect in Chaga's disease is due to trypanosome parasites (*Trypanosoma cruzi*), which infest the wall of the intestines. The parasites produce a toxin that destroys the intramural ganglion cells, leading to symptoms similar to those seen in Hirschsprung's disease.

Extrinsic autonomic nerves are also involved in the control of the colon. They synapse with neurones in the plexi to modulate the effects of the intrinsic innervation, and innervate the smooth muscle directly. Stimulation of the parasympathetic nerves increases motility, both via the interneurones and via their direct action on the muscle. Stimulation of the sympathetic nerves

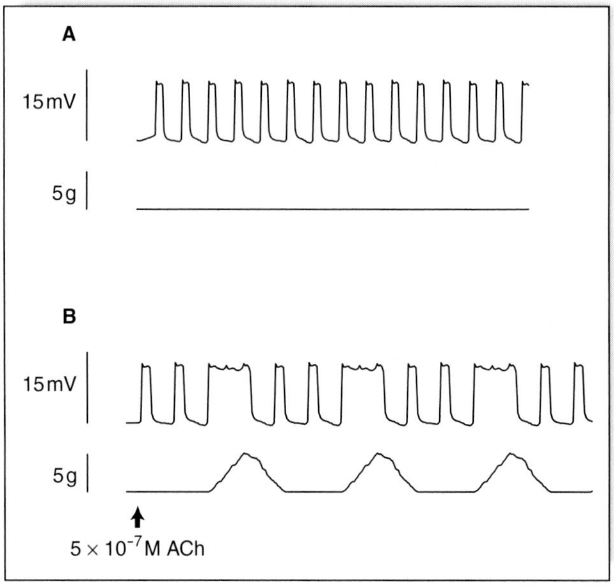

Fig. 10.7

Oscillating membrane potential (upper traces) and contractile activity (lower traces) in the circular smooth muscle of the colon. (A) Unstimulated muscle, (B) the effect of acetylcholine (ACh) (added at the arrow).

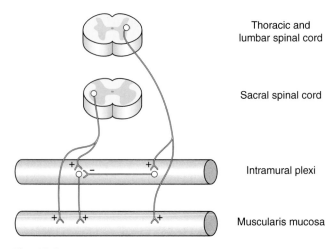

Fig. 10.8

A simplified scheme of control of motility in the colon.

inhibits motility via the interneurones in the plexi, but their direct action on the muscle causes increased contraction (Fig. 10.8). α-Adrenergic receptors are present at the synapses of sympathetic nerves, both in the plexi and on the muscle. The inhibitory interneurones in the plexi, with which the sympathetic nerves synapse, are not adrenergic (see above).

Reflex control

Distension of some regions of the colon causes relaxation in other parts. This is the colono-colic reflex. In addition other regions of the gastrointestinal tract can reflexly influence colonic motility. Thus a marked increase in motility in the large intestines occurs three to four times a day due to the gastro-colic reflex. This reflex is a response to food in the stomach, and it usually coincides with the ileo-gastric reflex (see Chapter 7). The gastro-colic reflex depends on the parasympathetic innervation of the colon, but the hormones gastrin and cholecystokinin (CCK) may also be involved.

Defaecation

Defaecation is a reflex response to the sudden distension of the walls of the rectum (Fig. 10.9) resulting from mass movements in the colon moving the faecal material into it. The reflex response has four components:

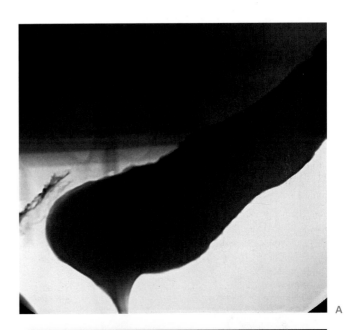

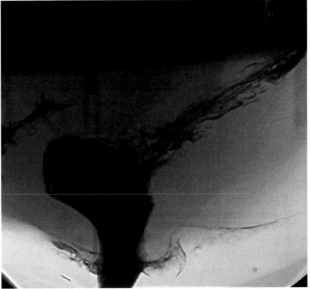

Fig. 10.9
An X-ray showing a rectum filled with contrast before (A) and during (B) contraction/defaecation.

Hirschsprung's disease Box 3

Motility

The importance of the intramural nerves in the control of motility in the colon becomes clear from the symptoms of Hirschsprung's disease. Loss of the ganglionic cells from a segment of the colon disrupts the coordinated propulsive activity of the organ, leading to severe constipation. Both excitatory and inhibitory neurones are affected.

An absence of excitatory cholinergic ganglion cells prevents segmental contractions and coordinated propulsion from taking place. However, the parasympathetic cholinergic fibres from the sacral spinal cord innervate the muscle directly and their activity results in sustained contraction, because modification of the contractile activity by inhibitory interneurones in the plexi can no longer take place. (Furthermore the adrenergic sympathetic nerve fibres can no longer act via inhibitory interneurones to augment the inhibition of the cholinergic nerves in the plexi.) Thus effective relaxation of the circular muscle is lost. Extrinsic sympathetic nerves also synapse directly on smooth muscle, and activation of the α-receptors on the smooth muscle cells by these nerves produces excitation and increased muscle tone. Thus both parasympathetic and sympathetic extrinsic influences lead to sustained tonic contraction of the smooth muscle in the aganglionic segment. The presence of the contracted segment results in blockage of the colon.

N.B. A well-known finding in Hirschsprung's disease is an elevated level of acetylcholinesterase in the narrowed segment. This is indicative of an abnormality of the cholinergic innervation.

1. increased activity in the sigmoid colon
2. distension of the rectum
3. reflex contraction of the rectum
4. relaxation of the internal and external anal sphincters (which are normally closed).

Control of defaecation

The caudal extremity is under nervous control. Defaecation is basically an intrinsic reflex mediated by impulses in the internal nerve plexi, which is reinforced by an autonomic reflex transmitted in the spinal cord. The reflex is integrated by the defaecation centre in the sacral spinal cord. However, defaecation is also regulated by higher centres. Figure 10.10 illustrates the pathways involved in the neural control of

defaecation. When faeces enter the rectum, distension of the wall activates pressure receptors. These send afferent signals that spread through the myenteric plexus to initiate peristaltic waves in the descending and sigmoid regions of the colon, and the rectum. These waves of contraction force the faeces towards the anus. As the wave approaches the anus, the sphincters are inhibited, and they relax. The external sphincter, which is innervated by somatic motor nerves, is under voluntary control. If the external sphincter is relaxed voluntarily when the faeces are pushed towards it, defaecation will occur.

This intrinsic reflex is augmented by an autonomic reflex. This involves parasympathetic nerve fibres in the pelvic nerves arising from the sacral spinal cord, which innervate the terminal colon. Thus activation of pressure receptors by distension of the rectum sends afferent impulses to the spinal cord (as well as to nerves in the intramural plexi). This results in impulses being transmitted in the parasympathetic nerve fibres to the descending colon, the sigmoid colon, and the rectum. The parasympathetic signals intensify the peristaltic waves, and augment the effect of the intrinsic neurones to cause increased motility, contraction of the rectum, and relaxation of the internal and external anal sphincters. Thus the parasympathetic reflex converts the weak intrinsic reflex to a powerful reflex. The sacral control centre also coordinates the other effects that accompany defaecation, including a deep inspiration, closure of the glottis, and contraction of the abdominal muscles, which forces the faeces downwards and extends the pelvic floor so that it pulls outward on the anus to expel the faeces. The reflex normally initiates contraction of the external anal sphincter, which temporarily prevents defaecation. The conscious mind then takes over, and either it inhibits the external sphincter to cause relaxation and allow defaecation to occur, or it keeps it contracted so that defaecation is resisted. Factors such as pain inhibit this relaxation, and this results in straining. If this becomes chronic it leads to dilation of the haemorrhoidal veins ('piles'), and may even prolapse the rectum through the anal canal.

The sensation of fullness of the rectum and the desire to defaecate often follows the ingestion of a meal. If the urge to defaecate is resisted, the sensation subsides, and the sphincters regain their normal tone. Therefore the reflex reactions to distension of the colon are transient.

The frequency of defaecation, and the time of day when it is performed, is a matter of habit. In two-thirds of healthy individuals it is between five and seven times a week.

In the human adult approximately 150 g of material are probably eliminated per day. Of this, two-thirds are

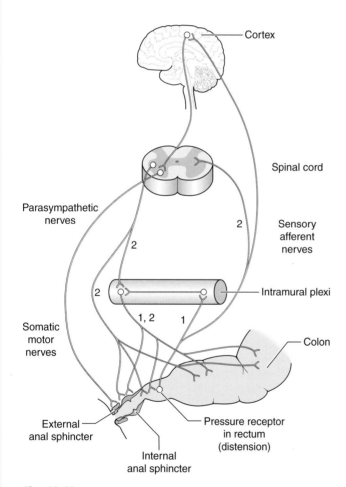

Fig. 10.10
A simplified scheme showing the neural control of defaecation. The basic reflex operates via the intramural plexi, and the spinal parasympathetic reflex reinforces the basic reflex. Control is also exerted by the conscious brain. Numerical labels: 1, components of the basic reflex, 2, components of the spinal sympathetic reflex.

water and one-third is solids. The solids are normally mostly undigested cellulose, bacteria, cell debris, bile pigments, and some salts. There is a high content of K^+ ions in the faeces, relative to the fluid entering the colon, as these ions are secreted by the walls of the colon. The brown colour of faeces is due to the presence of stercobilin and urobilin (see Chapter 6). The odour is caused mainly by products of bacterial fermentation. These include indoles, skatoles, mercaptans, and hydrogen sulphide.

Hirschsprung's disease Box 5

Defaecation reflex

The loss of reflex inhibition of the internal anal sphincter in Hirschsprung's disease illustrates the importance of the intramural nerves in the reflex control of defaecation. The innervation of the internal sphincter is defective in this condition and there is a fluctuating but mainly continuous contraction of the sphincter. The normal relaxation response of the sphincter muscle to distension of the rectum does not occur. This is because its relaxation normally depends on the presence of inhibitory fibres in the intramural plexi.

The basic defaecation reflex in response to distension of the rectum, depends on the transmission of afferent impulses to the intramural nerve plexi, and efferent impulses from these plexi to the muscle of the rectum and internal anal sphincter, to cause reflex contraction of the rectum and relaxation of the internal anal sphincter. This basic reflex cannot be operational if the ganglion cells are absent. Moreover the anal sphincter is innervated directly by parasympathetic cholinergic and sympathetic α-adrenergic nerve fibres. The activity in the extrinsic nerves normally reinforces the basic reflex via synapses with neurones in the plexi. However, in Hirschsprung's disease these influences cannot occur, and both the direct parasympathetic and the direct sympathetic innervation of the sphincter muscle cause contraction of the sphincter. In Hirschsprung's disease the sphincter remains contracted.

The response of the external anal sphincter is normal in Hirschsprung's disease as the somatic motor innervation is not affected.

Self-assessment case study: ulcerative colitis

A 22-year-old woman, who for the past 2 years had been experiencing intermittent attacks of diarrhoea and rectal bleeding, visited her general practitioner. She said the attacks lasted for several weeks each time, but there was complete remission of the symptoms between attacks. During the attacks she experienced lower abdominal cramps and sometimes felt feverish. The general practitioner thought the symptoms could be explained by the presence of any of a number of different conditions, including haemorrhoids, irritable bowel syndrome, and ulcerative colitis, and she decided to send the patient to see a specialist. The patient was referred to an outpatient clinic, and underwent sigmoidoscopy (direct visual examination of the rectum and distal sigmoid colon) and a radiographic examination of her abdomen. The provisional diagnosis of ulcerative colitis was made on the basis of the finding of inflamed and bleeding mucosa. A rectal biopsy specimen was taken during the procedure and sent to the pathology laboratory to confirm the diagnosis. A blood sample was taken for determination of plasma electrolytes, blood haemoglobin, and plasma albumen. The patient was prescribed corticosteroids, and these drugs ameliorated the symptoms of the disease within a week or so.

In ulcerative colitis, the mucosa of the colon is abnormal and inflamed (Fig. 10.11, page 186). In many ways the condition resembles Crohn's disease, although the latter more commonly affects the small intestine, whilst in ulcerative colitis the distal colon and rectum are always affected. Histological findings show that the inflammation is restricted to the mucosa and (to a lesser extent) the submucosa. Near the tips of the crypts are accumulations of polymorphonuclear cells (crypt abscesses). The epithelial cells in the crypts show evidence of degeneration (mucosal atrophy). Ulceration of the mucosa may also be evident. The aetiology of this disease is unknown, although it has been variously ascribed to infection, and to an abnormality of the immune system.

After studying this chapter and the details of this case, you should be able to answer the following questions:

① What would the sigmoidoscopy and radiography probably have shown?

② Why were the patient's plasma electrolytes determined?

③ Why was the patient's haemoglobin determined?

④ Why was the patient's plasma albumen concentration determined?

⑤ What could be the cause of the diarrhoea, and frequent bowel moments?

⑥ What is the rationale for treating this patient with corticosteroids?

Introduction

Understanding normal body function is the foundation of clinical practice. In this book the normal anatomy, physiology, and histopathology of the gastrointestinal tract has been applied to explain why different clinical conditions manifest their specific signs and symptoms. In the first ten chapters, clinical examples of diseases have been selected to highlight specific aspects of physiological gastrointestinal function. The final chapter provides an overview of gastrointestinal pathology and its manifestations.

The diseases described in this chapter are addressed anatomically under the headings: the oral cavity, the oesophagus, the stomach, the duodenum, the pancreas, the liver and biliary tract, the small bowel, and the large bowel. In addition to these sections three other clinical areas are addressed separately. These are:

1. Cancer of the gastrointestinal tract, which is the commonest cause of death from digestive tract disorders.
2. Abdominal pain, which is one of the most frequent causes of acute presentation to the health service.
3. Gastrointestinal surgery, which provides further insight into the functional importance of the components of the digestive tract.

Gastrointestinal malignancy

In the Western world, malignancy of the gastrointestinal tract accounts for approximately 10% of all deaths and 40% of deaths from cancer. Effective and even curative treatment is available for these tumours if they are diagnosed at an early stage. For these reasons, malignancies of the gastrointestinal tract must be considered at an early stage in the diagnostic process for any patient presenting with gastrointestinal symptoms (Table 11.1).

A number of general factors will influence the clinician as to the likelihood of any symptom being due to an underlying malignancy:

- The age of the patient
- The duration of symptoms
- The progression of symptoms
- Identifiable aetiological factors
- A family history of malignancy.

Solid tumours, including gastrointestinal cancers, occur in patients with increasing frequency with advancing years. They are rarely diagnosed in patients under the age of 50 years, but thereafter rapidly increase in frequency into the seventh decade of life. Symptoms may start in an insidious fashion, but often progress over a period of weeks or months. This is in contrast to acute infection, which often has a sudden onset of symptoms, or chronic inflammatory conditions which commonly display periods of exacerbation and remission.

Environmental factors may also alert the clinician to the underlying diagnosis. Thus a history of prolonged alcohol intake and chronic liver disease can alert the clinician to the possibility of a primary liver tumour (hepatoma).

The importance of dietary intake in causing gastrointestinal malignancies has long been recognised. In the Indian subcontinent chewing beetlenut is known to predispose to oral cancer, ingestion of pickles and salted fish in Japan is associated with an increased incidence of gastric cancer, and the high animal fat, low roughage diet of the Western world predisposes to colorectal cancer. More recently it has been recognised that many gastrointestinal malignancies develop because of an underlying inherited genetic predisposition.

Genetic predisposition may account for up to 20% of all colorectal cancer. In patients who are already predisposed to an inherited tumour, the tumours will tend to occur at an earlier age than in the general population. In addition the tumours may be multiple because the predisposition affects all the cells in the large bowel mucosa. A clinical history from the patient may reveal first-degree relatives affected by the same tumour, because they are usually inherited in an autosomal dominant fashion. The genetic defects that have led to

Table 11.1
Common gastrointestinal cancers

Site	Cases per annum England and Wales	Presenting symptoms
Large bowel	30 000	Alteration in bowel action
Stomach	12 000	Indigestion, epigastric pain
Pancreas	7 000	Jaundice, back pain, steatorrhoea
Oesophagus	5 000	Regurgitation, difficulty in swallowing (dysphagia)
Liver (hepatoma)	500	Features of chronic liver disease. A history of alcohol abuse or hepatitis

Forty per cent of all deaths from cancer in the Western world are attributable to gastrointestinal malignancy. Most early symptoms are due to the abnormal function of the organ.

the predisposition pertain to fundamental cellular functions. It is usual for these patients to be at risk of developing more then one type of tumour, and so a history of several different tumours in the same patient would also lead to the suspicion of an underlying inherited predisposition.

The most common tumours of the gastrointestinal tract affect its mucosal lining. These cells are presumed to be most at risk because of their high rate of proliferation. Moreover, these cells are constantly subjected to injury by ingested carcinogens. By comparison, tumours of the muscle wall, connective tissue, lymphatics or serosal surface of the bowel (peritoneum) are rare. The vast majority of gastrointestinal tumours are tumours of the glandular structures (adenocarcinomas), and develop from the glandular cells of the mucosal lining of the gastrointestinal tract. In the clinical setting, if a metastatic tumour deposit is identified, histological features of an adenocarcinoma would alert the clinician to look for a primary tumour in the digestive tract.

Symptoms of gastrointestinal malignancy

It is helpful to categorise symptoms of malignant disease into three groups:

- symptoms due to primary disease
- symptoms due to secondary disease
- symptoms due to non-metastatic manifestations of malignancy.

Primary disease

The symptoms of malignant disease of the gastrointestinal tract will depend upon the site and function of the part of the gastrointestinal tract that is affected. Carcinoma of the oesophagus will usually present with difficulty in swallowing (dysphagia), whereas adenocarcinoma of the colon will usually manifest with symptoms of a change of bowel habit. In addition to symptoms of disordered function, the site of the pain may also help to localise the tumour. Pancreatic adenocarcinoma often presents with back pain because of the retroperitoneal position of the pancreas, where a tumour of the liver may be associated with pain in the right side of the upper abdomen because of a localised inflammatory response in the overlying peritoneum (Fig. 11.1).

Secondary disease

One of the features of malignancy is the ability of the tumour to spread from the site of primary disease.

Colorectal cancer Box 1

Colon cancer

A 60-year-old woman presented to her general practitioner (GP) because of gastrointestinal symptoms. On direct questioning she said that the frequency of her bowel action had increased over the preceding weeks. In addition she had noticed some traces of blood in her stool on two occasions. She also complained that the consistency of her stool had changed and that she had not passed a formed stool in the preceding 2 weeks. No other person in the family had suffered any recent gastrointestinal upset and she had not suffered similar symptoms in the past. On specific questioning, she informed her GP that her father had died from colorectal cancer.

On examination, the GP found the patient to be anaemic, and her clothes were loose, indicating she had recently lost weight. Examination of her abdomen revealed an enlarged liver.

The GP was concerned that she may have an underlying colonic cancer and referred her to the hospital for further investigation. The consultant arranged a barium enema and a CT (computerised tomography) scan of her liver. The barium enema revealed a narrowing in the colon consistent with a carcinoma. The CT scan of the liver revealed a single metastasis in the right lobe. The diagnosis was explained to the patient and arrangements were made for surgery. At operation a left hemicolectomy was performed. This involved removal of the sigmoid and descending colon with its blood supply, and anastomosis of the splenic flexure to the recto-sigmoid junction. In addition, the right lobe of the liver, containing the metastasis, was removed.

Following operation, the patient made a slow but steady recovery. She returned to a normal diet on the sixth postoperative day. She did not become jaundiced following her operation.

This spread may occur via the lymphatics, the bloodstream or through the peritoneal cavity (transcoelomic spread). The lymphatic drainage of the gastrointestinal tract follows its arterial blood supply. Consequently, tumours of the stomach, small bowel or large bowel can spread via the lymphatics to the root of the coeliac artery, superior mesenteric artery, and inferior mesenteric artery respectively. As these lymph nodes are deep inside the abdominal cavity such spread is often initially undetected. The tumour may spread further up the thoracic chain and manifest as a swelling in the supraclavicular lymph nodes in the neck. Because the thoracic duct drains into the veins on the left

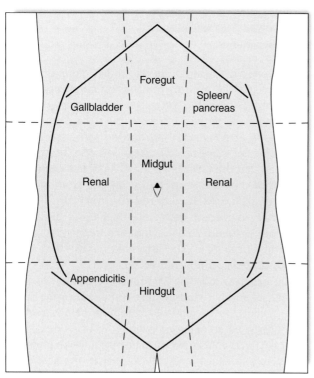

Fig. 11.1
Visceral pain is referred to its site of embryological origin. Parietal pain is more localised and is derived from inflammation of the overlying parietal peritoneum. The pointing pain in the right iliac fossa in appendicitis is typical of parietal pain.

side of the neck, an enlarged lymph node in the left supraclavicular region is always suspicious of lymphatic spread from an underlying gastrointestinal malignancy.

The venous drainage from the gastrointestinal tract is via the portal vein to the liver. For this reason most gastrointestinal malignancies can develop blood-borne metastases in the liver. Abdominal examination may reveal enlargement of the liver in the right sub-costal region and affected individuals may occasionally present with symptoms of pain or jaundice.

Non-metastatic manifestations of malignancy

Malignancy, particularly in its advanced stages, is associated with an increased metabolic rate. This is due in part to the rapid cell division and tumour growth, and also due to secreted proteins released from the tumour. This catabolic state results in loss of body weight and, in its advanced stages, visible loss of muscle mass. This can occur in the presence of a normal dietary intake, and is one of the most common non-metastatic manifestations of malignancy.

A further common finding is anaemia, due to bone marrow suppression. Because gastrointestinal malignancies usually disrupt the epithelial lining, which protects the gastrointestinal tract from injury, blood loss from the gastrointestinal tract is also common. The blood loss may be chronic and is often not clinically apparent. As the iron stores are depleted, red blood corpuscle maturation becomes impaired. An iron-deficient anaemia develops, in which the red blood cells are smaller (microcytic) and contain a reduced haem component (hypochromic).

Common gastrointestinal malignancies

In the Western world over half of deaths are accounted for by diseases of the cardiovascular system. The next most frequent cause of death is that of malignancy, which accounts for approximately 40% of all deaths. Gastrointestinal malignancies account for over 30% of all deaths from cancer, some 60000 deaths per annum in England and Wales alone. Unfortunately, although early tumours can often be cured by surgery, most patients present after the disease has spread and as a consequence treatment is less likely to be curable. The reserves of function in the gastrointestinal tract are such that radical resection of large sections are still compatible with a full and active life.

Carcinoma of the oesophagus

Carcinoma of the oesophagus affects approximately 5 per 100000 of the population per annum. Two-thirds of the tumours are squamous carcinomas and the rest are adenocarcinomas. This reflects the epithelial lining of the oesophagus, which is of squamous type. Adenocarcinomas are usually localised to the distal third of the oesophagus and probably develop from ectopic gastric mucosa.

The classical symptom is of difficulty in swallowing (dysphagia). The symptoms are slowly progressive, with patients describing difficulty in swallowing solids and often having altered their diet to compensate. Oesophageal tumours may enlarge into the lumen, but more often will infiltrate diffusely along and around the oesophageal wall (Table 11.2). The tendency for these tumours to grow along the wall of the oesophagus makes complete surgical resection difficult. Furthermore the lack of a serosal covering to the oesophagus enables direct extension of the tumour into the mediastinum. Involvement of the adjacent trachea and bronchi will result in respiratory problems. The oesophagus and rectum are the only two parts of the gastrointestinal tract that are not covered by a peritoneal coat, and tumours in these two loca-

Table 11.2
Oesophageal cancer

Symptom	Mechanism
Difficulty in swallowing (dysphagia)	The tumour may encase the oesophagus leading to narrowing or infiltration of the mucosal coat resulting in impaired motility
A history for many years of painful swallowing	It can develop following longstanding oesophagitis in the lower oesophagus
Weight loss	This may be due to alteration in diet secondary to difficulty in swallowing
Respiratory symptoms	Problems with swallowing will usually predate the development of metastatic disease. The patient may have symptoms from local infiltration of the organ such as the bronchi or trachea

tions commonly invade surrounding local structures. Spread into the lymphatic system may manifest with a palpable supraclavicular lymph node, and spread into the portal venous system results in the development of liver metastases. Because tumours of the oesophagus do not usually invade the lumen of the oesophagus, dysphagia is a late feature and as a consequence the tumour is rarely curable. Only 6% of patients survive for 5 years.

A number of aetiological factors are known to be associated with this tumour. The most frequent of these are heavy alcohol intake and smoking. These factors probably account for much of the variation in instance seen across different populations. A further interesting aetiological factor is that of acid reflux. Chronic oesophagitis associated with an incompetent gastro-oesophageal sphincter causes damage to the mucosa in the lower third of the oesophagus. This chronic injury appears to predispose to the development of adeno-carcinoma in the lower third of the oesophagus. These

Colorectal cancer Box 2

Treatment

Alteration in bowel habit is a common symptom of colonic cancer. It can be due to partial obstruction of the lumen of the large bowel or be the result of ulceration of the mucosal surface. Ulceration can also give rise to the symptoms of intermittent bleeding.

Colorectal cancer clusters in families in up to 20% of cases and so a family history of this disease is not uncommon in affected individuals. This is believed to be largely genetically determined, although the molecular basis in most families is not understood. Non-metastatic manifestations of gastrointestinal malignancies are more common in advanced disease and include weight loss and anaemia. The patient may have also been anaemic because of chronic gastrointestinal bleeding.

The GP was suspicious that the enlarged liver was due to metastatic disease, and in the light of the patient's large bowel symptoms the GP felt that a colorectal cancer was the most likely diagnosis. A double-contrast barium enema outlines the lining of the bowel, and infiltration by neoplasm creates a rigid narrowing that is easily visualised (Fig. 11.2). Computerised tomography is a useful way of defining abnormal areas of tissue in solid organs like the liver. The increased vascularity of metastatic tumours makes these easy to visualise on a CT scan (Fig. 11.3).

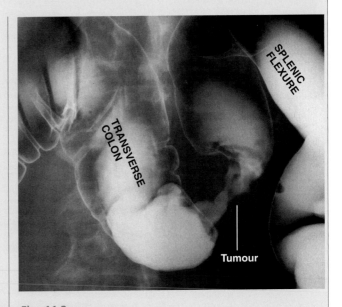

Fig. 11.2
An X-ray of the large bowel showing the large bowel lined with a coating of barium. A large tumour is visible at the splenic flexure. This encircles and narrows the lumen, creating the typical 'apple core' appearance.

different aetiological factors all result in a chronic injury to the oesophageal mucosa which over a period of time can lead to neoplastic change.

Gastric carcinoma (Table 11.3)

Gastric carcinoma is exceptional, in that its incidence has been in steady decline for the last 30 years, whilst other gastrointestinal tumours have increased in frequency with increased longevity. Despite this, it remains the third most common cause of death from gastrointestinal tumours in Western countries, and is a major health issue in Japan and Chile. Variation in populations are believed to be due to local environmental, mainly dietary, factors. Recognised dietary factors include spiced foods, dietary nitrates, as well as smoking and alcohol. *Helicobacter pylori* infection,

which is known to predispose to peptic ulcer disease, has also been implicated in gastric carcinomas. Conditions injurious to the gastric mucosa, such as pernicious anaemia and atrophic gastritis, are also associated with an increased incidence of subsequent neoplastic change. Symptoms due to the primary gastric tumour either arise as a consequence of ulceration of the mucosa, or from diffuse infiltration of the muscular wall. The ulcerating lesion has been classified as 'intestinal', whereas widespread infiltration of the muscle is classified as 'diffuse' type. Ulcerating tumours may present with pain from the injury to the mucosa, bleeding from erosion into underlying blood vessels, or peritonitis from perforation of the ulcer allowing gastric contents to leak into the peritoneal cavity. In contrast, diffuse gastric cancer often presents with a more insidious onset. The infiltrating nature of this tumour leads to a constricted stomach with a

---

Colorectal cancer Box 2 *continued*

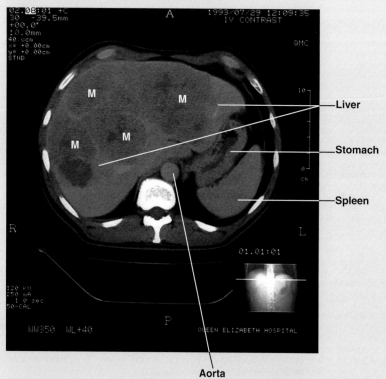

Fig. 11.3
CT scan showing a cross-section of the upper abdomen. Multiple opacities are seen in the liver due to blood-borne metastases (M) from a primary colonic cancer.

Surgical treatment required removal of the primary tumour, the draining lymph nodes, and the single metastasis in the liver. Because blood-borne metastases from colonic cancer preferentially spread to the liver, resection of these advanced tumours can still be curative for selected cases. It is important to exclude other sites of metastatic disease before undertaking such a procedure. The second most

common site of spread from colonic tumours is the lung, which is why the chest X-ray was reviewed prior to surgery.

Normal bowel function following segmental resection of the colon would be expected. No impairment of liver function would be anticipated following a limited resection so jaundice or fat malabsorption would not be anticipated.

Table 11.3
Gastric cancer

Aetiology	The storage function of the stomach makes it particularly susceptible to ingested toxins and dietary factors that can contribute to malignant change
Symptoms	
Bleeding	Ulceration of the tumour results in exposure of the submucosal vessels
Abdominal distension	Gastric tumours often spread from the serosal surface of the stomach creating peritoneal metastases. Leakage of extracellular fluid occurs in association with these lesions and gives rise to ascites
Weight loss	This is more a feature of advanced disease in gastric cancer because the tumours do not usually prevent the passage of ingested food (unlike oesophageal cancer)

grossly thickened wall (lienitis plastica). The nature of diffuse-type cancer mitigates against successful surgical resection. Unfortunately many gastric cancers present at an advanced stage. Patients may have an enlarged liver and associated jaundice due to blood-borne metastases. The disease may spread through the stomach wall onto the peritoneum causing ascites. In these situations the tumour is incurable.

Tumours of the pancreas

In common with other gastrointestinal tumours the majority of tumours of the pancreas are adenocarcinomas developing from the exocrine component of the organ. Because of the high concentration of endocrine cells in the pancreas, they are also the commonest site for endocrine tumours and account for 15% of pancreatic neoplasms. The site of the tumour in the pancreas and the nature of the cell type involved in the tumour will determine its presenting symptoms.

The rarer endocrine tumours will often present with symptoms due to hypersecretion of hormones. An insuloma or glucagonoma may present with hypoglycaemia or diabetes respectively, whereas a gastrinoma will present with intractable peptic ulceration and diarrhoea (Zollinger–Ellison syndrome). Adenocarcinomas often present with insidious symptoms of unexplained back pain and weight loss. The non-specific nature of these symptoms can delay diagnosis and as a consequence these tumours are often unresectable. Tumours that involve the head of the pancreas may present earlier because of obstruction to the common bile duct. The commonest symptoms are progressive jaundice due to obstruction of the bile duct, and steatorrhoea due to obstruction of the pancreatic duct and malabsorption of fat. Some early tumours of the head of the pancreas may be curable with radical surgery.

It has long been recognised that pancreatic cancer is associated with maturity onset diabetes. It was believed that the injurious process that caused diabetes resulted in subsequent tumour de192velopment. However, more recent studies have shown that pancreatic

Adenocarcinoma of the pancreas Box 1

Adenocarcinoma of the pancreas

A 70-year-old man presented to his GP with symptoms of vague upper abdominal pain, which he had noticed over the preceding weeks. From the clinical history, the doctor noted that the patient was a smoker. He suspected the symptoms may be due to peptic ulcer disease and prescribed a course of H₂ antagonists. The patient returned after 2 weeks without resolution of his symptoms. On this occasion the patient declared that the pain had spread to his back. The doctor considered the symptoms may be due to gallstones and arranged an ultrasound scan of the gallbladder. The ultrasound scan confirmed stones in the gallbladder, but also suggested that there was a degree of dilatation of the common bile duct. The serum bilirubin level was checked and was found to be elevated. These findings suggested that there was an obstruction at the lower end of the common bile duct and the GP referred the patient to a gastroenterologist.

At the hospital the patient underwent further investigations including blood glucose, CT scan of the upper abdomen including the pancreas, and endoscopic retrograde pancreatography (ERCP). His serum glucose was found to be mildly elevated, and the CT scan demonstrated a lesion in the head of the pancreas which was compressing the common bile duct. At ERCP, cytology brushings were taken from the pancreatic duct which subsequently supported the diagnosis of adenocarcinoma at the head of the pancreas. During the same procedure a short plastic tube (stent) was placed into the common bile duct to allow free drainage of bile from the liver.

Unfortunately, the tumour was found to be encasing the superior mesenteric artery and curative resection was not possible. Nonetheless, the patient's symptoms from obstructive jaundice were relieved with the stent and pain control was achieved by injection of the nerves in the coeliac plexus.

Adenocarcinoma of pancreas Box 2

Treatment

Abdominal pain that is localised to the upper abdomen can be caused by any structure derived from the foregut. This would include conditions affecting the stomach, gallbladder, or pancreas. Pancreatic diseases may involve the coeliac plexus which lies in close proximity and results in pain that also radiates through to the back.

Investigation of the upper abdomen frequently identifies gallstones, but these are often asymptomatic and may not be the cause of the pain. The bile duct passes through the head of the pancreas before entering the duodenum, and as a consequence tumours in this area can compress the duct and obstruct the flow of bile from the liver. This results in (obstructive) jaundice. The bile duct and pancreatic duct can be visualised by endoscopy. The tissue of the pancreas is best demonstrated by a CT scan of the upper abdomen (see Fig. 4.6 on page 64). At ERCP, cells that have been shed into the ducts can be sampled for microscopic evidence of neoplastic change (cytology). Because tumour tissue is generally friable this provides a useful method of diagnosis in less accessible tumours. A rigid plastic tube can be placed into the bile duct at endoscopy to relieve the obstruction (Fig. 11.4).

The superior mesenteric artery passes just posterior to the neck of the pancreas. This vessel supplies the whole of the midgut. It has to be preserved or the small bowel will be devascularised. If a tumour is involving this artery, surgical excision is impossible. Pain from advanced disease of the pancreas is often due to involvement of the nearby coeliac plexus of autonomic nerves. Injection of this region can safely obliterate the nerves and so help to reduce the pain.

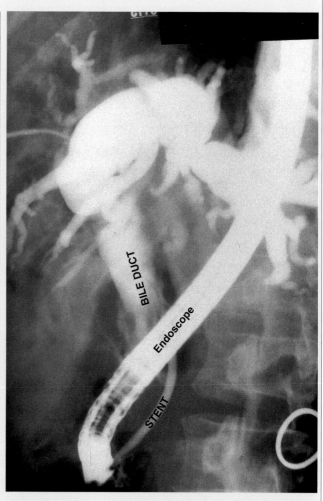

Fig. 11.4
A radio-opaque stent has been placed in the common bile duct using an endoscope, which has been passed via the stomach into the duodenum. The grossly dilated bile ducts have been made visible by the injection of contrast via the stent.

adenocarcinomas may secrete an anti-insulin factor that can cause diabetes, and removal of the tumour can be associated with restoration of normal glucose control. This could provide a future mechanism for earlier diagnosis of this condition.

Acute abdominal pain

Diagnosis of the cause of acute abdominal pain is one of the more challenging aspects of clinical medicine. Because of the lack of a somatic sensory nerve supply, identifying the diseased organ and the nature of the pathology requires a clear understanding of the anatomy, innervation, and physiological function of the different gastrointestinal structures. There are two sources of intra-abdominal pain. Pain may arise from stimulation of the autonomic afferent nerves innervating the abdominal organs. This results in poorly localised abdominal discomfort that manifests in the region of the corresponding somatic afferent nerve root. This is known as referred pain. Because the gastrointestinal tract is derived embryologically from a mid-line structure, pain is referred to the mid-line, usually anteriorly. This is seen in inflammation of the appendix, which derives its **autonomic** nerve

Acute appendicitis Box 1

Case history

A 20-year-old man called out his GP complaining of severe lower abdominal pain. On enquiry, the patient described a pain that had started insidiously and was initially centred around his umbilicus. He had first noticed it when he got out of bed, but had thought nothing of it. When he arrived at work the pain started to become more severe. He could not get comfortable and was unable to eat lunch. The pain shifted to the right lower abdomen and started to prevent him from walking. He returned home early and despite going to bed the pain persisted.

On examination, the GP found the patient to have a pyrexia and a tachycardia. Palpation of his abdomen revealed tenderness localised to the right lower quadrant. The pain was made worse on releasing pressure (rebound tenderness). The GP also tested the patient's urine but found no evidence of protein or blood. He contacted the local hospital which admitted the patient and as his symptoms and signs had not improved, proceeded to arrange for him to undergo an appendectomy. At operation the small bowel and omentum was adherent to an inflamed, swollen, necrotic appendix. Following operation the patient made a rapid recovery and was able to return home on the third postoperative day.

Acute appendicitis Box 2

Pathophysiology

The pain from the appendicitis often starts in the peri-umbilical region. As a midgut structure it derives an autonomic nerve supply from the level of T10, which is referred to the umbilicus. Once the inflammatory process in the wall of the appendix reaches the serosal surface, it causes secondary inflammation of the overlying peritoneum. This results in somatic pain, which becomes localised to the right iliac fossa. Any stretching of the peritoneum, which may be caused by movement or by palpation, will result in pain localising to the right lower quadrant. This inflammatory process also produces reactive changes in the overlying structures such as the small bowel and omentum, which become adherent. The inflammatory exudate, which is seen at operation as a purulent fluid in the peritoneal cavity, contains large numbers of white blood cells. Patients commonly describe a loss of appetite. This is believed to be due to the triggering of ileo-gastric reflex, which impairs gastric emptying. In addition there is a protective 'ileus', which reduces the peristaltic activity of the small bowel.

The appendix has an end artery supply, and inflammation through the wall of the appendix can easily result in thrombosis of the blood supply. This can cause gangrene in the wall and result in perforation of the appendix. Delaying the diagnosis and treatment of appendicitis is a common cause of peritonitis, because of perforation of the appendix wall. The doctor checked the patient's urine for evidence of a urinary tract infection which may have mimicked the symptoms of appendicitis. As there were no red blood cells or protein in the urine, a urinary tract infection was regarded as unlikely.

supply from the level of T10 (along with the rest of the midgut). Pain is therefore referred to the peri-umbilical region, which is innervated by **somatic** sensory nerves that enter the spinal cord at the same level (T10). Pain from the large bowel also refers to the mid-line, but to the infra-umbilical region. Pain from foregut structures (stomach and duodenum) is referred to the central upper abdominal region (epigastrium – see Fig. 11.1, page 190).

The second type of abdominal pain is due to inflammation of the overlying parietal peritoneum. This has its own somatic innervation and, therefore, results in well-localised pain over the area of inflammation. Appendicitis pain moves from the peri-umbilical region to the right lower abdomen region (right iliac fossa) once the inflammatory process in the appendix penetrates through the serosal surface causing inflammation of the overlying parietal peritoneum (Fig. 11.1).

The speed of onset of the pain can also help determine the nature of the organ involved. Very muscular structures with a narrow lumen will quickly cause severe pain if they become acutely distended. Thin-walled distensible structures will, however, give rise to a pain of more insidious onset. Pain due to distension

is initially due to stimulation of stretch receptors. As a consequence the pain is often cyclical in nature (colic). This contrasts with pain from inflammation of tissue, which gives rise to a persistent pain (such as pancreatitis).

Surgical resections

Most major surgical resections performed on the gastrointestinal tract are for the treatment of cancer. The fact that, following most procedures, patients are able to continue a normal and active life without nutritional support demonstrates the considerable amount of redundancy in the digestive system, and also its ability to adapt even after radical resections.

Major surgical resection of the oesophagus is usually undertaken for oesophageal carcinoma. Although this operation is rarely curative it provides remarkably good symptomatic relief from pain and obstruction, allowing the patient to return to a largely normal diet. Most tumours of the oesophagus involve the lower two-thirds. Removal of this portion of the oesophagus is possible. Restoration of continuity can be achieved by mobilisation of the stomach, which is brought into the chest and connected to the remaining oesophagus in the upper thorax. This is possible because the blood supply of the stomach is so plentiful that the right gastric vessels can be divided and the blood supply sustained on the left gastric artery. If a more radical resection of the oesophagus is required then a length of small bowel can be placed in the chest to be joined from the throat to the stomach. This requires re-anastomosis of the arterial supply and venous drainage as the superior mesenteric vessels (supplying the small bowel) are insufficiently long to reach into the upper thorax.

Replacement of the oesophagus will result in loss of normal peristalsis and so the patient will need to sit upright when eating. In addition there will be impairment of the motility and storage capacity of the stomach because of division of the vagal nerves. This requires the patients to eat smaller and more frequent meals to sustain their nutrition. This minor lifestyle adaptation is usually all that is required.

Removal of the antrum and pylorus of the stomach is undertaken for the complications of peptic ulcer disease and for carcinoma. This portion of the stomach mucosa contains the majority of the gastrin-secreting G cells, and as a result, resection dramatically reduces acid secretion in the stomach. In addition there is loss of the pyloric control of gastric emptying and reduced storage capacity. The stomach remnant can be reconnected to the proximal duodenum or the upper jejunum. This results in premature release of chyme from the stomach, in advance of the release of digestive juices from the gallbladder and pancreatic duct. The main consequence of this is impaired fat absorption and sometimes osmotic diarrhoea from incomplete digestion. Patients can usually control these symptoms by simple modification of their diet. The functional consequences of the loss of gastrin are not usually clinically apparent. An interesting, but relatively rare, complication of this operation is paradoxical hypoglycaemia following meals. The patient complains of symptoms of sweating and feeling faint soon after meals. This is due to inappropriate release of insulin from the pancreas in response to ingestion of food, but in advance of sufficient absorption of glucose from the gastrointestinal tract to counterbalance the insulin release.

Gastric carcinoma may require total gastrectomy in an attempt to cure the disease. In this case the jejunum is brought up to connect with the oesophagus, and the distal (the fourth part) of duodenum is re-joined to the jejunum more distally (Fig. 11.5). This anatomical rearrangement is necessary because the alkaline secretions from the gallbladder and pancreas would cause severe ulceration of the unprotected oesophageal mucosa if allowed to come into direct contact with it. Loss of the whole stomach does significantly impair the storage capacity of the digestive tract. As a consequence the patients must eat more frequent and smaller meals to maintain nutrition. Loss of acid secretion, pepsinogen, and gastrin all have surprisingly little effect on gastrointestinal function. However, loss of intrinsic factor does require replacement therapy by subcutaneous injection of vitamin B_{12}.

Removal of the gallbladder (cholecystectomy) is one

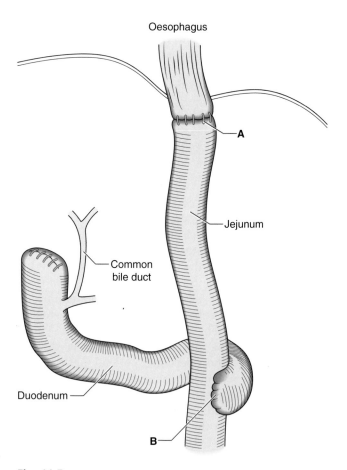

Fig. 11.5

The anatomical arrangement following a total gastrectomy, usually performed for a carcinoma of the stomach. The proximal jejunum (A) is joined to the oesophagus. The bile and pancreatic juice is directed away from the oesophagus by rejoining the fourth part of the duodenum to the mid-jejunum (B).

of the most common abdominal procedures performed in the Western world. The gallbladder is removed by division of the cystic artery and cystic duct, but the common bile duct is left intact to enable free drainage of bile from the liver into the duodenum. Loss of the storage reservoir for bile salts results in adaptation of bile salt present in the liver. Following surgery, the bile is present in higher volumes from the liver and is released continuously into the duodenum at a slow rate. On ingestion of a fatty meal, liver bile release increases rapidly which compensates for the lack of a gallbladder, and patients are able to tolerate meals with even a high fat content. There is an interesting secondary effect from this operation, that is the increased rate of bile uptake from the ileum into the enterohepatic circulation. This results in a higher proportion of secondary bile acids because of the increased circulation of the bile. There is some evidence to suggest that this may have a potentially carcinogenic effect on the large bowel and there is an association with an increased incidence of colorectal cancer.

Resection of the pancreas is a technically challenging procedure carried out both for inflammatory diseases of the pancreas (pancreatitis) and also for pancreatic cancer. Most pancreatic tumours arise in the head of the pancreas. When they are diagnosed at an early stage they can be treated successfully by removal of the head and neck of the pancreas. Because the pancreas receives a joint blood supply with the duodenum, it is necessary to remove the duodenum together with the head of the organ. This requires the common bile duct, tail of the pancreas, and stomach, to be re-joined with a loop of jejunum (Fig. 11.6). Safely joining the bowel to the pancreas is a hazardous procedure. This is partly because the tissue of the pancreas is soft and friable but also because activated digested enzymes released from pancreas interfere with the healing process at the anastomosis. Following this major procedure patients will have impaired fat and protein metabolism. This is not due to insufficient pancreatic secretion, but rather to premature stomach emptying without coordinated secretion from the pancreas and liver. It can be partially overcome by preservation of the pyloric sphincter (pylorus-preserving Whipple's procedure).

Total pancreatectomy is in one respect a safer operation, because anastomosis to the remaining pancreas is not required. It does, however, involve loss of all endocrine and exocrine secretions from the pancreas. For satisfactory digestion of food it is necessary to add pancreatic enzyme supplements to the diet. In addition these patients are diabetic, and because there is loss of both insulin and glucagon, control of their diabetes can be difficult.

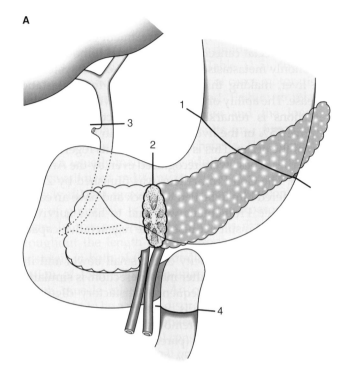

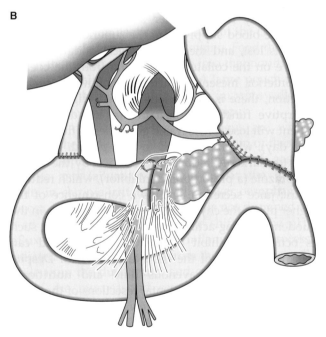

Fig. 11.6
The foregut anatomy before (A) and after (B) a partial pancreaticoduodenectomy (Whipple's resection). The stomach antrum is divided (1) along with the head of the pancreas (2), common bile duct (3) and the fourth part of the duodenum (4). The specimen is removed and the proximal jejunum joined to the stomach, bile duct and body of pancreas as shown. The operation is usually done for a carcinoma of the head of the pancreas.

Table 11.5
Oesophageal disease

Condition	Clinical features	Mechanism
Varices	Massive gastrointestinal haemorrhage, and haematemesis	Portal hypertension results in dilation and engorgement of the veins communicating between the portal and systemic circulation. Spontaneous haemorrhage occurs because of the raised venous pressure
	Features of cirrhosis	Chronic liver disease is associated with morphological changes in the hepatic architecture. This occludes venous drainage into the inferior vena cava, and results in portal hypertension
Infection	Associated with impaired immunity	The squamous epithelium of the oesophagus provides effective protection against infection. This can be impaired by immunosuppression
	Infection is often by organisms that are not normally pathogenic	Impaired immunity results in overgrowth of organisms that are commonly present in the oro-pharynx such as Candida (a yeast) or herpes simplex viruses
Oesophageal pouch (diverticulum)	The patient is usually elderly and complains of regurgitation of 'old' food	Weakness in the wall of the upper oesophagus allows the mucosa to bulge through the muscle coat. Because this sac is not enclosed by muscle it can't contract, so food can collect in it

Table 11.6
Oesophagitis

Aetiology	Reflux of gastric content into lower oesophagus
	Failure to clear luminal contents into the stomach

Symptoms	Mechanism
Pain	Inflammatory changes in the lower oesophageal mucosa
Dysphagia	Secondary fibrosis and narrowing of the lower oesophagus
	Impaired motility due to damage to underlying smooth muscle
Regurgitation	Blockage of the lumen. This may result from secondary neoplastic change
Weight loss	More common in the presence of neoplastic change

Investigation	
Endoscopy	Allows direct visualisation of the mucosa and biopsy for histological assessment
Barium swallow	Allows visualisation of the level of an obstruction, and also shows function of peristalsis

porto-systemic anastomoses at the lower end of the oesophagus become massively dilated in response to the raised venous pressure. These veins are thin-walled and bleed easily. Bleeding can be massive and life-threatening. The associated liver disease can complicate the situation because of impairment of coagulation. Optimal management requires occlusion of the veins by endoscopic ligation or sclerotherapy.

Infections of the oesophagus are surprisingly rare; the squamous epithelium is a highly effective barrier. Nonetheless, in the presence of impaired immunity, or obstruction and secondary stasis, infection can occur. Candidal fungal infection, seen as white plaques in the oesophagus, is a common infecting organism, particularly if patients have been on long-term antibiotics. Viral infections are also seen in the immune-compromised patient, notably herpes simplex and cytomegalovirus.

Stomach and duodenum

The most common clinical conditions in the stomach and duodenum involve the mucosa. The common benign conditions include acute and chronic gastritis, and peptic ulcer disease. Malignant disease in the stomach is an important site for gastrointestinal malignancy, but interestingly is relatively rare in the duodenum, as is the case for the rest of the small bowel. This observation indicates that the common aetiological factors involved in the development of peptic ulcers may differ from those that predispose to gastric cancer.

Acute gastritis is an inflammatory injury to the mucosa of the stomach, which is usually due to the ingestion of toxic substances such as drugs or bacteria in food. It is probably most commonly seen following alcohol ingestion. The condition is self-limiting and does not usually progress to chronic ulceration. Chronic gastritis, like other conditions that result in longstanding injury to the bowel mucosa, predisposes to malignant change. The aetiology of chronic gastritis is multifactorial but is best documented in pernicious anaemia. This is a familial disorder with a history of an affected relative in 30% of patients. Serum antibodies against gastric parietal cells and intrinsic factor are commonly found. Intrinsic factor antibody causes B_{12} deficiency. The condition is increasingly common in older patients who may present with (megaloblastic) anaemia or even neurological disorders caused by a lack of vitamin B_{12}. Approximately 1 in 12 affected patients will develop a carcinoma of the stomach, and for this reason regular surveillance endoscopy of the stomach is performed.

The reason some patients with acute mucosal ulceration may progress to chronic peptic ulcer disease has been a field of extensive investigation because of the high prevalence of this condition (Table 11.7). Environmental and genetic factors have been implicated. It has been shown that patients with duodenal ulcers tend to have a high basal level of acid secretion in the stomach. However, the overlap between the normal range and that seen in patients with peptic ulcer disease is considerable. A major development in understanding this condition followed the discovery of *H. pylori*. This organism is resistant to acid secretion and so can proliferate in the mucosa of the stomach and the duodenum. A strong association between this infection and chronic ulceration has now been established. Historically the treatment of peptic ulcer disease has centred on reducing acid secretion either by surgical or medical means in order to minimise the mucosal damage.

Modern therapy, however, focuses on clearing *Helicobacter* infection by the use of antibiotics. This treatment has been shown to result in a high percentage of ulcer healing and, importantly, a low incidence of recurrence of the disease. Historically, peptic ulcer disease was one of the most common reasons for intestinal surgery. The advent of medical therapy has revolutionised the management of this condition and surgery is now largely restricted to the treatment of complications from peptic ulcer disease. Because of the erosive nature of these ulcers they can result in catastrophic gastrointestinal haemorrhage, or perforation of the ulcer into the peritoneal cavity. These complications still require surgical intervention.

Hepatobiliary disease

Disorders of the hepatobiliary system include both diseases of the biliary tree and diseases affecting hepatocytes (Table 11.8). Diseases that primarily involve the hepatocytes impair liver function. This causes reduced production of serum proteins including albumin, and as a consequence leakage of fluid into the extracellular space by osmosis (oedema). The patient also develops an impaired immune status, resulting in a susceptibility to a range of infections. Derangement of the hepatocyte organisation can obstruct the drainage of the portal vein into the inferior vena cava and so produce a rise in pressure in the portal venous system. The combination of reduced protein production and raised portal pressure causes fluid to collect inside the abdominal cavity (ascites).

Disorders of the biliary tree can result in blockage of drainage of the bile into the duodenum. This manifests as jaundice. Chronic obstruction of bile flow can also produce (secondary) damage to the hepatocytes because of back pressure in the biliary system. It will primarily cause obstructive jaundice, which manifests with skin pigmentation, pale stools (due to the lack of bilirubin), and dark urine (due to the excretion of excess bilirubin by the kidneys).

Disorders of the biliary tree

The commonest disorder to affect the biliary tree is gallstone disease. This affects over 5% of the adult population in Britain. Whilst these stones remain in the gallbladder, they can be asymptomatic. Obstruction of flow of bile from the gallbladder into the common bile duct will, however, result in biliary colic when the gallbladder attempts to contract, and secondary infection in the gallbladder (cholecystitis). If the stones pass into the common bile duct they often lodge at the narrowing created by the ampulla of Vater, where the duct

Table 11.7
Peptic ulcer disease

Aetiology	*Helicobacter* infection of the mucosa impairs the protective mechanisms and allows secondary damage from the acid environment
Symptoms	**Mechanism**
Epigastric pain	Inflammatory reaction to chemical injury to the mucosa, notably hydrochloric acid and pepsin
Bleeding	Erosion of the submucosa exposes the underlying blood vessels which are then vulnerable to damage and secondary haemorrhage
Sudden severe epigastric pain	Further damage to the deeper muscle layers of the wall leads to fibrosis and ischaemia. If this is allowed to progress the ulcer can erode through the serosal surface leading to life-threatening peritonitis
Profuse vomiting	This is occasionally seen in chronic ulcers in the pyloric region and the duodenum because of the narrow lumen. Large ulcers in this region can cause obstruction to the outlet of the stomach

Table 11.8
Hepatobiliary disease

Condition	Features	Mechanism
Gallstones	Right-sided abdominal pain and shoulder tip pain	Gallstones may obstruct the flow of bile from the gallbladder. Pain is referred to the shoulder tip because of the level of autonomic innervation (C4). Abdominal tenderness is due to inflammation of the overlying parietal peritoneum
	Fever	The stagnant bile becomes infected (cholecystitis)
	Jaundice	Gallstones may pass from the gallbladder and lodge at the ampulla of Vater. This will obstruct the flow of bile from the liver
Acute hepatitis	Right upper quadrant pain	Swelling of the liver stimulates nerves in the liver capsule and overlying peritoneum
	Bleeding and bruising	Impaired coagulation results from failure to manufacture proteins required for the clotting cascade
	Reduced level of consciousness	Toxins build up in the systemic circulation because of failure of detoxification and excretion in the liver
Chronic hepatitis	History of previous liver damage	Most patients have suffered a clinical attack of acute hepatitis. Occasionally this is subclinical and passes unnoticed. This has been seen in hepatitis C infection from infected blood transfusions
Chronic liver disease (cirrhosis)	Jaundice	Failure to excrete bilirubin
	Oedema (fluid collecting in the extracellular space), swollen ankles, ascites	Failure of protein production reduces intravascular osmotic pressure and allows fluid to leak into the extracellular space

enters the duodenum. In this position they also obstruct the flow of bile from the liver and result in obstructive jaundice. This results in dark-coloured urine because of reflux of conjugated bile into the systemic circulation, and pale stools because of the absence of bile pigment in the faeces, as well as the classic yellow pigmentation of the skin, most easily seen in the sclera of the eyes. Common bile duct stones may, in addition, interfere with the flow of secretions from the pancreas, and cause acute pancreatitis. An interesting aspect of pain from the gallbladder is discomfort in the right shoulder. This is because it is partly derived embryologically from the diaphragm and shares its autonomic innervation via the phrenic nerve. These nerves enter the spine at the level of C4, along with sensory fibres from the shoulder tip.

The management of complications from gallstone disease is largely surgical. It involves the removal of any stones from the biliary tree in addition to removal of the gallbladder. In the Western world, the vast majority of gallstones form primarily in the gallbladder. In the Far East, where infections of the biliary tract are more common, the formation of stones primarily in the hepatic duct around the porta hepatis create considerable management problems because of their inaccessible position.

Obstruction to the flow of bile may result from fibrosis in the wall of the biliary tree. This is a rare dis-order known as primary sclerosing cholangitis. It is occasionally seen in association with inflammatory bowel disease, especially ulcerative colitis, and for this reason is believed to be of immunological aetiology. The chronic and progressive obstruction of the flow of bile results in secondary damage to the hepatocytes. There are currently no effective treatments for this disorder and the main therapy for advanced disease is liver transplantation.

Hepatocellular disease

Conditions that result in primary damage to hepatocytes result in acute hepatitis. This can be due to infections, usually viral (hepatitis A and B for example), or damage by drugs such as paracetamol, or by toxins such as alcohol. This can result in a range of presentations from mild sub-clinical liver injury to massive liver necrosis and hepatic failure. Any acute hepatitis can result in longstanding liver cell damage (chronic hepatitis). Progressive chronic liver cell injury results in disordered liver architecture associated with fibrosis and regenerative nodules. This is know as cirrhosis. This is an irreversible state resulting in impaired hepatic function encompassing bilirubin excretion, protein manufacture including immune function, and detoxification of drugs. This gives rise to the classic stigmata of chronic liver disease. Two important sequelae of cirrhosis are portal hypertension and liver cell tumours (hepatoma). The only therapeutic option for advanced cirrhosis is liver transplantation.

Nutrients from the gastrointestinal tract are transported via the venous system into the portal vein, which drains directly into the liver. Derangement in the liver architecture, commonly caused by cirrhosis, results in obstruction to the blood flow and a rise in portal venous pressure. This results in opening up of the collateral venous pathways and enlargement of the spleen (splenomegaly). The enlarged spleen traps circulating platelets leading to thrombocytopenia (low blood platelet levels). Collateral veins open up around the flaciform ligament, leading to the appearance of dilated veins around the umbilicus (caput medusae). The clinically important collateral pathway is the communication between the left gastric vein and azygous vein in the lower oesophagus. These dilated veins in the lower oesophagus (varices) are fragile and can burst spontaneously, leading to life-threatening haemorrhage. As the bleeding is often accompanied by thrombocytopenia and deranged clotting (because of the underlying cirrhosis), this can exacerbate the bleeding problem. Treatment requires ligation or sclerosis of the dilated veins, which can often be achieved endoscopically via the oesophagus. In the acute setting, direct balloon compression of the veins may be required. This is done using a specially designed tube (Minnesota tube), which can be passed from the mouth into the stomach.

The commonest malignant tumours of the liver in the West are metastatic cancer, often from primary cancers elsewhere in the gastrointestinal tract. Primary malignant tumours of the liver (hepatoma) are usually seen on a background of cirrhosis. These patients have a particularly poor prognosis as the reserves of liver function are often not sufficient to allow resection of the primary tumour.

Pancreas

Disorders of exocrine function of the pancreas are an important cause of malabsorption because of the central role of this organ in the digestion of fat and protein. Inappropriate activation of digestive enzymes in the pancreas can result in destruction of the organ with potentially catastrophic consequences. This secondary destructive process results in severe unrelenting epigastric pain, which usually radiates through to the back. The most important endocrine functions of the pancreas are the production of insulin and glucagon. Destruction of these islet cells results in diabetes. The pancreas has considerable reserves of function, and destruction of over 70% of the organ is required before clinical manifestation of diabetes or malabsorption becomes apparent.

Acute pancreatitis is a medical emergency, resulting in auto-destruction of the organ (Table 11.9). This process can be precipitated by bile duct stones, which disrupt free drainage of the pancreatic duct, or by acute alcohol ingestion, which is toxic to the organ.

The clinical presentation is often seen in middle-aged women (due to gallstone disease) and young men (following excessive alcohol ingestion). The destructive process results in severe upper abdominal pain, and is commonly associated with vomiting as a consequence of irritation of the overlying stomach. The autolysis causes a massive fluid and protein shift into the extracellular space, depleting the intravascular volume. This can lead to poor perfusion of the kidneys (renal failure),

Table 11.9
Acute pancreatitis

Aetiology	Autodigestion of the pancreas by secreted enzymes. Caused by toxic damage (e.g. alcohol) or by obstruction of secretions (e.g. gallstones)
Symptoms	
Epigastric pain	Local inflammation process damages autonomic nerves from the coeliac plexus
Vomiting	Local irritation of the stomach, which overlies the pancreas
Systemic damage	
Shortness of breath	There are massive fluid shifts into the extracellular space due to inflammatory injury and local release of digestive enzymes. Fluid leaks into the lung extracellular space and into alveoli (pulmonary oedema)
Hypotension	Loss of fluid from the vascular space. This results in underperfusion of many organs including the kidneys
Investigations	
Serum amylase	Inappropriately released into the system from the damaged pancreatic cells
CT scan	This will demonstrate swelling and destruction of the pancreatic gland and surrounding tissue
ERCP	This enables the pancreatic and bile ducts to be visualised and can demonstrate gallstones stuck at the ampulla of Vater (see Fig. 11.4, page 194). Stones can also be removed at this procedure

leakage of fluid into the lungs (pulmonary oedema), and generalised hypotensive shock. The key to treatment is prompt and rapid intravenous fluid replacement. Chronic pancreatitis is a related disorder, usually caused by excessive longstanding alcohol ingestion. In this disease the destruction of the pancreas is a slow and progressive disorder. Patients gradually develop steatorrhoea because of fat malabsorption, and diabetes because of injury to the islet cells. The destruction of the pancreatic tissue results in secondary calcification in the organ and cystic changes that are presumed to be due to obstruction of drainage of the small ductules in the gland. Successful management is largely reliant upon the patient ceasing to take alcohol.

Cystic fibrosis is a condition that is inherited in an autosomal recessive fashion, where both parents are carrying one defective gene. It is due to failure of the chloride pump at the duct cell surface. Before the genetics of the disease were fully understood, the diagnosis relied upon excessive sodium and chloride being found in the patients' sweat. Because this is such an important cellular mechanism, the consequences are widespread (Table 11.10). Newborn babies may be born with acute constipation due to meconium obstruction in the large bowel; this is known as meconium ileus. They may also have a failure in lung expansion because of difficulty in clearing secretions. This problem continues throughout life. Secretory problems in the pancreas result in obstruction of the duct and late pancreatic failure as well as the development of adult onset cirrhosis of the liver. The management of this condition has progressed rapidly over the last decade. Identification of the cystic fibrosis gene enables detection of carriers of the affected gene. Life expectancy has been prolonged by aggressive chest physiotherapy to help with secretory problems in the lungs, and respiratory failure can now be treated by lung transplantation. Gene therapy trials are now underway for this condition.

Small bowel conditions

The primary function of the small intestine to is absorb fluid and nutrients that are ingested. Tumours of the small intestine are surprisingly rare given the size of the organ, and as a consequence the most common conditions affecting the small bowel are concerned with alterations of function. The key functional unit in the small bowel is the mucosa, and malabsorption is invariably due to conditions that are injurious to the mucosal lining. These can be broadly divided into infective and non-infective causes (Table 11.11).

Improvements in living standards and hygiene in the Western world have reduced the frequency and clinical importance of gastrointestinal infections. An acute history of nausea, vomiting, and diarrhoea of sudden onset, often affecting a number of family members, implicates an infective cause. A range of viruses, bacteria, protozoa or toxins can be implicated.

Table 11.10
Pancreatic diseases

Condition	Features	Mechanism
Diabetes mellitis	Polyuria and polydipsia	Failure of insulin secretion results in a high blood sugar. This increases the osmotic potential of the filtrate and causes high urine volumes (polyurea). The hypovolaemia and raised serum osmolality stimulate thirst receptors (polydipsia)
	Coma	Deranged glucose and fatty acid metabolism results in a metabolic acidosis. Combined with hypovolaemia this causes a reduced level of consciousness, and death, if not treated promptly
Chronic pancreatitis	Longstanding alcohol abuse	Alcohol is toxic to the pancreatic gland
	Epigastric pain	Inflammation around the autonomic nerves in the coeliac plexus
	Weight loss and diarrhoea	Failure of exocrine function results in incomplete digestion
	Diabetes mellitus	Failure of islet cell function
Cystic fibrosis	Constipation	Failure in the Na/Cl exchange pump results in pancreatic failure and deranged fluid secretion/absorption in the gut. This manifests as mechanical obstruction in the neonate (meconium ileus) and constipation in later life
	Respiratory failure	Abnormal secretions in the alveoli and bronchioli result in airway obstruction and alveolar collapse. Neonates may suffer from impaired lung expansion and adults suffer recurrent respiratory infections

Table 11.11
Small bowel conditions

Condition	Clinical features	Mechanisms
Malabsorption Coeliac disease	Chronic diarrhoea, weight loss, anaemia. Most commonly in adults	Autoimmune disease of the small bowel. Malabsorption of fat results in bulky, pale, offensive smelling stools that often float in the toilet. Failure to absorb protein results in a net loss of protein from the body and loss of muscle bulk. Anaemia may result from failure to absorb folate and iron
Infection *Salmonella typhus*	Sudden profuse watery diarrhoea, which may be blood-stained. Associated with a high fever	The bacillus infection causes acute ulceration of the mucosa throughout the small and large bowel with associated loss of water and protein, resulting in watery diarrhoea. The ulcerated mucosa tends to bleed. The bacillus spreads through the bloodstream via the portal vein, infesting the liver and creating a marked inflammatory response with a high temperature
Cholera	Severe watery diarrhoea with loss of many litres of fluid each day	The vibrus cholera bacterium does not cause ulceration of the mucosa, but causes failure of the salt/water exchange pump allowing profuse amounts of water to pass into the bowel lumen. This results in watery diarrhoea because the colonic mucosa is unable to reabsorb the high volume. Protein loss is not seen
Ischaemia	Abdominal distension, bleeding from the bowel, and abdominal pain	Impaired blood supply damages the mucosa first because of of its large oxygen requirement and high cell turnover. This results in mucosal ulceration and venous bleeding. The ischaemic bowel loses its normal contractility, resulting in bowel dilatation and abdominal distension

Diagnosis can often be made by culture of the liquid diarrhoea. Key to the successful management of acute infections is the replacement of salts and fluid by the oral route, or, if necessary, the intravenous route. Blood-stained diarrhoea is most likely to be due to a bacterial organism, such as *Salmonella*, and will benefit from appropriate antibiotic therapy. Most infections in Britain today are due to viruses or toxins, and are self-limiting. Cholera remains a major killer worldwide, though improvements in water supply and sewerage have helped to control this infection. *Salmonella* remains an important bacterial infection even in the West, and in the 1990s reports of infection by poultry products received considerable media attention. Chronic sub-clinical infections can occur, usually in the biliary tree. As a consequence, members of the public who handle food and food products continue to be a source of outbreaks of this infection.

Crohn's disease

The cause of chronic symptoms of diarrhoea can be more difficult to ascertain. Crohn's disease provides a good example of chronic small bowel disease (Table 11.12). Although it is relatively rare, with an incidence in the UK of approximately 1 in 10 000, Crohn's disease is a chronic condition with periods of remission and exacerbation, and patients are frequent presenters to the health services. They develop classical symptoms of diarrhoea and abdominal pain, associated with weight loss.

This chronic granulomatous disease can affect any part of the gastrointestinal tract, but most commonly involves the terminal ileum. Genetically determined predisposition is known to play a part in this condition, but a wide range of aetiological factors have been implicated. These include viral infection, microbial infection, dietary, and vascular factors. None of these have been established as causative in the condition and the aetiology is likely to be multifactorial.

The inflammatory process in Crohn's disease affects the full thickness of the bowel wall. As a consequence, ulceration and secondary fibrosis can result in blockage of the lumen. As the inflammatory process penetrates to the external surface of the bowel (serosa), local abscess formation and perforation into other loops of bowel or other organs, such as the bladder, can occur (fistula). A combination of medical treatment to control the disease, and surgical treatment to deal with its

Table 11.12
Crohn's disease

Aetiology	Multi-factorial: genetic predisposition has been established through family studies, but no specific genetic defect has been identified. Microbiological flora, superimposed infection, and dietary factors have all been implicated. These factors may exert their effect on a genetically predisposed population
Symptoms	**Mechanism**
Abdominal pain/weight loss	Usually from (incomplete) blockage to the passage of food through the small bowel due to narrowing of the lumen. Malnutrition results from reduced nutritional intake, in addition to impaired absorption and protein loss from the diseased mucosa
Diarrhoea	Fluid and protein loss from the ulcerated mucosa is the primary cause. Secondary bacterial overgrowth proximal to the obstruction compounds the symptoms
Fatigue	Anaemia is a common feature of this condition. Poor nutrition combined with chronic bleeding from the ulcerated mucosa results in an iron deficiency. The terminal ileum is commonly involved in this disease and impaired resorption of intrinsic factor may result in B_{12} deficiency
Localised abdominal swelling	Intra-abdominal abscesses are a common feature of this condition. Because the whole thickness of the bowel wall is involved in the inflammatory process deep ulcers or fissures can perforate through to the serosal surface
Painful mouth ulcers and anal canal ulcers	The condition can affect any part of the digestive tract.
	As the mouth and anal canal are the only regions with a somatic innervation, these lesions are locally painful

complications, is required. At present there is no curative therapy.

Coeliac disease

Coeliac disease is a rare condition that affects the mucosa of the small bowel and, like Crohn's disease, also results in malabsorption. It does not, however, cause ulceration or stricture formation. It is caused by a sensitivity to gluten in the diet. Symptoms are usually completely relieved by adoption of a gluten-free diet.

Like Crohn's disease, there is known to be an inherited predisposition to coeliac disease, with up to 20% of siblings being affected. The genetic determinants of this condition are as yet undefined. The classical histological features are of villous atrophy, which is most marked in the proximal small bowel, associated with a chronic inflammatory infiltrate. Although the disease may present at any age, it is most commonly seen in the third and fourth decades, suggesting that the sensitivity to gluten is in part acquired. In addition to chronic diarrhoea, the most prominent symptoms are weight loss and fatigue, due to malabsorption.

Acute ischaemia

Acute ischaemia of the gastrointestinal tract is a medical emergency. Ten per cent of the cardiac output flows to the gastrointestinal tract. Interruption of this bloodflow first affects the mucosal layer of the bowel. Fluid collects in the submucosa resulting in oedema and the mucosal cells quickly start to slough into the lumen. This results in blood-stained diarrhoea. These changes are reversible because the mucosa has regenerative properties. It can be associated with a fever, due to an associated bacteraemia, because of disruption of the mucosal barrier. Persistence of the ischaemic episode will result in secondary damage to the bowel wall by digestive enzymes. Resolution of the ischaemia at this stage can result in secondary fibrosis and stricturing. Ischaemia that persists beyond a few hours results in loss of integrity of the bowel wall (perforation) and ultimately leakage of intestinal contents into the peritoneal cavity (peritonitis), which can be fatal. Acute ischaemia of the gastrointestinal tract is a relatively rare event because of the extensive collateral circulation between the mesenteric arteries. Complete occlusion of the superior mesenteric artery, either by thrombosis or an embolic event, may still not lead to infarction because of the collateral blood supply of the coeliac axis and the inferior mesenteric artery. Ischaemia is more frequently a result of localised venous occlusion. This is most commonly seen when the bowel is twisted or trapped in a hernia sac. In this situation the arterial pressure is high enough to continue to perfuse the loop of bowel, but the venous drainage which is at a lower pressure is occluded. In this situation, back pressure into the capillary beds results in ischaemia by secondary obstruction to arterial flow.

Infective diarrhoea

Intestinal infections (Table 11.11) have historically been a major cause of morbidity and mortality, and continue to be so in underdeveloped countries. The main causes of death are dehydration and electrolyte loss, making infants and the elderly particularly susceptible.

Cholera is due to infection of the gastrointestinal tract by *Vibrio cholera* and continues to be an important infection in developing countries because of contamination of the drinking water. The symptoms of profuse watery diarrhoea are as a consequence of the blockade of the sodium exchange pump by the enterotoxin. Fluid loss can be as high as one litre per hour and rapidly results in hypovolaemic shock, acute renal failure and metabolic acidosis.

In contrast, *Salmonella typhi* and *Shigella* infections directly damage the mucosa of the gastrointestinal tract. *Shigella* infections result in moderate amounts of diarrhoea associated with a high fever. Damage to the bowel mucosa also results in protein and microscopic blood loss. *Shigella dysenteriae* has more effect on the large bowel mucosa, and is associated with frank blood loss in the stool, because the blood is not degraded by proteinases as when it occurs in the small bowel. *Salmonella typhi* infections can be transmitted from contaminated water or food and, like *Shigella*, directly invade the small intestinal mucosa. This initial infection is not, however, directly toxic to the mucosal cells and the organisms spread to the liver via the mesenteric blood supply. Here a secondary incubation period is followed by a clinical bacteraemia. The accompanying inflammatory reaction to this infection results in ulceration of the bowel mucosa, producing diarrhoea, bleeding, and fever. As a consequence of the direct damage to the mucosa, the diarrhoea results in protein loss in addition to salt and water loss. Because these infecting organisms have a different mechanism of action, the incubation period for each infection varies. A cholera infection will manifest symptoms within 12 hours, but a *Shigella* infection will usually take several days. Because of the secondary incubation period, a *Salmonella* infection has an incubation period of about 10 days.

Amoebic dysentery remains an important cause of infective diarrhoea in the tropics. It is caused by the ingestion of food and water contaminated by the cysts of *Entamoeba histalytica*. The cysts develop into trophoziotes, which invade the mucosa of the colon and can penetrate all the layers of the intestinal wall. This results in ulcer formation and secondary blood-stained diarrhoea. As is the case with many intestinal infestations, some individuals fail to develop invasive disease and remain asymptomatic carriers. The condition can mimic ulcerative colitis because of the mucosa ulceration, but the diagnosis is readily established from biopsy of the ulcer or from examination of fresh stools for the presence of cysts. The condition is readily treated by antibiotics. Because the ulcers penetrate the full thickness of the bowel wall, secondary stricture formation in the large bowel can be seen following treatment.

Large intestine

The most important disease of the large bowel is that of colorectal cancer. Nonetheless, benign disorders of the large bowel also form an important group of clinical disorders (Table 11.13). All large bowel disease results in alteration of bowel habit. The key symptoms are that of a change in bowel habit, which may be either diarrhoea or constipation, together with rectal bleeding and lower abdominal pain. Inflammation of the mucosa of the large bowel usually results in diarrhoea. The important causes are diverticulitis, ulcerative colitis, and infection.

Diverticular disease has a high prevalence in the Western world. This is believed to be due to a low fibre diet, which results in raised intraluminal pressure in the large bowel. This in time leads to muscle hypertrophy in the wall of the colon and pulsion diverticula in the wall of the bowel (Fig. 11.7). The diverticula are out-pouchings of the mucosa through the muscle coat of the colon. Without a muscle coat these little mucosal sacs are unable to empty, and faecal residues become lodged in the sac, predisposing the individual to secondary infection. Colonic diverticulae are present in 30% of the population aged 55 years and over, but the majority are asymptomatic. Complications occur because ulceration of the mucosa in the wall of the diverticulum results in bleeding, or obstruction to the neck of the diverticulum results in abscess formation with or without perforation into the peritoneal cavity. These complications are only seen in about 1 in 50 patients with diverticular disease, but when they do occur they can be life-threatening.

Obstruction to the flow of faecal contents in the large bowel is life-threatening, because the ileocaecal valve, lying at the proximal end of the colon, creates a closed loop that can only decompress by perforation of the colon. Perforation usually occurs at the caecum where

Table 11.13
Large bowel disease

Condition	Features	Mechanism
Diverticular disease	Central, lower, abdominal pain	Referred pain from the embryonic hind gut. Muscle hypertrophy in the wall of the bowel results in spasms of pain (colic)
	Fever	The diverticulum can become obstructed and infected. This results in a small abscess in the wall of the colon
	Generalised abdominal pain and tenderness	Rupture of the diverticulum into the peritoneal cavity can cause generalised intraperitoneal infection. (Peritonitis)
Ulcerative colitis	Diarrhoea and bleeding	Ulceration of the large bowel mucosa results in failure to absorb water from the lumen, and bleeding from the submucosal vessels
	Abdominal distension	Mucosal failure results in loss of peristalsis and a functional obstruction. The proximal bowel can dilate and even perforate causing peritonitis (toxic megacolon)
Dysentery	May follow foreign travel	Infection from ingestion of contaminated food or water
Entamoeba histolytica	Blood-stained diarrhoea	Ulceration of the mucosa results in water/protein loss and bleeding from the submucosal vessels

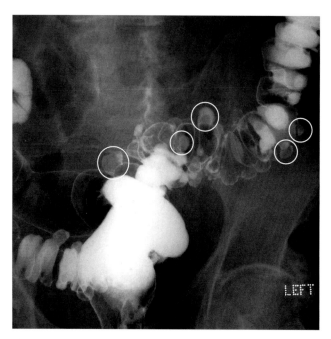

Fig. 11.7
An X-ray of the large bowel, which has been coated with barium. Moderate diverticular disease is apparent in the sigmoid colon. This shows up as small out-pouches filled with barium (circled).

the wall is thin and distends easily. Colorectal cancer is the commonest cause of large bowel obstruction, but obstruction of a diverticular abscess or scarring in the wall of the colon following acute diverticulitis can also cause this problem. The treatment is surgical, and requires resection of the obstructing segment, and where possible, reconstitution of the bowel continuity by anastomosis to the rectum.

Ulcerative colitis

This is an inflammatory condition that is limited to the mucosa of the large bowel. Its incidence has been estimated at approximately 2% per annum in the West, but the vast majority of these patients have disease that is mild and limited only to the rectal mucosa. In a small proportion of cases the inflammation extends throughout the large bowel mucosa and can result in a more florid illness. The aetiology of this condition is not known, but like Crohn's disease it is believed to be due to a sensitivity to environmental factors that have yet to be identified. There is an underlying genetic predisposition in at least a proportion of cases. It is interesting to note that ulcerative colitis and Crohn's disease may be seen in the same family, suggesting common aetiological factors.

Extensive mucosal damage results in watery, blood-stained diarrhoea. Infective causes of diarrhoea should always be excluded. Diagnosis is by histological examination of mucosal biopsies. As is the case elsewhere in the digestive tract, extensive ulceration of the mucosa can result in bacteria migrating from the lumen into the portal system. Although the condition is limited to the mucosal lining of the bowel, acute florid attacks will result in transmural inflammation and can lead to secondary perforation and peritonitis. Treatment requires fluid and salt replacement and antibiotics to control any secondary infection.

Immune suppressive therapy is used to damp down the inflammatory destruction. In a small percentage of patients, medical treatment is unsuccessful and emergency surgery with removal of the large bowel (colectomy) is required. Longstanding disease also increases the risk of secondary colorectal cancer in these patients and occasionally a prophylactic colectomy is necessary to prevent malignant disease developing. Advances in surgical techniques have enabled the development of ileo-anal anastomosis, which reconstitutes bowel continuity and avoids the formation of a permanent stoma in many of these patients.

ANSWERS

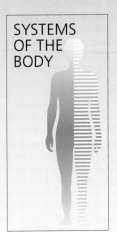

SYSTEMS
OF THE
BODY

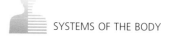

ANSWERS

Chapter 1
Self-assessment case study

① What sort of diet would the patient's diet sheet indicate? Can you explain why?

The diet would involve a low calorie regime, in which the fat and carbohydrate are reduced so that fewer calories are provided in the food than the normal requirement for a relatively inactive adult man (approximately 2500 kilocalories).

② Which other measures could the patient adopt to help him lose weight? Explain why.

A programme of exercise. Weight loss is due to more calories being lost as energy, than are taken into the body in the food. Exercise increases energy output.

③ What do you understand by the 'alimentary' regulation of hunger?

Regulation by factors in the gastrointestinal tract; the functional activity of the oral cavity; emptiness of the stomach lowers the blood glucose which causes hunger contractions via the vagus nerve; distension of the stomach and intestines signals satiety via mechanoreceptors in the walls of the tract; the chemical composition of food in the duodenum (e.g. fat).

④ Which nutrients are involved in the 'nutritional' regulation of food intake?

Glucose, amino acids, lipids.

⑤ What defects in the hypothalamus could lead to hyperphagia (overeating), albeit in rare cases?

A tumour of the hunger centre or a lesion of the satiety centre.

⑥ What is the function of the satiety centre?

It inhibits the 'hunger' centre in the hypothalamus, probably when blood glucose levels increase after a meal.

⑦ What do you understand by appetite? Which areas of the central nervous system are involved in its control?

Appetite is a desire for specific foods. It is probably under the control of the amygdala and cortical areas of the limbic system.

⑧ Can you give an example of a drug which could be prescribed for this patient if other measures prove unsuccessful?

Amphetamines. However, this usually results in loss of approximately only 10% of weight.

Self-assessment questions

① Which structures outside the gastrointestinal tract provide important digestive juices?

The salivary glands, the pancreas, and the liver.

② Which physiological process is central to the functioning of the digestive system, and why?

Absorption. All other processes subserve it.

③ What are the major components of the faeces?

Undigested residues, substances excreted by the liver, cell debris, bacteria.

④ What are the major functions of the splanchnic circulation?

(1) It supplies the organs of the gastrointestinal tract with oxygen and nutrients. (2) It acts as a store of blood which can be diverted to other regions of the body when the need arises (for example, to skeletal musculature during exercise). (3) It carries nutrients from the small intestine to the liver via the portal vein and so into the systemic circulation.

⑤ What are the main determinants of the rate of transport of a substance by passive diffusion?

The concentration gradient, the electrical gradient, the permeability, and the surface area.

⑥ How does active transport differ from passive transport?

It is more rapid, it requires energy, it is unidirectional, it is temperature-dependent, it can be inhibited by metabolic inhibitors, and it is saturable.

⑦ How does Ca^{2+} trigger the contraction of smooth muscle?

It combines with calmodulin-Ca^{2+} binding protein complex which then activates inactive myosin light-chain kinase. This catalyses the phosphorylation of myosin. The phosphorylated myosin interacts with actin, and ATP is split to provide the energy for contraction.

⑧ What are 'pacemaker' cells in the gastrointestinal tract?

Specialised smooth muscle cells, mainly in the longitudinal layer. They are located in close proximity to autonomic nerves and respond to released transmitter by depolarisation or hyperpolarisation of their membranes. Action potentials set up in these cells are propagated throughout neighbouring smooth muscle cells, via nexuses.

⑨ Which regions of the gastrointestinal tract are innervated by the vagus nerve?

All regions from the mouth to the first part of the transverse colon.

⑩ Which types of neurone are present in the enteric nervous system?

Excitatory and inhibitory interneurones, autonomic motor neurones, sensory neurones.

⑪ Which regions of the gastrointestinal tract are innervated by somatic motoneurones?

The mouth, pharynx and upper oesophagus, and the external anal sphincter.

⑫ What is the difference between 'open' and 'closed' APUD cells?

Open APUD cells have a luminal membrane which can sense the contents of the lumen. Closed APUD cells do not have a luminal membrane; information is conveyed to them via neurones or by hormones or paracrine factors.

⑬ What is meant by the cephalic phase of control of the digestive system?

The response to the approach of food, or food in the mouth.

⑭ What is meant by the intestinal phase of control of the digestive system? Which hormones are involved in the control of pancreatic and gastric secretions during this phase? What are the major stimuli for the release of these hormones? In what ways do they affect the release of gastric juice and pancreatic juice?

The phase of control mediated by the volume and composition of chyme in the small intestine, mainly in the duodenum. The major hormones involved are secretin, cholecystokinin (CCK) and GIP. The major stimulus for secretin release is acid in the duodenal chyme and the major stimulus for CCK and GIP release is fat in the duodenal chyme.

Chapter 2
Self-assessment case study

① Would you expect damage to the inferior dental nerve to affect the patient's ability to chew? Explain your answer, indicting the mechanisms involved in the regulation of the bite.

Chewing depends on activation of periodontal receptors which results in impulses in sensory nerve fibres in the inferior dental nerve being transmitted to the chewing centre. (In practice, chewing is not usually a problem following such nerve damage.) Regulation of the bite is via stimulation of tooth pulp and periodontal ligament receptors, which transmit tactile information to the brainstem. These inputs modify the activity of the chewing pattern generator. They stimulate the opening centre and inhibit the closing centre. This results in jaw opening. Impulses from the closing centre then inhibit the opening centre and the jaw closes.

② Would you expect damage to the lingual nerve to affect the patient's ability to chew?

The tongue moves the food around in the mouth to aid chewing. Therefore if the tongue is anaesthetised the process of mastication could be impaired. (In practice this is not usually a serious problem.)

③ Would you expect the patient to have difficulty in swallowing? Explain your answer.

The swallowing reflex is initiated when the tongue moves the food bolus to the back of the mouth where it activates pressure receptors in the pharynx. In practice, swallowing is usually not seriously affected after such nerve damage, because only a small part of the musculature is likely to be affected.

④ Would you expect the patient to have a dry mouth? Explain your answer.

The lingual nerve innervates the submandibular and sublingual salivary glands. However, between meals the mouth is kept moist by saliva from the smaller glands in the oral and buccal mucosa. When food is eaten or at the approach of food, over half of the increased flow comes from the parotid glands. Thus interference with flow of saliva is not a serious problem after unilateral lingual nerve damage accompanying a wisdom tooth extraction.

⑤ Would you expect the nerve damage to affect the patient's speech?

Articulation of many sounds depends on fine control of the movements of the muscles of the tongue. These reflexes partly depend on tactile information from the tongue. However, in practice, unilateral damage to these nerves accompanying wisdom tooth extraction does not affect speech to any significant extent.

⑥ Would you expect damage to the lingual nerve to have affected the patient's sense of taste? Explain your answer.

Some nerve fibres in the lingual nerve carry sensory information from the taste buds on the tongue (via the chorda tympani). In practice, loss of some taste sensation on one side of the tongue is not a serious problem.

⑦ Would you expect the loss of pain sensation to be a problem for this patient? Explain your answer.

This can be a serious problem because the patient could damage his tongue by biting it without realising it. He may also burn the tongue and other tissues in his mouth by drinking liquid that is too hot.

⑧ Why was the patient's lower lip numb?

Because the inferior dental nerve innervates the lower lip, and this nerve was damaged.

Self-assessment questions

① How does the ionic composition of saliva in the acinus compare with that of blood plasma?

It is approximately isotonic with blood plasma as it is an ultrafiltrate of plasma.

② How does the ionic composition of (a) unstimulated and (b) stimulated saliva in the mouth compare with that of blood plasma? In what situations would you expect the rate of flow to be increased?

The saliva in the mouth is usually hypotonic because Na^+ is extracted from it faster than K^+ is added to it. The concentration of Na^+ is lower than in blood plasma in both cases and the concentration of K^+ is higher than in plasma in both cases. However, the concentration of Na^+ is higher in stimulated saliva than unstimulated saliva as there is less time for extraction of the ion from the saliva at high flow rates. The concentration of K^+ is somewhat higher in unstimulated than stimulated saliva. The flow would be stimulated when a meal is being eaten, or at the approach of food.

③ How does the pH of saliva in the mouth during a meal compare with that of unstimulated saliva? Why is the altered pH at high rates of flow important for the functions of the mouth?

The pH of stimulated saliva is higher due to its higher HCO_3^- concentration. The high pH enables salivary α-amylase which has an alkaline pH optimum to act. It also neutralises acid in food, which might erode tooth enamel.

④ What are the mechanisms involved in bringing about the changes in concentration of ions as saliva flows down the ducts?

There are active transport processes in the duct cell membranes. These actively extract Na^+ ions from the saliva and actively add K^+ ions to the saliva. The transport processes have the greatest impact at low flow rates when the saliva is in contact with the duct cells for a relatively longer time.

⑤ Why is it important for the sense of taste for a low concentration of (a) Na^+ ions and (b) HCO_3^- ions to be present in the saliva in the mouth?

(a) The salt submodality of taste depends on the concentration of Na^+ in the saliva which stimulates the taste buds. (b) The sour submodality depends on H^+ ions (or pH). HCO_3^- ions neutralise the H^+ ions with the formation of undissociated H_2CO_3 molecules.

213

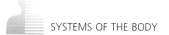
What tests would be performed on the sample?
Chymotrypsin or trypsin content, fat content.

Self-assessment questions

① What exocrine cell types are present in the pancreas? What is the composition of each type of juice secreted?
Acinar cells, centroacinar cells, duct cells. Enzyme-rich from the acinar cells, bicarbonate-rich from the centroacinar and duct cells.

② Can you describe the cellular mechanisms involved in the secretion of alkaline pancreatic juice? How is the CFTR involved in this process?
Bicarbonate is formed via dissociation of carbonic acid which in turn is formed from the reaction of CO_2 with H_2O. The HCO_3^- is transported across the luminal membrane in exchange for Cl^- ions, on the CFTR in the membrane.

③ Can you describe the cellular mechanisms of secretion of pancreatic enzymes? What part of this process is under physiological regulation by hormones?
Enzymes are synthesised on the endoplasmic reticulum, and released into the cisternae. Buds break off and move towards the luminal surface of the cell. At the level of the Golgi apparatus they fuse together to form condensing vacuoles. These become more and more densely staining as they approach the surface. At the surface the membrane of the condensing vacuole fuses with the cell membrane and the contents of the vesicle are exocytosed. The fusion and exocytosis are under the control of CCK which stimulates Ca^{2+} influx into the cell. This triggers exocytosis.

④ How is the secretion of each components of pancreatic juice controlled by food in (a) in the mouth, (b) in the stomach, (c) in the duodenum?
(a) Touch and taste and approach of food cause impulses in the vagus nerve which increase the secretion of both enzyme-rich and alkaline juices. (b) Peptides in the stomach, and distension cause the release of gastrin which stimulates both enzyme-rich and alkaline fluids. (c) Acid in the duodenum causes the release of secretin which stimulates the alkaline secretion, and fat in the duodenum causes CCK release which stimulates the enzyme juice secretion. The duodenal phase is the most important.

Chapter 6
Self-assessment case study

① How is a therapeutic dose of paracetamol normally metabolised in the liver?
It is conjugated to form soluble glucuronide or sulphate derivatives. These can then be excreted in the bile.

② Why are high levels of paracetamol toxic to the liver?
In high concentrations it is metabolised by P-450 mixed-function oxidases, to the reactive metabolite N-acetyl-p-benzoquinone imine. When glutathione is depleted these intermediate forms build up and cause hepatocyte cell death. A dose of approximately

10g of paracetamol is sufficient to produce hepatic necrosis.

③ Why was intravenous acetylcysteine administered?
Paracetamol can be conjugated to form sulphates, as well as glucuronides. This reaction requires glutathione. Acetylcystine increases glutathione synthesis in the liver and this increases the conjugation of paracetamol to paracetamol sulphate which can be excreted. Glutathione itself is not used because it does not readily penetrate the liver.

④ Why did the patient suffer a relapse after she appeared to have recovered?
The relapse was due to hepatotoxic effects of paracetamol metabolites which take more than 24 hours to inflict significant damage to hepatocytes.

⑤ Why did the patient appear jaundiced after her relapse?
The liver was damaged and therefore bilirubin could not be excreted in the bile, and consequently it accumulated in the blood. This would be predominantly unconjugated bilirubin, because of the widespread liver cell damage.

⑥ Why were the patient's serum prothrombin and transaminase levels excessively high?
Transaminases are inappropriately released from the dying hepatocytes. Liver cell failure results in lack of clotting factor production, which results in increased prothrombin time.

⑦ How can we explain the patient's aggressive behaviour?
Encephalopathy accompanies hepatic necrosis. This is due to increasing levels of toxic substances in the blood as a result of the inability of the liver to detoxify and excrete them.

⑧ Why was an EEG performed, and what was it likely to have shown?
An EEG can be used to monitor the encephalopathy, because of the effects of the toxins on the central nervous system.

⑨ Why was a liver transplant necessary?
The ability of the liver to recover function is well recognised, but in this case over 80% of the hepatocytes must have been irreversibly damaged.

⑩ Why were serum bilirubin levels, prothrombin time, and serum albumin levels, monitored after the transplantation?
As the new liver becomes functional the bilirubin levels fall because the liver regains its ability to sequester it from the blood and excrete it into the bile. The process of excreting the bilirubin takes several weeks, but the production of clotting factors and albumin is seen within hours. Prothrombin time and albumin levels are therefore more sensitive tests for monitoring transplant function.

⑪ Would forced diuresis or renal dialysis have been useful in this patient?
No. These procedures do not increase the excretion of paracetamol or its metabolites as the compounds bind tightly to tissues.

⑫ Can you suggest why alcohol ingestion should be avoided if paracetamol has been taken for a headache?
Alcohol is an enzyme inducer and therefore it enhances

the formation of toxic metabolites of paracetamol. Thus the combination of a normally safe dose of paracetamol and a high level of blood alcohol can lead to liver damage. This combination is particularly dangerous if there is underlying liver disease (as can be the case in an alcoholic).

Self-assessment questions

① What are the special features of the liver's blood supply?
Oxygenated blood in the hepatic artery is only 20% of the blood supply. The rest arrives in the portal vein which carries nutrients absorbed from the intestines.

② What are the functions of alkaline bile secreted from the duct cells?
It helps, together with other alkaline juices, to provide the correct pH for micelle formation and enzyme action by neutralising acid in the small intestine.

③ How is the alkaline secretion controlled?
By secretin released into the blood in response to the presence of acid in the duodenum.

④ What are the excretory functions of the hepatocytes?
Uptake of metabolites and xenobiotics, and their detoxification and conjugation, and secretion of conjugated metabolites into the blood or the bile.

⑤ How is the hepatocyte secretion controlled?
Mainly via the levels of bile acids in the blood.

⑥ What are the functions of Kuppfer cells?
They phagocytose cell debris and other substances.

⑦ What are the functions of the gallbladder?
Storage and concentration of bile, and controlled release of bile into the duodenum.

⑧ How do cholesterol gallstones form in bile? What factors predispose an individual to develop cholesterol stones?
Microcrystals of cholesterol precipitate out of the bile and these coalesce to form gallstones. The factors responsible are a low bile acid pool, or a high cholesterol:bile acid ratio in the bile.

⑨ What causes pigment stones to form in bile in some individuals?
Excessive formation of bile pigments in haemolytic anaemias, or deconjugation of bilirubin glucuronide in the biliary tract causing the bile to become supersaturated with unconjugated pigment, which precipitates out. Unconjugated bilirubin forms insoluble calcium bilirubinate.

⑩ What is meant by 'the enterohepatic circulation'?
Absorption of bile salts in the ileum, uptake by the liver, resecretion by the liver, release into the small intestine, re-uptake by the ileum, and so on.

⑪ What purpose does deconjugation of metabolites and drugs serve?
It makes them more polar and therefore more easily excreted.

⑫ What determines whether a compound is excreted by the liver or by the kidney?
Molecular size. The cut-off point above which compounds are excreted in the bile is approximately 500 Da.

Chapter 7
Self-assessment case study

① Why are abnormally high amounts of Cl^- lost in the faeces?
The exchanger transports Cl^- out of the lumen, in exchange for HCO_3^-. If the exchanger protein is absent Cl^- is lost in the faeces.

② How does this defect result in diarrhoea?
The high concentrations of electrolytes present in the lumen cause water to be transported by osmosis into the lumen (osmotic diarrhoea).

③ Is the fluid likely to be due to the absence of the exchanger in the small intestine or the large intestine, or both? Explain your answer.
The absence of the exchanger in the jejunum is less important than its absence in the ileum and colon, because water is transported as a consequence of Na^+/glucose and Na^+/amino acid co-port mechanisms in the jejunum but these co-port systems are not numerous in the ileum and not present in the colon. So the osmotic forces in the ileum and colon cause water malabsorption.

④ Why was it not necessary to include glucose in the oral replacement fluid?
The transport of water as a consequence of the Na^+/glucose co-port mechanism is not affected in this condition, and can be operating optimally. As the mechanisms which are absent operate in the distal small intestine and colon, glucose would not be helpful.

⑤ Can you explain the development of alkalosis in the child?
The exchanger protein which is missing transports Cl^- into the blood in exchange for HCO_3^- which is transported into the lumen. If the exchanger is absent, HCO_3^- accumulates in the blood and causes alkalosis.

⑤ Why were the child's faeces acid?
The Na^+/H^+ exchange system transports Na^+ into the blood in exchange for H^+ which is transported into the lumen. This is normally neutralised by the HCO_3^- transported into the lumen in exchange for Cl^-, but in this case it is lost in the faeces.

⑥ What is the basis of the oral replacement therapy with KCl and NaCl?
The child's plasma Cl^- was low because of the absence of the Cl^-/HCO_3^- exchanger, and the inhibition of the Na^+/H^+ exchanger. The K^+ was low because K^+ is transported into the lumen down its concentration gradient. If water accumulates in the lumen, as in diarrhoea, this gradient will favour transport into the lumen. The oral replacement therapy will correct the hyponatraemia, the hypokalaemia and the hypochloraemia.

Self-assessment questions

① How does cholera toxin cause diarrhoea?
It activates adenyl cyclase to increase intracellular cAMP which elicits a massive secretion of water and electrolytes from the crypt cells in the jejunum.

② How is the small intestine specialised for absorption?
Folds of Kerkring, villi, microvilli all increase the surface

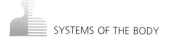

ANSWERS

area compared to a simple cylinder of the same dimensions.

③ What determines water absorption in the small intestine?
It is transported down the osmotic gradient set up by the absorption of other substances, notably Na^+, Cl^-.

④ Can you describe three special mechanisms for the absorption of Na^+ ions in the small intestine?
Co-port with glucose or galactose, co-port with neutral amino acids, the operation of the Na^+/H^+ exchanger.

⑤ Can you describe the four major mechanisms of diarrhoea?
Stimulation of secretion of the crypt cells which overwhelms the absorptive capacity of the colon, inhibiton of Na^+ absorption, osmotic diarrhoea, increased intestinal motility.

⑥ Why is the small intestine longer after death?
Tonus keeps it partially contracted in the normal individual.

⑦ What is the MMC?
It is a complex type of motility in the small intestine which occurs in cycles, even in the empty small intestine. It involves contraction of a group of segments of the intestine. The contractions last approximately 10 minutes. They start in the stomach and progress to the terminal ileum. In the human the frequency is approximately once every 1.5 hours.

⑧ What measures can be taken to alleviate constipation?
Treatment with laxatives that include lactulose or poorly absorbed salts which cause a relative osmotic diarrhoea, or increased indigestible, bulk-forming substances such as bran, in the diet, which become hydrated, and thereby decrease the viscosity of the luminal contents (to increase flow through the gastrointestinal tract) and stimulating motility.

Chapter 8
Self-assessment case study

① Why was steatorrhoea present in this patient?
This was due to fat malabsorption in the proximal small intestine, resulting in loss of fat in the faeces.

② What are the likely causes of diarrhoea in coeliac disease?
High concentrations of unabsorbed nutrients in the chyme would lead to osmotic diarrhoea. However, the delivery of large amounts of fat into the colon can result in the production of hydroxylated fatty acids by colonic bacteria. These can act as cathartics.

③ What is the cause of malabsorption of nutrients in this condition?
Damaged villi and loss of enterocytes leads to reduced surface area for absorption. Fat malabsorption is exacerbated if bile and pancreatic juice secretion is affected by deficiency of CCK and secretin. The digestion of other nutrients, and consequently their absorption, would also be affected if pancreatic juice secretion were defective.

④ Why was iron-deficiency anaemia present?
Iron is absorbed in the upper small intestine, the region that was diseased in this patient.

⑤ If the duodenum and proximal jejunum were the only regions of the small intestine involved, which nutrients are likely to be malabsorbed?
The absorption of hexoses, amino acids, fat, fat-soluble vitamins, folate, and Ca^{2+} ions could be impaired as they are all absorbed in the upper small intestine.

⑥ What problems result from deficiencies of these nutrients?
(1) Weight loss and fatigue due to malabsorption of fuels such as carbohydrates and fat, and malabsorption of amino acids required for synthetic reactions, (2) anaemia and fatigue due to iron or folate malabsorption, (3) osteomalacia or osteoporosis as a result of vitamin D malabsorption, and Ca^{2+} malabsorption, and the formation of Ca^{2+} soaps with unabsorbed fatty acids, (4) bleeding from nose, gastrointestinal tract, vagina, and ureters, as a result of vitamin K deficiency. This could exacerbate the anaemia.

⑦ How would a defect in CCK and secretin release affect the functioning of the digestive system?
As these hormones control the secretion of pancreatic juice and bile, the secretion of these digestive juices would be reduced. As pancreatic juice contains the major digestive enzymes, most complex nutrients will be digested only slowly. Bile acids are required for fat digestion and absorption, so these processes would be affected by deficiency of bile as well as deficiency of pancreatic juice.

⑧ Why was the patient's clotting time measured?
To determine if she was deficient in vitamin K.

⑨ Is milk intolerance likely to be a complication in this condition?
Yes, because lactase may be deficient, as this enzyme is present in the enterocyte brush border in the proximal small intestine.

⑩ Why were the patient's blood electrolyte concentrations measured?
There can be severe loss of electrolytes in diarrhoea (see Chapter 7).

Self-assessment questions

① Which enzymes are available for starch digestion in the digestive tract?
Salivary and pancreatic α-amylases, glucoamylase, α-1,6,glycosidae, sucrase, maltase, isomaltase, lactase.

② How is glucose absorbed in the enterocyte?
Secondary active transport. A carrier, SGLT1, transports glucose and Na^+ into the cell, utilising, as the driving force, the Na^+ gradient set up by the pumping of Na^+ out of the cell at the lateral border. Glucose leaves the cell via the GLUT2 carrier in the basolateral membrane.

③ Which products of protein digestion are absorbed in the small intestine?
Amino acids, dipeptides, tripeptides.

④ What is the mechanism of vitamin B_{12} absorption in the ileum?
It forms a complex with intrinsic factor, and the complex binds to a receptor. The vitamin is probably then split off the complex, to enter the cell by an active transport mechanism.

⑤ What are the roles of vitamin D in the process of Ca^{2+} absorption?

It stimulates the synthesis of the Ca^{2+} binding proteins present in the mucosal membrane and the cell cytosol. It also stimulates the activity of the Ca^{2+} pump in the basolateral border of the cell.

⑥ In which forms can iron be absorbed in the small intestine?

Fe^{2+} and haem.

⑦ What is the role of xanthine oxidase in iron absorption?

It is the enzyme which catalyses the release of Fe^{2+} from haem, with the concomitant formation of apoprotein.

Chapter 9
Self-assessment case study

① What metabolic processes would have been occurring to enable this man to maintain his plasma glucose levels?

Glycogenolysis in liver and (indirectly via lactate production and gluconeogenesis) glycogenolysis in muscle and gluconeogenesis from amino acids, lactate, and glycerol.

② Why is it important that plasma glucose levels do not fall too far?

Because the nervous system is an obligatory utiliser of glucose during the initial phase of fasting. Later it can adapt to utilise keto acids.

③ Would you expect the man's plasma insulin levels to be low?

They would be at the basal level.

④ Would you expect the man's acid–base status to be disturbed? Explain your answer.

He would probably have a metabolic acidosis due to the production of ketone bodies and fatty acids, but respiratory and renal compensation would be occurring.

⑤ Would you expect this man to be excreting glucose and ketone bodies in his urine? Would acetone be detectable on his breath?

He would be unlikely to be excreting glucose and ketone bodies in his urine, but acetone could probably be detected on his breath.

⑥ Would you expect the man's plasma glucagon level to be high or low? Explain your answer.

Glucagon levels would be high initially, as low glucose stimulates glucagon secretion from the pancreatic α-cells. However, after a few days of fasting it returns to normal. Thus in this man the levels of glucagon would not be elevated.

⑦ Would it be advisable for the rescued man to drink a concentrated solution of glucose?

If a lot of concentrated glucose solution is drunk it would pass too quickly into the small intestine and cause osmotic diarrhoea, and the man could become dehydrated. The rapid absorption of glucose could cause him to suffer from a rebound hypoglycaemia, and he might faint. However isotonic or hypotonic solutions would help.

⑧ What treatment would you recommend for the starving yachtsman?

Isotonic fluid containing some glucose for a while.

Self-assessment questions

① What is the major fuel used by most tissues of the body in the absorptive state?

Glucose.

② What are the direct actions of insulin in (a) the liver, (b) the muscle, and (c) adipose tissue?

(a) Stimulation of glycogenesis, and inhibition of glycogenolysis, lipolysis, and proteolysis, (b) stimulation of glucose uptake, glycogenesis, and inhibition of glycogenolysis, and proteolysis, (c) stimulation of glucose uptake, inhibition of lipolysis.

③ What are the secondary effects of insulin?

By increasing glucose uptake into a tissue, it increases reactions whereby glucose is metabolised in that tissue, by a mass action effect.

④ How is glucose transported into muscle and adipose tissue?

In the presence of insulin stimulation it is mainly via the GLUT4 glucose transporter. In the basal state it is mainly via the GLUT1 transporter.

⑤ What is meant by the 'feedback' control of plasma glucose by insulin?

High glucose stimulates insulin release. High insulin then promotes glucose uptake into tissues and lowers the blood glucose, thereby removing the stimulus for insulin release.

⑥ What is the mechanism whereby insulin increases glucose transport into adipose tissue and muscle?

It binds to a receptor. This activates the tyrosine kinase activity of the receptor, which by an unknown mechanism causes translocation of the cytoplasmic GLUT4 into the plasma membrane. Glucose is transported into the cell by the transporter.

⑦ What are the glucose-supplying processes which occur in the postabsorptive state?

Glycogenolysis in liver, and gluconeogenesis from amino acids, glycerol (via lipolysis), and lactate (via muscle glycogenolysis) in liver.

⑧ What are the glucose-sparing processes which occur in the postabsorptive state?

Lipolysis leading to free fatty acid and ketone body production.

⑨ What are the major distinguishing features of (a) IDDM, (b) NIDDM?

(a) Low plasma insulin, fatty acids and ketone bodies, acidosis, polyuria, glucosuria, ketonuria, polydipsia, (b) high plasma fatty acids, polyuria, glucosuria, polydipsia. Insulin initially may be high, or normal. The tissues are insensitive to insulin.

⑩ How do adrenaline and glucagon promote glucose-sparing reactions in the postabsorptive state?

They stimulate the rate-limiting step (triacylglycerol conversion to diacylglycerol) in lipolysis.

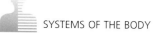

GLOSSARY

abetalipoproteinaemia – a rare autosomal recessive disorder characterised by a low plasma level of betalipoprotein.

aborally – in a direction away from the mouth.

achalasia – a motor disorder in which a muscle is unable to relax, particularly the lower oesophagus and the lower oesophageal sphincter (cardiospasm).

achlorhydria – lack of hydrochloric acid secretion in gastric juice.

acholic – absence of bile secretion.

adenocarcinoma – a malignant tumour of the glandular epithelium (e.g. colonic mucosa).

aetiology – the study of the causes of a disease.

aganglionic – displaying an absence of ganglionic cells.

amorphous – without visible structure.

anaemia – a reduction in total blood haemoglobin.

anastomosis – a connection between two vessels or a surgical joining of two bowel segments to allow flux of the contents from one to the other.

aneurysm – a localised dilatation of the wall of a blood vessel.

anorexia nervosa – a condition in which the desire for food is lost.

antidiuretic – a substance which diminishes urine production.

aphagia – a condition in which there is an inability to swallow.

ascites – a fluid collection in the peritoneal cavity.

atony – a lack of contractile function.

atrophy – wasting or shrinking (of an organ or tissue).

autoimmune – pertaining to the development of an immune response (antibody production) to the body's own tissues.

bacteriostatic – tending to restrain the reproduction of bacteria.

benign – non-malignant (pertaining to tumours).

bilirubinuria – the presence of bilirubin in the urine.

calculus – an abnormal stone formed in tissues by an accumulation of mineral salts.

cathartic – a (purgative) medicine which increases evacuation of the bowels.

caveolae – invaginations of the cell membrane extending into its cytoplasm.

chloridorrhoea – excessive loss of chloride ions in the faeces.

cholangitis – a bacterial infection of bile in the bile duct.

cholecystectomy – removal of the gall bladder.

cholecystitis – infection (of bile) in the gall bladder.

cholelithiasis – the presence of gall stones.

cholephilic – attracted to bile; easily dissolved in bile.

cholestasis – interruption of bile flow.

cirrhosis – a progressive inflammatory disease in the liver where there is an increase in non-functioning tissue and disruption of the architecture.

colectomy – removal of part of the large bowel (colon).

colic – cyclical intra-abdominal pain owing to dysfunctional peristalsis of the intestine.

colitis – inflammatory disease of the colon.

colostomy – a surgically created opening of the colon in the wall of the abdomen.

computed tomography (CT) scanning – a radiographic scanning procedure where the detailed structure of a tissue is revealed by densitometry. The body is imaged in cross-sectional slices and the computer quantifies the X-ray absorption by the tissues.

congestive heart failure – a pathological condition that reflects impaired cardiac pumping of the left and right ventricles.

constipation – difficulty in passage of stools or infrequent passage of stools.

cytopemsis – vesicular transport.

deglutition – swallowing.

diarrhoea – an abnormal increase in stool liquidity and in daily stool volume.

diuresis – increased production of urine.

diverticulitis – infection in one or more diverticula, usually of the sigmoid colon.

diverticulosis – the presence of pouch-like herniations (diverticula) in the muscular layer of the colon, especially the sigmoid colon.

dysaesthesia – altered perception of oral sensation.

dysphagia – difficulty in swallowing.

ectasia – dilatation of a duct, vessel or hollow viscus, usually resulting from obstruction to flow or degenerative changes of the wall.

ectopic – present in an abnormal location (e.g. in pregnancy).

embolus – a substance (usually dislodged atheroma or blood clot) lodged in a blood vessel, which blocks the flow of blood.

emetic – a substances which causes vomiting.

emollients – substances which alter the consistency (of the faeces).

encephalopathy – any disease or degenerative condition of the brain.

endocytosis – process whereby a molecule or particle becomes surrounded by the cell membrane and engulfed into the cell in a vesicle.

endogenous – originating within the tissues.

endoscopic retrograde pancreatography (ERCP) – a procedure employing a combination of fibre optic endoscopy and radiography to investigate the presence of biliary and pancreatic disease.

endoscopy – visual examination of a hollow organ (e.g. the gastrointestinal tract) by insertion of an endoscope (an illuminated optical instrument).

enteritis – inflammation of the intestines.

epigastric – in the upper central abdominal region.

excoriation – an injury to the surface of the body, e.g. a scratch.

exocytosis – the process by which vesicles release their contents by fusing with the cell's plasma membrane.

exogenous – originating from outside the tissues.

extrinsic – originating (usually situated) outside the tissue.

exudate – a fluid that has oozed out of a tissue and so has a high protein content.

fenestrae – pores.

fibrosis – proliferation of fibrous connective tissue.

fistula – an abnormal passage from an internal organ to the body surface or between two organs.

gastrectomy – surgical removal of the stomach.

glucagonoma – a glucagon-secreting tumour of the pancreatic islet cells.

glucostatic theory – control of feeding via blood glucose levels.

glycosuria – glucose in the urine.

granuloma – a chronic inflammatory lesion characterised by accumulation of macrophages.

gustation – taste.

haemodynamics – the study of the physical aspects of the blood circulation.

haemolytic – causing the red blood cells to break down and release haemoglobin.

haemorrhoid – a submucosal swelling in the anal canal caused by congestion of the veins of the haemorrhoidal plexus.

hemicolectomy – surgical removal of part of the large bowel with restoration of continuity.

hepatitis – an inflammation of the liver.

hepatoma – a primary tumour of the liver.

homeostasis – constancy of the internal environment of the body.

hydrophilic – attracted to, and easily dissolved in, water.

hydrophobic – not attracted to, and insoluble in, water.

hyperaemia – increased (regional) blood flow.

hyperbilirubinaemia – an abnormally high concentration of bilirubin in the plasma.

hyperglycaemia – increased plasma glucose.

hyperinsulinaemia – increased plasma insulin.

hyperkeratosis – overgrowth of the cornified epithelium layer of the skin, e.g. a wart.

hyperketonaemia – an abnormally high level of ketone bodies in the plasma.

hyperplasia – abnormal growth of a tissue owing to an increased rate of cell division.

hypertension – chronically increased arterial blood pressure.

hypertonic – containing a higher concentration of effectively membrane-impermeable solute particles than normal (isotonic) extracellular fluid.

hypertrophy – enlargement of a tissue or organ because of increased cell size rather than increased cell number.

hypoalbuminaemia – decreased plasma albumin.

hypocalcaemia – decreased plasma calcium.

hypochromia – a low haemoglobin concentration in the erythrocytes.

hypoglycaemia – low plasma glucose.

hypoinsulinaemia – low plasma insulin.

hypokalaemia – decreased plasma K^+ concentration.

hypotension – low blood pressure.

hypotonic – containing a lower concentration of effectively non-penetrating solute particles than normal (isotonic) extracellular fluid.

hypovolaemia – low blood volume.

hypoxia – deficiency of oxygen (in a tissue).

idiopathic – of unknown cause.

ileitis – inflammatory disease of the ileum.

ileus – loss of peristalsis in the small bowel, usually following surgery, that results in a functional obstruction.

inanition – loss of weight.

inspissated – thickened.

insulinoma – a tumour of the insulin-secreting cells of the pancreas.

intrinsic – originating within the tissue.

ischaemia – decreased supply of oxygenated blood to an organ or structure.

isosmotic – having the same total solute concentration as extracellular fluid.

isotonic – containing the same number of effectively non-penetrating solute particles as extracellular fluid.

jaundice – yellowish discolouration of the skin, mucous membranes and sclerae owing to deposition of bilirubin.

ketoacidosis – acidosis accompanied by an accumulation of ketones in the body.

leukocytosis – an increase in the number of white blood cells, usually in response to infection.

lipolysis – breakdown of lipids.

lipostatic theory – control of feeding by lipid metabolites.

lithotripsy – shattering of (gall or kidney) stones by ultrasound waves.

macrocytic – high mean cell volume (usually pertaining to red blood cells).

malignancy – a tumour with the ability to invade and spread to other tissues and organs.

mastication – chewing.

meconium – greenish material which fills the intestines of the fetus and forms the first bowel movement in the newborn.

meconium ileus – obstruction of the small intestine in the newborn by impaction of meconium (usually in cystic fibrosis).

megacolon – a massively enlarged colon.

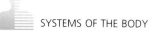

megaloblast – an abnormally large, nucleated, immature erythrocyte present in large numbers in pernicious anaemia or folate-deficiency anaemia.

metastasis – the process by which tumour cells spread to distant parts of the body.

microcytic – characterised by the presence of cells with low mean cell volume (usually pertaining to red blood cells).

myogenic – pertaining to (cardiac and smooth) muscle that does require nerve impulses to initiate and maintain a contraction.

necrosis – localised tissue death in response to disease or injury.

neoplasm – an abnormal new development of cells (a tumour).

nexus – gap junction; a zone of apposition between two cells where action potentials can be conducted between the cells.

oedema – accumulation of excess fluid in interstitial spaces.

olfaction – smell.

orad – in a direction towards the mouth.

osmolality – total solute concentration per unit weight of solvent (water).

osmolarity – total solute concentration of a solution.

osteopaenia – a reduction in bone mass.

pancreatitis – inflammatory disease of the pancreas.

paracrine – relates to an agent that exerts its effects on cells near its site of secretion (by convention, excludes neurotransmitters).

parenteral – relating to treatment other than through the digestive system (e.g. by intravenous administration).

parietal cells – oxyntic cells; acid-secreting cells of the stomach.

periodontal – pertaining to the area around the teeth.

peritonitis – inflammatory disease of the peritoneum, often secondary to perforation of the bowel.

pinocytosis – endocytosis when the vesicle encloses extracellular fluid or specific molecules in the extracellular fluid that have bound to proteins on the extracellular surface of the plasma membrane.

polydipsia – excessive drinking (usually seen in hyperglycaemia).

polyuria – high urine output.

prophylactic – an agent used to prevent the development of a disease.

purgative – a strong medication used to promote evacuation of the bowels.

pyroplasty – division of the pyloric muscle to allow easier emptying of the stomach.

roughage – non-digestible dietary fibre, important to promote gut motility.

ruga – a fold of mucosa in the stomach.

satiety – cessation of the feeling of hunger.

scintigraphy – a clinical procedure consisting of the administration of a radiolabelled agent with a specific affinity for an organ or tissue of interest, followed by determination, with a detector, of the distribution of the radiolabelled compound.

sclerosis – hardening of a tissue, especially by the overgrowth of fibrous tissue.

sclerotherapy – a technique using sclerosing solutions to cause obliteration of pathological blood vessels (as in the treatment of haemorrhoids).

secretagogue – a substance that regulates the release of a secretion.

sigmoidoscope – a rigid tubular instrument used for direct visualisation of the rectal and sigmoid colonic mucosa.

somatic – pertaining to one of two major divisions of the peripheral nervous system, consisting of sensory neurones concerned with sensation from the skin and body surface and motor neurones to the skeletal muscles, the other division being the autonomic nervous system.

splenomegaly – enlargement of the spleen.

steatorrhoea – a condition where the faeces have a high fat content.

stenosis – a narrowing or constriction of a tube (e.g. bowel) or aperture (e.g. ampulla of Vater).

stent – a short plastic tube.

submodality – subclass of a stimulus which evokes a sensory response.

submucosal – beneath the mucosa.

tetany – a maintained contraction.

thrombocytopaenia – deficiency of thrombocytes (blood platelets).

thrombocytosis – an abnormal increase in the number of thrombocytes (blood platelets).

thrombus – a clot which attaches to the wall of a vessel.

tonic – undergoing continuous muscular activity.

toxaemia – presence of bacterial toxins in the blood plasma.

transcoelomic – spreading through the peritoneal cavity.

transudate – fluid that has leaked out of a tissue, usually because of increased osmotic/hydrostatic pressure and therefore having a low protein content.

vagotomy – division of the vagus nerves.

varices – dilated veins, usually of the oesophagus, owing to raised portal vein pressure.

vasoconstriction – constriction of blood vessels.

vasodilator – a substance which causes dilatation of arterioles.

viscera – body organs (e.g. liver, pancreas).

xenobiotic – an organic substance which is foreign to the body (e.g. a drug or an organic poison).

xeraphthalmia – a disturbance of epithelial tissues.

xerostomia – dry mouth.

INDEX

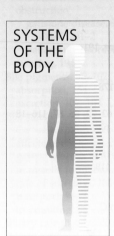

FIGURE ACKNOWLEDGEMENTS

Fig. 1.2 Based on a figure from Vander A. J., Sherman J. H., Luciano D. S. 'Mechanisms of body function' 1e New York: McGraw-Hill 1970. Reproduced with permission from McGraw-Hill Companies.

Fig. 2.4(B) Based on a figure from Morimoto F., Takada T. 'Neurophysiology of ingestion'. Elsevier Science 1993. Reproduced with permission from the publishers.

Fig. 2.7 Based on a figure from De Lorenzo A. J. D. In: Zotterman Y. (Ed.) 'Olfaction and taste'. Elmsford, NY: Pergamon Press 1963. Reproduced with permission from the publishers.

Fig. 2.14 Based on information in Thaysen J. H. American Journal of Physiology 1954; 178: 155.

Fig. 2.18 Based on a figure from Christensen J., Wingate D. L. (Eds) 'A guide to gastrointestinal motility'. Oxford: John Wright 1983. With permission from Butterworth Heinemann, a division of Reed Education & Professional Publishing Ltd.

Fig. 3.1(B) Based on a figure from Schulze-Delrier K. et al. In: Roman C. (Ed.) 'Gastrointestinal motility'. Lancaster: MTP Press, 1984.

Fig. 5.9 Based on a figure from Gorelick F. S., Jamesen J. D. In: Johnson R. L. (Ed.) 'Physiology of the gastro-intestinal tract.' Vol. 2. New York: Raven Press 1981.

Fig. 6.9 Based on a figure from Coleman R. Biochemical Transactions 1987; 15: 685–805. Reproduced with permission from the author. © The Biochemical Society.

Fig. 6.15(A) Based on a figure from Basmijian J. V., Stoneker C. E. 'Grant's Method of anatomy' 11e. Williams and Wilkins 1989.

Table 7.3 Based on information from Schanker L.S. 'Absorption of drugs from the rat colon.' Journal of Pharmacology and Experimental Therapeutics 126(4): 283–290.

Fig. 7.10 Based on information from Hogben C. A. M., Tocco D. J., Brodie B. B., Schanker L. S. 'On the mechanism of intestinal absorption of drugs.' Journal of Pharmacology and Experimental Therapeutics 125(4): 275–282.

Fig. 8.7(A) Based on a figure from Turk E., Wright E. M. Journal of Membrane Biology 1997; 159: 2. With permission from Springer-Verlag.

Fig. 8.7(B) Based on a figure from Thorens B. Annual Reviews in Physiology 1993; 55: 593. With permission from Annual Reviews www.AnnualReviews.org.